Biosensor Technologies for Prostate Cancer

Shriyansh Srivastava
Molakpogu Ravindra Babu
Shashank Shekhar
Editors

Biosensor Technologies for Prostate Cancer

Early Detection and Precision Diagnosis

Springer

Editors
Shriyansh Srivastava
Department of Pharmacy
School of Medical and Allied Sciences
Galgotias University
Greater Noida, Uttar Pradesh, India

Molakpogu Ravindra Babu
Department of Pharmacy
School of Medical and Allied Sciences
Galgotias University
Greater Noida, Uttar Pradesh, India

Shashank Shekhar
Department of Radiotherapy
AIIMS, Gorakhpur
Gorakhpur, Uttar Pradesh, India

ISBN 978-981-95-8643-1 ISBN 978-981-95-8644-8 (eBook)
https://doi.org/10.1007/978-981-95-8644-8

This Springer imprint is published by the registered company Springer Nature Singapore Pte Ltd.
The registered company address is: 152 Beach Road, #21-01/04 Gateway East, Singapore 189721, Singapore

I dedicate this book to my greatest inspiration, my father, ***Sanjay Srivastav****, and my strongest support, my mother,* ***Pushpa Srivastava****, who always believed in my potential. They planted the seeds of knowledge in my mind and nurtured them with unwavering love, guidance, and care.*

I also dedicate this work to my younger brother, ***Romil Srivastav****, and my beloved sister,* ***Soumya Srivastava****, whose constant presence fills my life with joy, encouragement, and motivation.*

Finally, I offer my heartfelt gratitude to all teachers who teach with passion and patience, shaping young minds and inspiring dreams that drive progress and discovery.

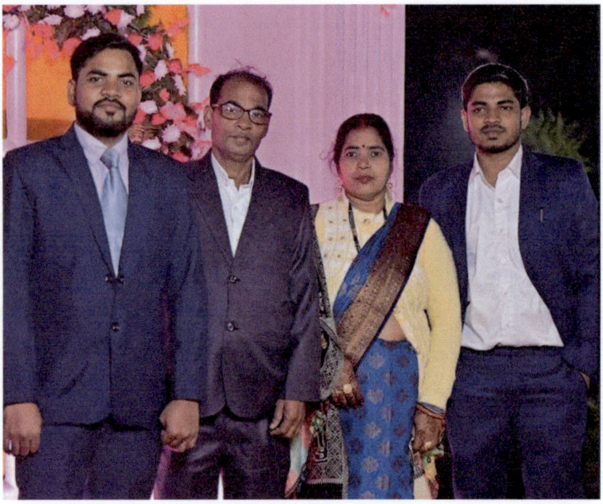

Shriyansh Srivastava

Preface

Prostate cancer remains one of the most prevalent malignancies affecting men worldwide, and early detection plays a decisive role in improving treatment outcomes and survival rates. Clinicians widely use conventional diagnostic tools such as prostate-specific antigen (PSA) testing and tissue biopsy; however, these methods often yield false-positive or false-negative results, leading to unnecessary invasive procedures or delayed clinical intervention. Such limitations highlight the urgent need for more reliable, sensitive, and patient-friendly diagnostic approaches.

Recent advances in biosensor technology have transformed the landscape of prostate cancer diagnosis. Biosensors enable rapid, highly sensitive, and accurate detection of disease-specific biomarkers, offering a powerful alternative to traditional diagnostic techniques. Researchers and clinicians increasingly recognize biosensors as a transformative tool for early detection and personalized disease monitoring. Despite this progress, the field lacks comprehensive resources that integrate biosensor development with clinical translation.

This book addresses that gap by presenting state-of-the-art research, fundamental design principles, and real-world clinical applications of biosensors in prostate cancer diagnosis. It provides healthcare professionals, researchers, and biomedical engineers with a clear and practical understanding of how biosensor technologies enhance early detection, improve diagnostic precision, and minimize reliance on invasive testing. By elucidating the critical role of biosensors in prostate cancer detection, this book empowers readers to advance research efforts and implement innovative diagnostic solutions in clinical practice.

Greater Noida, Uttar Pradesh, India — Shriyansh Srivastava
Greater Noida, Uttar Pradesh, India — Molakpogu Ravindra Babu
Gorakhpur, Uttar Pradesh, India — Shashank Shekhar

Acknowledgments

I gratefully acknowledge all the contributors for sharing their valuable insights and thoughtful inputs, which significantly enriched this book. I especially thank Rahul Kumar and Sakshi Patel for their dedicated contributions and support.

Shriyansh Srivastava

Contents

Introduction to Prostate Cancer

1

Shriyansh Srivastava

Abbreviations

ADT	Androgen deprivation therapy
AI	Artificial intelligence
BPH	Benign prostatic hyperplasia
CT	Computed tomography
CZ	Central zone
DRE	Digital rectal examination
HIFU	High-intensity focused ultrasound
mCRPC	Metastatic castration-resistant prostate cancer
mpMRI	Multiparametric MRI
MRI	Magnetic resonance imaging
PSA	Prostate-specific antigen
PZ	Peripheral zone
QoL	Quality of life
SCC	Squamous cell carcinoma
TRUS	Transrectal ultrasound
TZ	Transition zone

S. Srivastava (✉)
Department of Pharmacy, School of Medical and Allied Sciences, Galgotias University, Greater Noida, Uttar Pradesh, India

S. Srivastava et al. (eds.), *Biosensor Technologies for Prostate Cancer*, https://doi.org/10.1007/978-981-95-8644-8_1

1.1 Introduction

Prostate cancer is a common diagnosis among men and a significant concern for society. It begins in the prostate gland and can grow slowly or quickly, spreading quickly [1]. Even though advanced prostate cancer does not seem like much, it can cause serious problems with urination and reproduction that can be deadly. As adult populations age, lifestyle changes occur that exacerbate the disease. This is why awareness, screening, and early intervention are crucial for reducing death rates [2]. It is the fifth most prevalent cause of cancer-related deaths globally and the second most common malignancy diagnosed in men. Globally, approximately 1.4 million new cases and 375,000 deaths occur annually, according to GLOBOCAN 2020 [3]. In countries where screening is routinely performed, such as North America, Australia, and Western Europe, the incidence rates are highest. In contrast, Asia and some parts of Africa have lower rates, often due to underdiagnosis and healthcare problems [4]. However, prognosis depends on the stage of disease at diagnosis, with more than 98% of 5-year survival rates for localized cases in high-income countries. For that, treatment allows the survival rate to be at 90%, but it comes down to 30% if cancer has spread to other regions; thus, it is imperative to detect it early. Kapil Jaju, a researcher studying infectious diseases [5]. Although prostate cancer remains a global health problem with increasing incidence attributed to longer life expectancy and changing lifestyle factors, incidence decrease is noted among developing countries of Asia and the population >40 years [6]. However, this means that survival rates are good in cases where they are detected early; however, the variations in access to healthcare are enormous. Continuing research to increase knowledge, pushing for more awareness, and increasing the efficiency of screening and treatment strategies are the only ways the world can fight prostate cancer and help patients endure. As illustrated in Fig. 1.1, prostate cancer encompasses complex factors from epidemiology and diagnosis to clinical impact and future therapeutic strategies. Prostate cancer is a kind of cancer that starts in the tissues of the prostate, a gland located under the bladder in the male reproductive system. The seminal fluid, which nourishes and supports sperm contained in the prostate, is produced by the prostate in the male reproductive system [7]. When aberrant cells proliferate in the prostate and are not eliminated by the body, prostate cancer develops. Among males worldwide, it is one of the most often diagnosed malignancies, particularly in older persons [8]. Some prostate cancers are slow-growing and do not present as major health threats; others, though, are aggressive and need immediate medical treatment [9]. Prostate cancer is important for public health, healthcare resources, and patient quality of life. Prostate cancer management involves awareness, screening, and early detection, because early detection and appropriate treatment can be of tremendous benefit to patients [10]. Despite showing high incidence and mortality rates worldwide, particularly in the third world, prostate cancer is the second most frequently diagnosed cancer in men and one of the leading causes of cancer-related death [11]. A high incidence is primarily reported from high-incidence regions, particularly North America, Western Europe, and Australia, which is due to the high screening rates prevalent in those regions and the associated increase in lifetime

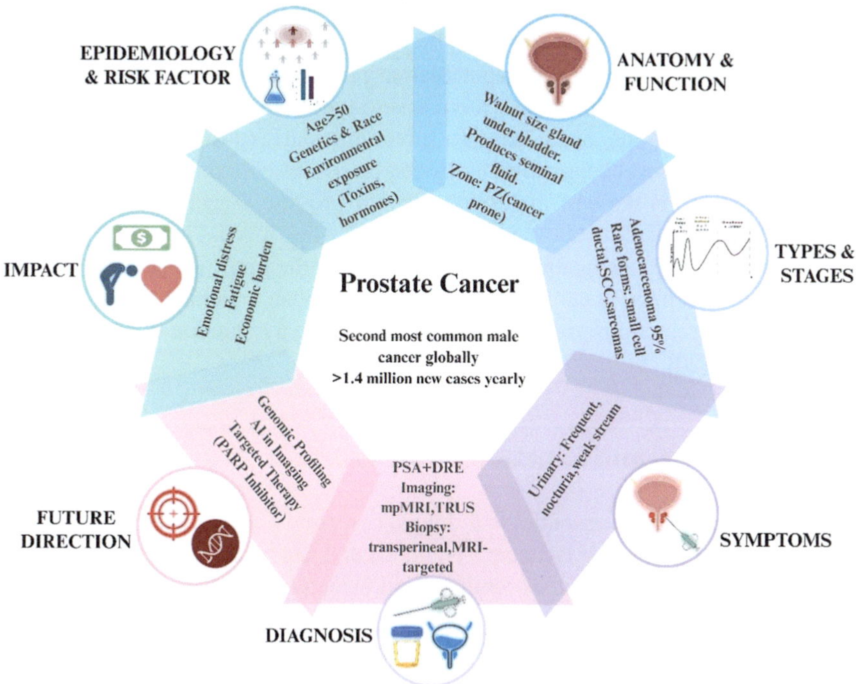

Fig. 1.1 Prostate cancer: epidemiology, pathophysiology, and clinical perspectives

[12]. Rising cases are being observed in moderate-incidence regions, including certain parts of South America and Asia, as people age or adopt different lifestyles [13]. However, low-incidence areas, such as parts of Africa and Asia, have fewer cases due to possible genetic differences, but underdiagnosis, as well as limited access to healthcare, may lead to a high degree of underreporting [14]. However, prostate cancer is no small headache worldwide, and these variations are an indication that it is time for greater awareness, better early detection tools, and more treatment breakthroughs to stem the course of the disease and improve patients' health.

1.1.1 Risk Factors and Epidemiology

The global epidemiology of prostate cancer operates on several risk factors that predispose the prostate to developing cancer. In most cases, age is the most common factor, with cases being diagnosed in men over 50 [15]. In addition, genetics and family history are also important; men with a family member nearby (father or brother) who had prostate cancer have a higher risk of having it. This would suggest a hereditary aspect [16]. Susceptibility is further influenced by ethnicity and race: Compared to Asian or Caucasian males, African American men are far more likely to acquire severe prostate cancer. Testosterone and other androgens have a role in cancer cell growth due to this [17]. Additionally, they attribute the illness to lifestyle choices and dietary habits. For example, they link a diet heavy in red meat and saturated fats and low in fruits and vegetables to prostate cancer, and they correlate obesity and a sedentary lifestyle to more severe types of disease [18]. Research is required to confirm the links between environmental exposure to carcinogens, chemicals, toxins, and occupational risks and an increased risk of prostate cancer. Regular screening is the best method to identify prostate cancer early enough for successful treatments. Prostate cancer is identified when it is not symptomatic [19]. Understanding these risk factors in detail, along with their prevalence in the public, can help develop effective public health policies, establish screening guidelines, and inform future research programs, ultimately leading to a reduction in prostate cancer worldwide [20].

1.2 Anatomy and Function of the Prostate

The prostate gland is an essential and crucial component of the male reproductive and urinary systems [21]. It is a man's gland located just below the bladder and surrounding the urethra; it produces seminal fluid, which nourishes and carries sperm. Males' prostates are vital to their general health and are susceptible to a number of diseases, such as prostate cancer, prostatitis, and benign prostatic hyperplasia (BPH) [22]. Understanding the structure, function, and age-related changes of the prostate is crucial for the early identification and treatment of prostate disorders [23]. However, age-related changes and conditions like BPH and prostate cancer can affect the prostate gland, which is situated at the base of the bladder. To detect early and intervene early, we have to understand its anatomy, function, and the importance of PSA testing to begin with [24]. Prostate health management can be accomplished proactively with screening and treatment that are advancing to lower the burden of prostate-related disorders and to improve outcomes of patients.

1.2.1 Structure and Role of the Prostate Gland

The walnut-shaped prostate is composed of both muscle and glandular tissue. For example, it is separated into many zones [25] (Fig. 1.2). *Peripheral zone (PZ):* Prostate cancer generally begins in this part of the prostate; it is the largest region, known as the peripheral zone (PZ). *Central zone (CZ):* It surrounds the ejaculatory ducts and is less frequently affected by cancer. *Transition zone (TZ):* Benign prostatic hyperplasia (BPH) usually develops in the area called the transition zone (TZ).

The prostate, functionally, is involved in the production of seminal fluid that accounts for about 30% of semen volume. This fluid is made up of proteins, zinc, and enzymes that help sperm survive and move [26]. In addition, the gland's muscular fibers also assist in propelling semen down the urethra during ejaculation. The prostate undergoes physiological changes as men age, and there are some factors that can affect the health of a man [27]. The gland grows from puberty into

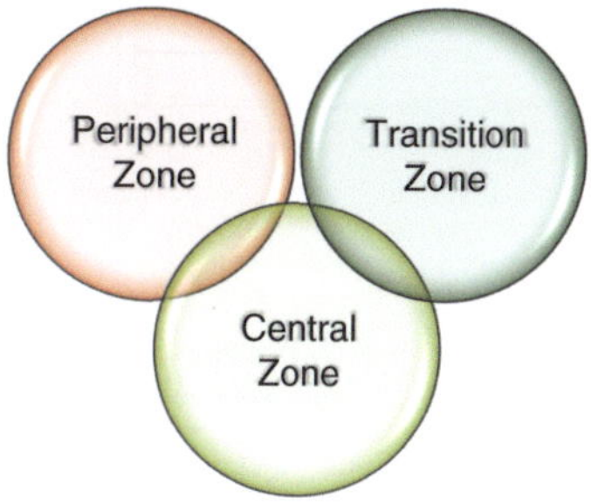

Fig. 1.2 Role of the prostate gland in many areas

adulthood in the presence of male hormones, most importantly testosterone and dihydrotestosterone (DHT). Men often begin to notice benign prostatic hyperplasia (BPH) or an enlargement of the prostate by middle age, which can obstruct the urethra and cause urinary symptoms, like frequent urination, weak stream, and lack of emptying of the bladder [28]. Prostate cancer is also associated with an elevated risk of aging, especially in men older than 50, who need to start screening and detection early.

1.2.2 Prostate-Specific Antigen (PSA) and Its Importance

Prostate-specific antigen (PSA) is a protein that the prostate produces and that aids in the liquefaction of semen. Elevated PSA levels indicate prostatic problems, including BPH, prostatitis, or prostate cancer, despite the fact that the circulation normally contains trace quantities of PSA [29]. PSA testing is a widely used screening tool for prostate cancer and will help to find the disease in its early stages. While PSA levels may be high with cancer, additional causes of elevated PSA include infection, inflammation, or recent medical procedures [30]. PSA testing is still important despite its limitations, however, especially for older men, those with blood relatives at risk, or those of African descent [31]. PSA is more effective for early detection when used with DRE and imaging testing.

1.3 Classification of Prostate Cancer

There are several ways that prostate cancer can develop and spread, making it a diverse condition [32]. The importance of knowing its classification, staging system, and distinction between the two categories of aggressive and indolent forms of the disease will determine prognosis and lead you to choosing the best treatment [33]. Prostate cancer is a complex disease with multiple subtypes with different biological behavior and treatment approaches (Table 1.1) [34]. Adenocarcinoma is the most common type and the one most often manageable with early detection, but other carcinomas, such as small cell carcinoma, squamous cell carcinoma, transitional cell carcinoma, and sarcomas, require special treatment strategies [35].

Table 1.1 Classification of prostate cancer

Type of prostate cancer	Frequency	Origin	Aggressiveness	Key characteristics	References
Adenocarcinoma	Most common (>95%)	Glandular cells of the prostate	Varies (slow-growing to aggressive)	Most cases are detected via PSA testing	[37]
Acinar adenocarcinoma	Most common subtype	Acini (small glandular pouches)	Generally slow-growing	Usually detected early via PSA	[37]
Ductal adenocarcinoma	Rare (<5%)	Prostatic ducts	More aggressive than the acinar type	Often diagnosed at an advanced stage	[38]
Small cell carcinoma	Very rare (<1%)	Neuroendocrine cells	Highly aggressive	Poor response to hormone therapy, rapid progression	[39]
Squamous cell carcinoma (SCC)	Extremely rare	Epithelial cells of the prostate	Highly aggressive	Does not respond to hormone therapy, rapid progression	[37]
Transitional cell carcinoma (TCC)	Rare	Urethral lining and bladder cells	Moderate to aggressive	Linked to bladder cancer, urinary symptoms	[37]
Sarcomas and other rare forms	Extremely rare	Soft tissues of the prostate	Highly aggressive	Includes leiomyosarcoma, rhabdomyosarcoma	[37]

Therefore, it is crucial to be aware of these differences to make an accurate diagnosis, select the appropriate treatment, and enhance the patient's outcome. A renewed focus on ongoing research into the molecular features of prostate cancer will help the development of precision medicine and personalized medicines for the disease [36].

1.3.1 Adenocarcinoma (Most Common Type)

In almost 95% of cases, adenocarcinoma is the most common kind of prostate cancer. The glandular cells of the prostate, which produce the seminal fluid, make up this structure [40]. Although most adenocarcinomas progress at a slow rate and remain local for many years, certain forms could be aggressive and spread quickly. There are two main subcategories of adenocarcinoma. The most prevalent kind of prostate cancer is called prostate acinar adenocarcinoma; it originates in the acini, the small glandular passages within the prostate. It is seldom detected late and is normally identified initially through a blood test for prostate-specific antigen (PSA), typically before symptoms occur [41]. This subtype is often slow-growing, making it challenging to monitor with active surveillance or treatment, such as radiation or surgery.

1.3.2 Ductal Adenocarcinoma (Rare but Aggressive)

Ductal adenocarcinoma, although it is less common and more aggressive, originates from the prostatic ducts rather than the acini. It is a tiny portion of prostate adenocarcinomas that are marginally more likely to spread outside the prostate early on [42]. It is usually found at an advanced stage, which makes treatment more challenging because the symptoms develop rapidly and may not be apparent for some time. On the other hand, ductal adenocarcinoma needs stronger treatment, such as surgery, radiation, and systemic therapies, to improve patient outcomes [43].

1.3.3 Small Cell Carcinoma (Neuroendocrine Prostate Cancer)

Small cell carcinoma of the prostate is a rare and aggressive type of prostate cancer that makes up less than 1% of all cases. It comes from neuroendocrine cells, which are cells that can make hormones [44]. Small cell carcinoma does not need testosterone to grow, unlike most prostate cancers, which start in glandular tissue. It is also considered "androgen independent," meaning it does not respond to standard androgen deprivation therapy (ADT). This cancer grows and spreads very fast, and often metastasizes to the lymph nodes, bones, liver, and lungs early, before a diagnosis is possible [45]. Because of its aggressive nature, small cell carcinoma is generally diagnosed at a late stage, which decreases the prognosis, and the treatment options are limited. Unlike other types of prostate cancer, small cell carcinoma does not usually result in higher PSA levels, which makes early detection very difficult [46]. Small cell carcinoma is dissimilarly treated in comparison to standard prostate cancer treatments. Given its tendency to behave as fulfilling, its treatment mainly consists of systemic chemotherapy with platinum-based regimens like cisplatin and etoposide [47]. Radiation treatment can be used for local cases, and in some cases, combination treatments including surgery or immunotherapy can be applied. Because of its hard-to-treat aggressive behavior and its hormone therapy resistance, early detection is very significant yet challenging. Further research into targeted treatments and biomarker-based screening may help patients with this rare and deadly form of prostate cancer [48].

1.3.4 Prostate Squamous Cell Cancer

Squamous cell carcinoma (SCC) of the prostate is very rare and is the most aggressive of all prostate cancers, representing fewer than 1% of all prostate cancers. Absent adenocarcinoma, which develops from glandular cells, SCC develops from flat, epithelial cells that both cover the prostate [49]. As a non-glandular tumor, it acts contrary to the usual prostate cancers and is more aggressive by the rule. One of the characteristics of this cancer is rapid growth and a high risk of metastasis. It usually grows rapidly and invades and spreads into the surrounding tissues, reaching nearby bones, bladders, or other organs before being diagnosed [50]. Unlike adenocarcinoma, SCC does not cause the production of prostate-specific antigen (PSA); thus, routine PSA screening for early detection is unsuccessful [51]. On the other hand, most cases are diagnosed late in the progression, making the survival rate low and treatment limited. In addition, because of PC cells' lack of growth sensitivity to PC standard remedy therapies, including androgen deprivation therapy (ADT), it is a major problem in treating planar cell carcinoma. Since SCC cannot grow from the hormone testosterone, hormone-repressing medications that are effective against adenocarcinoma are ineffective against this type [52]. Management of SCC of the prostate will usually require an aggressive multimodal treatment, which involves the following: *Surgery (radical prostatectomy)*: usually done in the localized situation to remove the prostate and stop the cancer from spreading; *Radiation therapy*: alone or in conjunction with surgery to destroy the cancer cells and the rate of progression; *Chemotherapy*: in advanced or metastatic cases, given since systemic treatment is needed for aggressive tumors. Because prostate squamous cell cancer is rare, there is not much evidence for the optimal management of such cases, complicating the treatment of patients [53]. None of these is an early sign; diagnosis, however, remains difficult. Nevertheless, progress in imaging techniques and molecular research, as well as improvements, will often become visible and lead to a better cure.

1.3.5 Transitional Cell Carcinoma (Urothelial Cancer of the Prostate)

Transitional cell carcinoma develops from urothelial cells, which line the prostate and bladder, although bladder cancer remains its main association. The clinical presentation of this prostate cancer is very uncommon because it develops initially in the urinary tract transitional epithelium before metastasizing to the prostate tissue [54]. Like bladder cancer, it displays histological characteristics that lead to blood in the urine, together with urinary blockage symptoms and pelvic area discomfort. The diagnosis of transitional cell carcinoma requires medical professionals to perform cystoscopy alongside biopsy examinations and imaging tests [55]. Treatment choices for this illness need to consider both stage and spread levels and involve doctors performing radical cyst prostatectomy, along with chemotherapy and radiation therapy. Patients with this cancer type often need care from multiple specialists because bladder cancer also exists frequently in these cases, thus requiring urologists and oncologists to create a treatment plan [56].

1.3.6 Sarcomas and Other Rare Variants

Sarcomas and other rare variants: extremely uncommon and typically more aggressive than conventional adenocarcinomas. Sarcomas of the prostate begin in mesenchymal cells instead of epithelial cells, which makes them separate entities from the more common adenocarcinoma variant [57]. Patients develop these tumors when they experience quick urinary difficulties along with pelvic mass and perineal distress. Healthcare providers detect this condition through biopsy tests, together with MRI or CT scanning [58]. Sarcomas need aggressive medical intervention with radical procedures combined with chemotherapy drugs and radiation therapy because they demonstrate intense aggression. Early detection, together with intervention, becomes essential for better outcomes because sarcomas lack the responsiveness to hormone therapy, which characterizes the treatment of adenocarcinomas [59].

1.4 Staging Systems (TNM Categorization and Gleason Score)

Prostate cancer staging is essential for assessing the extent of the disease and planning treatment [60]. The primary staging systems are as follows:

T (tumor) This tells you how big and wide the main tumor is. T1: Imaging or a physical exam cannot find the tumor; T2: The tumor is only in the prostate; T3: The tumor is outside the prostate; T4: The tumor has spread to nearby tissues like the bladder or rectum.

N (nodes) This indicates whether the cancer has spread to the lymph nodes in the affected area. N0: No lymph nodes are involved; N1: Cancer has spread to lymph nodes that are close by.

M (metastasis) This investigates whether the patient has developed cancer in other parts of the body. M0: no distant metastasis; M1: distant metastasis (i.e., bones, lungs, liver).

Gleason score The Gleason grading system involves examination of samples of prostate cancer under a microscope to determine the aggressiveness level. The grading procedure assigns a score ranging from 2 to 10 by adding the quantities of the two major tumor types [61]. *Low grade (≤6):* atypical, slow-growing neoplasm; *intermediate grade (7):* moderately aggressive behavior; *high grade (8–10):* These aggressive tumors have a significant metastatic propensity in the body.

1.4.1 Comparison of Aggressive and Indolent Variants

Due to the variation in the disease characteristics of prostate cancer that present themselves differently, they must be treated in certain ways [62]. The major criteria used to distinguish the aggressive prostate cancer and its less aggressive indolent one include the following:

Aggressive Prostate Cancer In case of a Gleason score between 8 and 10, together with 3-T4, N1, M1 TNM stage, and rapid prostate-specific antigen (PSA) doubling time, prostate cancer is aggressive. The ability of the disease to distribute cancer cells in the body creates more opportunities for tumor growth in the bones, lungs, or liver. Recommendations for aggressive behavior in prostate cancer include early medical attention [63]. Patients with prostate cancer may consider radical prostatectomy, chemotherapy, radiation therapy, or androgen-deprivation hormone therapy as treatment options. When the disease spreads to other parts of the body, clinicians administer systemic treatments, including immunotherapy and targeted medications [64]. The treatment of advanced prostate cancer is determined by the stage of diagnosis and the effectiveness of the treatment [65]. To handle the condition efficiently, patients should be monitored on a constant basis and should be examined periodically to adjust treatment based on disease progression and treatment reactions.

Indolent Prostate Cancer This is a type of prostate cancer that is characterized by slow development and low risk and would rarely spread beyond the prostate gland. The classification of the disease takes into consideration Gleason scores of 6 or less, T1 to T2 stage tumors, which did not invade the lymph nodes (N0) or distant locations (M0). A steady increase in PSA levels may be observed [66]. The prostate cancer of low-risk type is usually not symptomatic for a number of years, making timely medical treatment, as a rule, unnecessary because of the low level of risk to the health of a patient [67]. Active surveillance is the suggested approach for dealing with low-risk prostate cancer. The reason behind this is that it involves routine tests, computerized examinations, and the use of biopsies occasionally to examine any indication of progression [68]. Active monitoring of patients can help delay the occurrence of potential adverse effects, which are less likely to occur in cases of surgery and radiation therapy, unless the cancer is stable. Once the disease turns violent [69], the medical staff might consider alternative methods of managing the disease, including surgery, radiation, and hormone therapy. Continued advancement in molecular profiling and imaging technologies provides physicians with an increased number of options to measure risk, which enables them to provide individual patients with the highest possible treatment.

1.5 Causes and Risk Factors of Prostate Cancer

The subsequent part examines all causes of the formation of the evaluated health status [70]. Awareness of different variables affects the performance of early disease diagnoses and evidence-based management techniques.

1.5.1 Genetic and Hereditary Factors: Decoding the Inherited Predisposition

The genetic makeup of a person is a major determinant of their vulnerability to different health-related conditions, although the exact effect of the same might not be well understood [71]. This part looks at the far-reaching effects that inherited genes have on the development of diseases. *Polygenic architectures*: This model studies the consistency of the occurrence of diseases obtained by the overall impact of multiple genes that cause insignificant effects to increase susceptibility rates [72]. GWAS, a novel genomic method, currently demonstrates an intricate web of genes that involve genes that do not have a major effect in themselves. PRs are genetic tests that involve the use of probability to determine the likelihood of an individual falling ill [73]. Multifactorial inheritance examines the valuable connection between natural predisposition and the surrounding environment. Certainly, given certain genetic predispositions, individuals are more susceptible to health problems after exposure to certain stress factors within the environment or certain lifestyle decisions occur [74]. There are many reasons why science has investigated this dynamic area of gene–environment interaction: The epigenetic modifications have been shown to be important mediating factors. Epigenetics examines the interaction between genes and the environment and studies how heritable molecular tags modify genes by the organization of environment-induced mechanisms that do not change the original DNA sequences [75]. The mechanism of histone modification, DNA methylation, and non-coding RNAs might result in an individual with the same genetic background to develop divergent disease pathways [76]. *Pharmacogenomics*: treatment based on genetic composition. This topic demonstrates how certain drugs react to genetic variation in individuals [77]. This development of pharmacogenomics implies a lot in patient-centered medicine because the healthcare practitioners can use genetic data to select the most effective drug and reduce the adverse effects to a minimum [78]. *Personalized genomics*: It uses uncommon variants and has become popular in research due to the fact that GWAS is effective in identifying common risk variants, yet uncommon, unique genetic variations require further investigation [79]. The discovery of novel technologies to sequence whole genomes and exomes assists scientists in discovering rare variations that provide families and individuals with better prognostic diagnostics. Genetic counseling proves useful because it assists individuals in comprehending their findings in tests and determining the risks faced in their families, which allows them to make wise health and reproductive decisions [80]. Researchers should develop measures that will protect the privacy of the genetic information of people, develop guidelines to avert genetic discrimination, and secure the responsible use of predictive genetic information.

1.5.2 Lifestyle and Dietary Factors Provide Modifiable Strategies to Maintain Health and Prevent Illness

The personal daily eating habits, physical activity programs, stress control, and medication use have a significant influence on personal health outcomes, altering the susceptibility to different health disorders [81]. This part discusses how lifestyle factors can be utilized as useful evidence of the etiology of diseases. *Chronic inflammation*: Long-term systemic inflammatory syndrome is associated with dietary habits based on processed food, saturated fats, and refined sugars, coupled with inactivity and chronic stress, triggering low-grade systemic inflammation [82]. Explain protein-based mechanisms, the role of the inflammatory cytokines and chemokines, and their impact on various chronic medical disorders. *Metabolic dysregulation*: The evaluation will examine the effect of lifestyle practices on the basic metabolic activities, starting with glucose homeostasis, which is interrelated with lipid metabolism and energy balance [83]. Discuss the relevance of insulin resistance, dyslipidemia, and obesity in connecting unhealthy lifestyle decisions and an increased risk of getting sick. *Oxidative stress and antioxidant defense mechanisms*: Discuss the distinction between antioxidant defense mechanisms and the generation of reactive oxygen species (ROS) [84]. The body of older individuals can be susceptible to sickness because of oxidative stress caused by pollution of the environment through smoking and diets that are low in antioxidants. *Gut microbiota*: The gut microbiota varies depending on lifestyle components such as nutrition, mental health, and drug use, which alter the amount of bacteria in the intestines [85]. Explore how both way communication of intestinal microbiota with various physiological mechanisms can be used to adjust immunity and metabolism and to change neurobehavioral health. *Physical activity*: Determine the benefits of physical activity to the body, particularly in terms of weight and many other health-related benefits that are not directly linked to calories burned. Assess cardiovascular functions concerning the insulin sensitivity, immune activity, regeneration of nerve cells, and the decrease in chronic inflammation, because these biological processes have such effects. Research the physiological effects of sustained stress and lack of sleep. Explain how the activation of the hypothalamic–pituitary–adrenal (HPA) axis triggers the secretion of stress hormones, which eventually result in long-term changes in immunological reactions, cardiovascular activities, and metabolism [86]. The discussion should pay more attention to the methods of stress management and the habits of good sleep.

1.5.3 Environmental and Occupational Exposures: The External Factors Affecting Health

The environment in which we work and the physical, chemical, and biological substances that surround us present us with diverse elements that influence our health and predispose us to illnesses [87]. In everyday life and in the workplace, people are exposed to numerous physical, chemical, and biological agents that may have an impact on their physical, mental, and health conditions and increase their risk of illness. There are numerous sources of air pollution, including car emissions, industrial wastes, and indoor air pollution. It damages our lungs and leads to heart ailments, nervous system issues, and cancer [88]. The discussion will involve the transmission of adverse outcomes by particulate matter, gaseous pollutants, and ultrafine particles through reviewing their cellular and molecular pathways. Another problem that can impact the health of the citizens is water contamination. Professional investigators examine how industrial contamination of businesses combines with agricultural waste products and disease-causing microorganisms that can cause infections, developmental disorders, and chronic diseases [89]. All people must understand the importance of ensuring that the environment has good water quality and also has good sanitation systems. *Chemical exposures*: Individuals are exposed to a considerable amount of man-made and natural chemicals at the workplace and in products during daily life [90]. The chemical hazards analysis requires consideration of the endocrine disruptor behavior, carcinogenicity effects, neurotoxicity, immunotoxicity, and especially, the strategies of exposure minimization. People are advised to distinguish between two types of radiation exposure, that is, the ionizing exposures (including the medical imaging devices, and nuclear sources) and the non-ionizing exposures (including the electromagnetic fields of the electronic devices) [91]. Radiation sources may damage DNA, lead to cancer, and alter the body's reaction to stress, which can be diminished through appropriate safety measures. Emphasize occupational risks across different professions by examining the specific hazards associated with workplace exposures and the physical demands of each occupation. All employees must be aware of the hazards of being near dust, solvents, heavy metals, fumes, ergonomic stressors, and accidents in the workplace and how to wear protective equipment and act according to safety regulations [92].

1.6 Symptoms and Early Warning Signs

People need to be able to recognize signals from their bodies in order to get medical help and treatment on time. This section gives a full analysis of the signs of illness, from the first signs that are hard to notice to the more obvious signs that come later. By recognizing these signs, people can get medical help right away, which increases their chances of getting better.

1.6.1 Recognize Urinary and Sexual Symptoms as Early Indicators and Subtle Alterations

The development of urinary and sexual features is a critical warning sign of early detection of this condition [93]. Even though such symptoms can be present in less severe conditions, it is important to be keen on diagnosis owing to their importance. *Increased urinary frequency (Pollakiuria)*: The symptoms of Pollakiuria are an increase in the frequency of urination during the day and at night without any alteration in the volume of urine [94]. Investigate the possible causes of the bladder pressure and the pain in the urinary tract. *Urgency*: The abrupt need to urinate that cannot be delayed. The condition can lead to a strong urge to urinate. Research the neural systems and brain tissues that cause this feeling in the human body. *Nocturia*: Patients experience the necessity to wake up several times during the night to urinate. The frequency of nocturnal urination plays two roles in patient evaluation; a few instances are normal, whereas frequent instances have to be addressed with medical attention. Determine possible causes of changes in fluids, hormonal reactions, and underlying pathophysiology [95]. *Weak or intermittent urinary system*: The urinary stream is difficult to start or presents irregular flow patterns [96]. It also does not express itself, and it does not break in midstream and restart. Discuss the physical deformities and functional impairment that may lead to the given disorders. For example, straining to urinate: The patient has urine retention or must strain his muscles before he or she begins to urinate [97]. The condition seems to be caused by a blocked urinary tract or difficulty with emptying. *Incomplete bladder emptying*: After urination, the bladder might not be emptied completely, and this will cause an urge to withhold the urination [98]. Failure to empty the bladder to full capacity may result in frequent urination and increase the chances of developing urinary tract infections. During their menstrual cycle, patients who have *dysuria* report burning or pain during that period. Consider both inflammatory and infectious diseases as etiologies. *Hematuria* can be classified into two groups based on the observability of blood in the urine: microscopic hematuria, where blood can only be seen under a microscope, and gross hematuria, where blood is actually visible, and the urine is red [99]. The analysis of hematuria should be done in a fast manner since any blood in the urine should undergo professional testing to determine the cause.

1.6.2 Sexual Symptoms: Impact on Function and Comfort

The urinary and sexual symptoms vary in people, and the differences between them are significant [100]. Depending on personal experiences of menopause, the degree of urinary and sexual changes is negligible to significant. The diagnosis requires a full medical history and physical examination, as urinary and sexual symptoms are frequently observed with other diseases. *Erectile dysfunction (ED)*: It is a health condition whereby men find it difficult to achieve or maintain a good erection to engage in sexual contact that is satisfactory [101]. The paper examines how the vascular, neurological, hormonal, and psychological variables affect the development of erectile dysfunction. Painful ejaculation (*Dysorgasmia*) is a condition characterized by painful ejaculation during or after the sexual release. Medical workers should examine the presence of inflammatory or obstructive afflictions of the reproductive canal. *Decreased ejaculate volume*: Reduced ejaculate volume is present in cases where a reduced amount of semen is emptied during sexual climax. An altered functioning of the glands can be the cause of this syndrome [102]. *Hematospermia* (blood in the ejaculate): The condition might not necessarily mean a serious problem, but it is necessary to check with a doctor in order to rule out possible dangerous diseases [103]. *Changes in libido (sexual desire)*: The sexual appeal of an individual may be less because of changes in hormones and the physical and mental impact of the medical disorder.

1.6.3 Advanced Disease Manifestations: Indicators of Progression and Systemic Involvement

The disease progresses to advanced stages where severe symptoms are manifested, and therefore, they need to be treated in specific ways to ensure that patients have the best possible outcome. The deep bone pain is characterized by long-term pain mainly affecting the back, hips, ribs, and pelvis, and it sometimes indicates metastatic disease, which usually increases in intensity with body movement or even during rest [104]. The recurrent or increasing lower back pain accompanied by symptoms of radiating pain may indicate that the disease is deteriorating in the region or an issue with the nerves. Engagement of the locals and inflammation can lead to pressure-related symptoms, i.e., perineal pain or discomfort [105]. Systemic effects like weight loss that occur as a result of increased metabolic demands and deep fatigue are systemic manifestations that often occur due to a combination of inflammation, anemia, and metabolic changes that affect the body [106]. Anemia, which is characterized by a lack of red blood cells, causes fatigue, dyspnea, and weakness, which can be explained by the involvement of bone marrow, therapeutic procedures, or chronic inflammation. Pressure or blockage in the lymphatic system causes edema in the legs or ankles. Approved bowel movement disruption, including constipation or incontinence, occurs due to compression of nerves or involvement of tissues next to them [107]. Nerve symptoms such as numbness, tingling, and weakness of legs or feet when pressure is put on the spinal cord or peripheral nerves tend to manifest [108]. Swollen lymph nodes in the groin and other parts of the body may mean that cancer has spread to the lymphatic tissues. The diverse nature of advanced illness leads to differing symptomatology among patients, as the progression of the disease and specific patient factors affect symptom expression [109].

1.6.4 When to Get Medical Help: Identifying Warning Signs and Taking Quick Action

In the early stages, prostate cancer grows without causing any symptoms, which makes it hard for people to notice it in their daily lives. Table 1.2 indicates that a medical evaluation is warranted when certain symptoms manifest during the progression of prostate cancer [110]. Medical results are enhanced due to prompt intervention upon the emergence of these warning indicators.

1.6.4.1 When to Seek Medical Evaluation

An individual exhibiting these symptoms should consult a medical professional for evaluation, since several illnesses other than prostate cancer may elicit comparable symptoms. Digital rectal exams and the routine delivery of prostate-specific antigen testing are crucial for the early detection of prostate cancer, particularly aimed at individuals with elevated risk [117]. The American Cancer Society recommends

Table 1.2 Symptoms that signal warning signs of prostate cancer and indicate when to seek medical attention

Category	Symptoms/Details	Sources	References
Urinary changes	More frequent urination, particularly throughout the night (nocturia) A weak or irregular urine stream or trouble starting to urinate A sensation of incomplete bladder emptying Urgency or pain during urination	Zero Cancer, Hackensack Meridian Health, NHS	[111, 112]
Hematuria and hematospermia	Blood in the urine or semen (appearing pink, red, or cola-colored)	Mayo Clinic, American Cancer Society	[113]
Erectile and ejaculatory issues	Difficulty achieving or maintaining an erection Painful ejaculation or decreased volume of ejaculate	Johns Hopkins Medicine, Prostate Cancer UK	[114]
Persistent pain	Unexplained pain in the back, hips, pelvis, or bones (potentially indicating advanced disease)	Hackensack Meridian Health	[115]
Systemic symptoms	Unintended weight loss Fatigue or generalized weakness	Urology Health, Cleveland Clinic, Wikipedia	[116]

that persons consider prostate cancer screening at the following intervals: The screening commencement age for average-risk male patients should be 50; for men who have been recognized as high risk, such as African American men and those whose family relatives were diagnosed before the age of 65, prostate cancer screening should begin at age 45; prostate cancer screening for male patients is warranted at age 40 if they have several first-degree relatives diagnosed at an early stage.

1.6.4.2 Advancements in Detection and Treatment

Recent improvements in prostate cancer diagnosis and treatment have made it much easier to find the disease early and get personalized care. Multiparametric MRI (mpMRI) offers high-resolution imaging to identify suspicious areas, thereby improving biopsy accuracy [118]. Genomic testing looks at genetic markers to figure out how aggressive a cancer is, which makes it possible to create personalized treatment plans. Localized therapies such as cryotherapy and high-intensity focused ultrasound (HIFU) specifically target malignant areas while minimizing damage to adjacent healthy tissue [119]. Immunotherapy and targeted therapy also prove to be promising as an attempt to combat cancer cells in a more efficient manner with the aid of the body's immune system and special medications. Education constitutes knowing the symptoms of prostate cancer and screening early to detect the disease and treat it successfully [120]. Attending the doctor immediately after the symptoms appear will ensure prompt treatment and availability of the latest advancements in the treatment of prostate cancer, which will result in improved outcomes and improved quality of life.

1.7 Screening and Diagnosis

The treatment of prostate cancer is important and needs early diagnosis, as well as an increase in the number of those who will survive. Screening procedures are involved in the early detection of cancer, and it is most treatable at this stage, and diagnostic treatments are used to confirm the presence of cancer and the extent of its badness [121]. The detection and screening of prostate cancer have been developed to a higher level, integrating improved imaging, genetic testing, and AI-based approaches [122]. Although PSA testing and DRE are standard screening procedures, new procedures in place of the standard, such as mpMRI, biomarker analysis, and molecular diagnostics, are more accurate and reduce the number of unnecessary tests. Early and proper diagnosis results in timely and proper treatment, hence better patient outcomes [123].

1.7.1 PSA Testing

PSA is a protein produced by both benign and cancerous cells of the prostate. One popular blood test that aids in the early detection of prostate cancer is the PSA test. *Indications for PSA testing*: routine screening among men over 50 years;

pre-screening (at the age of 40–45 years) in men with a family history of prostate cancer or in African Americans; monitoring response to treatment in patients with a diagnosis. *Limitations of PSA testing*: PSA levels can rise in non-malignant diseases such as benign prostatic hyperplasia (BPH) and prostatitis; there is a risk of false positives and resultant unnecessary biopsies and distress; certain prostate cancers are not of high PSA production, thus leading to false negatives.

1.7.1.1 Digital Rectal Examination (DRE)

During a DRE, a medical professional monitors the prostate gland by inserting a gloved, lubricated finger into the rectum. *Advantages of DRE*: It can detect abnormalities such as asymmetry, nodules, or induration; it is beneficial in identifying prostate cancers with normal PSA levels. *Limitations of DRE*: It cannot detect cancers deep within the prostate; it is generally used in conjunction with PSA testing to increase diagnostic sensitivity.

1.7.2 Imaging Techniques (MRI, Ultrasound, Biopsy)

Multiparametric MRI (mpMRI) has transformed the diagnosis of prostate cancer with its detailed images of the prostate and the ability to mark suspicious regions that need to be biopsied. *Advantages of mpMRI*: It enhances the detection of clinically significant prostate cancer; it avoids unnecessary biopsies by identifying low-risk lesions; it guides targeted biopsy procedures for precision diagnosis. *Limitations of MRI*: It is costly and not readily available; it needs skill to comprehend; it may give false negatives in some situations. *Ultrasound (Transrectal Ultrasound—TRUS)*: To direct prostate biopsies and measure prostate volume, TRUS is frequently utilized. *Advantages of TRUS*: It is widely available and relatively inexpensive; it can guide systematic prostate biopsies. *Limitations of TRUS*: It has a limited ability to differentiate between benign and malignant tissues; it is less accurate than mpMRI in detecting prostate cancer. *Prostate biopsy*: The most reliable way to confirm prostate cancer is with a biopsy. To perform the surgery, small tissue samples from the prostate are taken for histological examination [124]. There are three different categories of biopsy methods (Fig. 1.3). It also has certain drawbacks; it is an intrusive operation that has a risk of infection and bleeding; occasionally, the sampling error may lead to underdiagnosis, and sometimes, it may miss clinically significant cancer if not properly targeted [125].

1.7.3 Emerging Diagnostic Approaches

1.7.3.1 Biomarker-Based Testing

Novel biomarkers and genetic assays are being explored to improve prostate cancer diagnosis beyond PSA testing. The Prostate Health Index (PHI), integrating PSA, free PSA, and [−2] proPSA, enhances the precision of cancer diagnosis [126]. The 4 K score test evaluates four distinct PSA-related proteins to determine cancer risk,

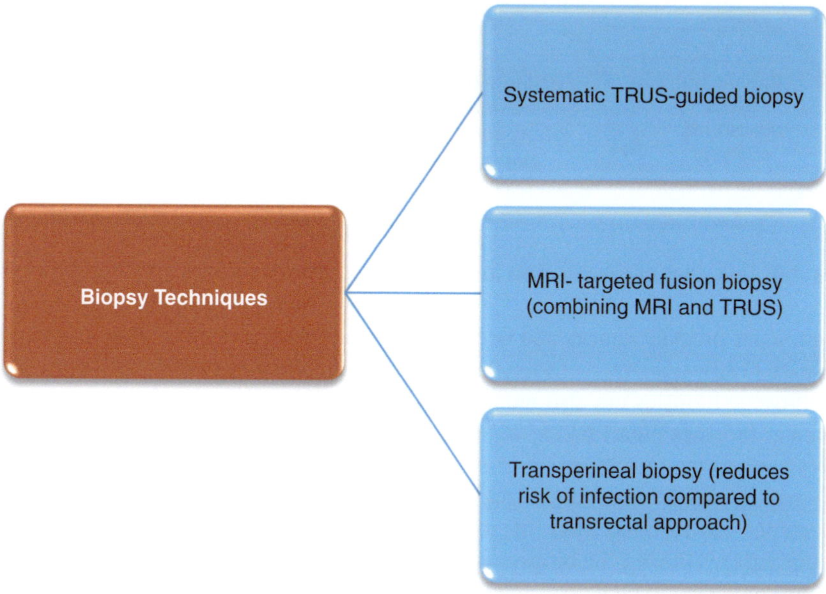

Fig. 1.3 Three distinct types of biopsy techniques

whereas the urinary PCA3 test identifies prostate cancer antigen 3, which is highly specific to prostate cancer. These evaluations improve diagnostic accuracy and enable risk stratification [127]. Genomic tests are noteworthy in determining the aggressiveness of a cancer. The "Decipher Test" considers the probability of spread, and the Prolaris Test considers the probability of worsening. The tests offer huge information about the molecular characteristics of prostate cancer, so that they can be treated in a customized manner [128].

1.7.3.2 Artificial Intelligence (AI) in Prostate Cancer Diagnosis

Artificial intelligence (AI) is transforming the way we diagnose prostate cancer, providing us with powerful tools that will enhance the effectiveness and accuracy of other diagnostic methods. It can be used in the interpretation of medical images, to verify the accuracy of biopsy procedures, and in the examination of samples in pathology [129]. Medical imaging AI algorithms are being trained to play a crucial role in the processing of magnetic resonance imaging (MRI) and ultrasound data [130]. These algorithms could learn with a lot of pictures, and this allows it to discover intricate patterns and issues that one may not easily see with their eyes (Fig. 1.4). AI can assist in dividing the prostate gland into sections, identifying suspicious lesions by their texture, shape, and contrast enhancement patterns, and predicting Gleason scores that are significant in determining the aggressiveness of a cancer in MRI [131]. AI may conduct real-time analysis, point out the areas of concern, and reduce the number of unnecessary biopsies during ultrasonic imaging. The inputs of AI to radiologists can enhance the specificity of detecting clinically

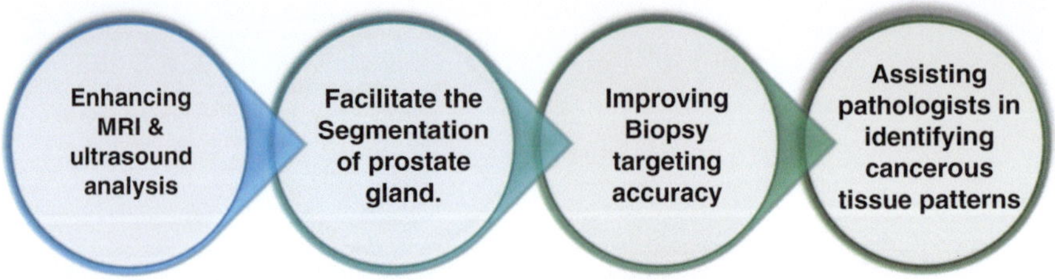

Fig. 1.4 Utilization of AI technology in the diagnosis of prostate cancer

significant prostate cancer and decrease the chances of over-detecting an indolent disease [132].

Prostate biopsies are also much more accurate with the help of AI. Normal systematic biopsies entail taking random samples around the various sections of the prostate and may exclude cancerous areas. Intelligent computer systems based on AI may be used to direct the targeted biopsies using advanced MRI data [133]. Such machines can fuse the MRI images obtained prior to surgery with real-time ultrasound images during the biopsy, which enables urologists to direct the tumors that AI has indicated to be worrisome during the biopsy. This narrow technique makes it more likely that higher tumors will be found and makes it easier to put patients into the right risk group [134].

1.8 Impact of Prostate Cancer on the Patient's Life

Prostate cancer is one of the most common types of cancer among men worldwide, and it has a significant effect that goes beyond the reasonable size of the disease. Table 1.3 [135], which presents the diagnosis and treatment of prostate cancer, places a heavy burden of physical and emotional costs on patients and their families, negatively affecting the quality of life and causing significant economic and social impacts on individuals and healthcare systems [136].

1.8.1 Physical and Emotional Burden

The physical consequences of prostate cancer manifest themselves in a significant number of ways, beginning with difficulty in peeing, pain, and difficulty in gaining an erection. Diagnostic tests, including biopsies, might be painful and dangerous. Prostate cancer can be treated using hormone therapy, radiation therapy, chemotherapy, and surgery, although all of them can have adverse effects [138]. These can result in urinary incontinence, bowel dysfunction, sexual dysfunction, fatigue, and bone pain that can have a significant impact on the physical health and life of a person. Prostate cancer does not just affect the body, but also the emotions of the victims to a large measure. The fear and panic of a cancer diagnosis, the uncertainty

Table 1.3 Effect of prostate cancer on the patient's quality of life

Domain	Key aspects	Effects	References
Physical and emotional burden	Physical effects	Urinary difficulties, pain, erectile dysfunction, and side effects from treatment (incontinence, bowel dysfunction, fatigue, bone pain)	[137]
	Emotional impact	Anxiety, depression, uncertainty about prognosis, and distress due to physical and sexual health changes	
	Family and caregiver impact	Emotional stress, anxiety, helplessness, and a need for psychological support	
Effects on quality of life (QoL)	Physical well-being	Reduced energy level, fatigue, limited mobility, and chronic pain	[115]
	Social relationships	Withdrawal from social interactions, intimacy issues, alters family dynamics	
	Emotional well-being	Stress, self-esteem issues, fear of recurrence, and ongoing monitoring anxiety	
	Sexual health	Erectile dysfunction, loss of intimacy, and psychological distress	
Economic and social implications	Financial costs	Direct costs (treatment, medication, consultations) and indirect costs (lost wages, caregiving expenses)	[116]
	Healthcare system burden	High resource demand for screening, treatment, long-term management, and research funding needs	
	Social challenges	Responsibilities for caregiving, changes in family roles, and the need for community and support networks	

of the prognosis and treatment results, and the suffering brought on by the side effects of treatment may cause severe psychological trauma [139]. Patients can develop feelings of desperation, anxiety, changing self-esteem, and loss of body system and sexual functioning. The emotional strain can be transmitted to the spouses and even to the family members, where they may feel anxious, tense, and helpless as they help their loved one [140]. To manage these emotional issues, one should be forthright with each other and should be in a position to access psychiatric assistance.

1.8.2 Impact on Life Quality

The associated physical and mental complications associated with the occurrence of prostate cancer pose significant implications on the overall quality of life (QoL) of the patient [141]. The effect is evident in diverse aspects, including physical, social, mental, and sexual health. As a side effect of the treatment, urinary incontinence and erectile dysfunction may have a significant impact on the self-esteem of the man, his relationship with his wife, and his social activities [142]. It may be difficult to even do the routine chores and reduce your overall energy, which may deteriorate your quality of life. Besides, mental health and social bond can deteriorate due to the mental pain associated with the condition and its management. Patients can step aside from social life because of physical impairments or mental trauma [143]. The uncertain development of the disease and the constant need to follow and possibly receive further treatment can increase chronic stress and anxiety, thus decreasing the quality of life even more [144]. It is agreed that quality of life (QoL) is a crucial component of prostate cancer treatment, and it should be improved and measured. Interventions, which assist in managing the side effects and psychological interventions, are of particular significance toward enhancing patient outcomes.

1.8.3 Economic and Social Implications

Diagnosis and treatment of prostate cancer have significant implications for an individual and society collectively. Patients and their families could also encounter high direct medical expenses, relating to consultations, diagnostic tests, treatments, medications, and additional care [145]. Diagnosis and treatment of prostate cancer have significant implications for an individual and society collectively. Direct medical expenses may be substantial for consultations, diagnostic tests, treatments, and drugs, as well as additional care for patients and their families [146]. Moreover, the long-term care of survivors of prostate cancer, including recurrence monitoring and treatment of late side effects, is also an additional cost to the overall healthcare expenditure. Prostate cancer has social impacts on a family and communities. When one of the family members is ill, this can alter the way things are done at home and leave spouses or other family members to take care of them, which in turn affects the way individuals interact. Community-based programs and support networks play a crucial role in providing emotional, physical, and informational support to patients and their families, helping to mitigate some of the social challenges associated with the condition [147]. This knowledge of these economic and social impacts is critical to formulating holistic approaches to the management and care of prostate cancer.

1.9 Current Trends and Future Perspectives

1.9.1 Advances in Research and Treatment

The future of research and therapy of prostate cancer in 2025 is that the trends are changing at a very high rate. Much focus is made on creating more customized and less invasive methods [148]. The advances in imaging technology, particularly PSMA-PET scans, are contributing to the fact that it is becoming easier to diagnose and stage the diseases, which can give information about how widely they have spread and how they recur. New types of drugs, like Lutetium-177 PSMA radioligand treatments, show promise in treating metastatic castration-resistant prostate cancer (mCRPC), sometimes even before chemotherapy [149]. The advancement of novel combination medicines, including PARP inhibitors paired with androgen receptor inhibitors, is broadening treatment options for advanced illnesses. Focal therapy, designed to target just the malignant regions inside the prostate, is now being studied to reduce adverse effects [150]. Current research on immunotherapy aims to increase the immune system's ability to recognize and combat prostate cancer cells.

1.9.2 Role of Personalized Medicine

By 2025, the treatment of prostate cancer will depend more on personalized therapy. Genetic testing for germline and somatic mutations is becoming increasingly common, facilitating the identification of males at elevated risk, informing treatment choices, and predicting responses to certain medications [151]. The presence of BReast CAncer gene (BRCA) or other mutations in homologous recombination repair genes can qualify patients for PARP medicines. Risk stratification instruments that incorporate genetic and genomic data are being refined to more accurately assess cancer aggressiveness and inform decisions between active surveillance and prompt intervention [152]. Molecular biomarkers and artificial intelligence are being investigated to determine which patients may derive the greatest benefit from specific therapies, including adjuvant androgen therapy.

1.9.3 Future Directions in Prevention and Care

By 2025, future efforts to prevent and treat prostate cancer will focus on finding the disease earlier and more accurately, giving less aggressive treatment to people who are at low risk, and getting better results for people who are in later stages. Research into dietary and microbial metabolites is exploring potential prevention strategies [153]. Risk-adjusted screening methodologies, potentially incorporating genetic risk scores and novel biomarkers, aim to identify high-risk individuals at an earlier stage. For localized prostate cancer, there is a growing preference for conservative management, such as active surveillance, particularly for intermediate-risk disease, to delay or avoid treatment and its associated adverse effects. The invented imaging and customized treatment will probably enhance the focused therapy approaches [154]. In high-grade prostate cancer, the emphasis is on the struggle of therapy resistance and new immunotherapeutic approaches, as well as on the quality of life of patients with the metastatic disease based on the improved quality of symptom control and supportive therapy [155]. It is believed that the use of artificial intelligence in the diagnosis, treatment planning, and monitoring of prostate cancer will have a significant effect on prostate cancer treatment in the future.

1.10 Conclusion

Medicine proves that prostate cancer is a very common type of cancer that men contract worldwide. It also presents significant issues in the epidemiologic criteria, clinical practice, and social aspects. This chapter gave the reader the basic information about prostate cancer by outlining its basic attributes, examining its prevalence, its risk factors, and its methods of diagnosis and treatment. A study of the structure of the prostate glands, which included the study of the TNM stage classification systems and Gleason grading systems, showed that effective diagnostic organizations are useful in helping healthcare professionals to choose appropriate treatments. PSA and DRE are significant methods through which prostate cancer can be detected at an early stage, when it is most likely to be treated. To learn the regularities of prostate cancer development, scientists examined various risk factors such as genetic predisposition, individual choices, and environmental factors. They were studied using clinical research on the medical and psychological impacts of the disease on the health of patients, as well as the financial and social costs of the disease. Integrating the studies of biomarkers with images and accurate medicine will enable the establishment of proper diagnoses and provide individual treatment opportunities. The fundamental concepts of the development of new plans in the treatment of prostate cancer are based on the application of technology in the examination of the disease and the prioritization of patients. The introductory concepts will be utilized as the background information in the further discussions. The introduction provides a simple insight into prostate cancer, and it becomes easier to discuss the approaches to treating the disease and how to take care of the patients.

1.11 Summary

Prostate cancer is one of the most common stages of cancer in men worldwide, and more so in those above 50 years. This chapter was very detailed on the anatomy of the disease, risk factors, classification, symptoms, diagnosis, and new methods of treating the disease. The importance of better imaging and biopsy, the growing importance of artificial intelligence and precision medicine, and the usefulness of early detection using PSA tests and DRE were all in the spotlight. Socioeconomic, emotional, and physical impacts of prostate cancer were addressed, and future perspectives and research trends in personalized care and current trends were discussed. By being aware of these things, the researcher and the medical professionals can successfully treat prostate cancer and develop new methods of treating prostate cancer.

Glossary

Adenocarcinoma A type of cancer that forms in glandular tissues, most commonly in the prostate.

Biopsy A procedure where tissue samples are taken for diagnostic examination.

Digital rectal examination (DRE) A manual exam to assess prostate abnormalities via the rectum.

Gleason score A grading system to determine prostate cancer aggressiveness.

Hormone therapy (ADT) Treatment that reduces levels of male hormones to control cancer growth.

Metastasis Spread of cancer to distant organs or tissues.

MRI Magnetic resonance imaging, used for detailed visualization of the prostate.

Neuroendocrine tumors Rare prostate cancers originating from hormone-secreting cells.

PSA (prostate-specific antigen) A protein produced by the prostate, elevated in prostate conditions.

Transperineal biopsy A type of biopsy accessed through the perineum to reduce infection risk.

References

1. Gandaglia G, et al. Epidemiology and prevention of prostate cancer. Eur Urol Oncol. 2021;4(6):877–92.
2. Descotes J-L. Diagnosis of prostate cancer. Asian J Urol. 2019;6(2):129–36.
3. Rawla P. Epidemiology of prostate cancer. World J Oncol. 2019;10(2):63.
4. Barlow M, et al. Ethnic differences in prostate-specific antigen levels in men without prostate cancer: a systematic review. Prostate Cancer Prostatic Dis. 2023;26(2):249–56.
5. Storås AH, Fosså SD, Ursin G, Andreassen BK. Survival trends for patients with primary metastatic prostate cancer before and after the introduction of new antitumor drugs. Prostate Cancer Prostatic Dis. 2023;26(1):53–8.
6. Bass EJ, et al. A systematic review and meta-analysis of the diagnostic accuracy of biparametric prostate MRI for prostate cancer in men at risk. Prostate Cancer Prostatic Dis. 2021;24(3):596–611.
7. Kawada T, et al. Diagnostic performance of prostate-specific membrane antigen positron emission tomography–targeted biopsy for detection of clinically significant prostate cancer: a systematic review and meta-analysis. Eur Urol Oncol. 2022;5(4):390–400.
8. Seetharaman A, et al. Automated detection of aggressive and indolent prostate cancer on magnetic resonance imaging. Med Phys. 2021;48(6):2960–72.
9. Kilic M, Madendere S, Vural M, Koseoglu E, Balbay MD, Esen T. The role of the size and number of index lesion in the diagnosis of clinically significant prostate cancer in patients with PI-RADS 4 lesions who underwent in-bore MRI-guided prostate biopsy. World J Urol. 2023;41(2):449–54.
10. Twilt JJ, et al. Evaluating biparametric versus multiparametric magnetic resonance imaging for diagnosing clinically significant prostate cancer: an international, paired, noninferiority, confirmatory observer study. Eur Urol. 2025;87(2):240–50.
11. Kimura T, Sato S, Takahashi H, Egawa S. Global trends of latent prostate cancer in autopsy studies. Cancers (Basel). 2021;13(2):359.
12. Nowroozi A, et al. Global and regional quality of care index for prostate cancer: an analysis from the Global Burden of Disease study 1990–2019. Arch Public Heal. 2023;81(1):70.
13. Zi H, et al. Global, regional, and national burden of kidney, bladder, and prostate cancers and their attributable risk factors, 1990–2019. Mil Med Res. 2021;8:1–15.
14. Zhang W, et al. Global burden of prostate cancer and association with socioeconomic status, 1990–2019: a systematic analysis from the global burden of disease study. J Epidemiol Glob Health. 2023;13(3):407–21.

15. Chowdhury-Paulino IM, Ericsson C, Vince R Jr, Spratt DE, George DJ, Mucci LA. Racial disparities in prostate cancer among black men: epidemiology and outcomes. Prostate Cancer Prostatic Dis. 2022;25(3):397–402.
16. Berenguer CV, Pereira F, Câmara JS, Pereira JAM. Underlying features of prostate cancer—statistics, risk factors, and emerging methods for its diagnosis. Curr Oncol. 2023;30(2):2300–21.
17. Craig EL, et al. Statins and prostate cancer—hype or hope? The epidemiological perspective. Prostate Cancer Prostatic Dis. 2022;25(4):641–9.
18. Qiu H, Cao S, Xu R. Cancer incidence, mortality, and burden in China: a time-trend analysis and comparison with the United States and United Kingdom based on the global epidemiological data released in 2020. Cancer Commun. 2021;41(10):1037–48.
19. Huang J, et al. Global trends of prostate cancer by age, and their associations with gross domestic product (GDP), human development index (HDI), smoking, and alcohol drinking. Clin Genitourin Cancer. 2023;21(4):e261–70.
20. Du J, et al. Quantifying suicide risk in prostate cancer: a SEER-based predictive model. J Epidemiol Glob Health. 2025;15(1):1–13.
21. Hashemi M, et al. Anatomy and function of prostate. In: Prostate cancer: molecular events and therapeutic modalities. Springer; 2024. p. 3–21.
22. Ryman-Tubb T, et al. Comparative pathology of dog and human prostate cancer. Vet Med Sci. 2022;8(1):110–20.
23. Tao L, Ma L, Xie M, Liu X, Tian Z, Fei B. Automatic segmentation of the prostate on MR images based on anatomy and deep learning. In: Proceedings of SPIE – the International Society for Optical Engineering; 2021. p. 115981N.
24. Lin Y-H, et al. Anterior fibromuscular stroma-preserved endoscopic enucleation of the prostate: a precision anatomical approach. World J Urol. 2023;41(8):2127–32.
25. Prins GS. Developmental estrogenization: prostate gland reprogramming leads to increased disease risk with aging. Differentiation. 2021;118:72–81.
26. Moura F, et al. Structural and ultrastructural morphological evaluation of Giant anteater (Myrmecophaga tridactyla) prostate gland. Biology (Basel). 2021;10(3):231.
27. Cannarella R, Condorelli RA, Barbagallo F, La Vignera S, Calogero AE. Endocrinology of the aging prostate: current concepts. Front Endocrinol (Lausanne). 2021;12:554078.
28. Fiard G, et al. Cellular senescence as a possible link between prostate diseases of the ageing male. Nat Rev Urol. 2021;18(10):597–610.
29. Guzmán-Esquivel J, et al. The impact of doxycycline as an adjunctive therapy on prostate-specific antigen, quality of life, and cognitive function in metastatic prostate cancer patients: a phase II randomized controlled trial. Pharmaceutics. 2025;17(4):404.
30. Dejous C, Krishnan UM. Sensors for diagnosis of prostate cancer: looking beyond the prostate specific antigen. Biosens Bioelectron. 2021;173:112790.
31. Zhang S, Tang X, Zang L, Zhao L. Carbon quantum dots (CQDs)-sensitized CdS/CuInS2 heterojunction as a photoelectrochemical biosensing platform for highly sensitive detection of prostate-specific antigen. Talanta. 2024;272:125811.
32. Hanson ED, et al. Body composition, physical function and quality of life in healthy men and across different stages of prostate cancer. Prostate Cancer Prostatic Dis. 2021;24(3):725–32.
33. Wasim S, Lee S-Y, Kim J. Complexities of prostate cancer. Int J Mol Sci. 2022;23(22):14257.
34. Hu L, Zhou D-W, Guo X-Y, Xu W-H, Wei L-M, Zhao J-G. Adversarial training for prostate cancer classification using magnetic resonance imaging. Quant Imaging Med Surg. 2022;12(6):3276.
35. Twilt JJ, van Leeuwen KG, Huisman HJ, Fütterer JJ, de Rooij M. Artificial intelligence based algorithms for prostate cancer classification and detection on magnetic resonance imaging: a narrative review. Diagnostics. 2021;11(6):959.
36. Hassan MR, et al. Prostate cancer classification from ultrasound and MRI images using deep learning based explainable artificial intelligence. Futur Gener Comput Syst. 2022;127:462–72.
37. Parimi V, Goyal R, Poropatich K, Yang XJ. Neuroendocrine differentiation of prostate cancer: a review. Am J Clin Exp Urol. 2014;2(4):273–85.

38. Chow K, et al. Ductal variant prostate carcinoma is associated with a significantly shorter metastasis-free survival. Eur J Cancer. 2021;148:440–50. https://doi.org/10.1016/j.ejca.2020.12.030.
39. Demirtaş A, et al. Small cell prostate carcinoma: a case report and review of the literature. Case Rep Urol. 2013;2013:387931. https://doi.org/10.1155/2013/387931.
40. Zhang S. Adenocarcinoma. In: Diagnostic imaging of lung cancers. Springer; 2024. p. 3–49.
41. Siech C, et al. Life expectancy in rare histological prostate cancer subtypes. Int J Cancer. 2024;156:2311.
42. Cabanillas G, Montoya-Cerrillo D, Kryvenko ON, Pal SK, Arias-Stella JA III. Collecting duct carcinoma of the kidney: diagnosis and implications for management. In: Urologic oncology: seminars and original investigations. Elsevier; 2022. p. 525–36.
43. Ranasinha N, et al. Ductal adenocarcinoma of the prostate: a systematic review and meta-analysis of incidence, presentation, prognosis, and management. Bjui Compass. 2021;2(1):13–23.
44. Wee CE, Costello BA, Orme JJ, Quevedo JF, Pagliaro LC. Chemotherapy with atezolizumab for small cell or neuroendocrine carcinoma of the prostate: a single institution experience. Prostate. 2021;81(13):938–43.
45. Gopalan A, Al-Ahmadie H, Chen Y, Sarungbam J, Sirintrapun SJ, Tickoo SK, et al. Neuroendocrine differentiation in the setting of prostatic carcinoma: contemporary assessment of a consecutive series. Histopathology. 2022;81(2):246–54.
46. Kanayama M, Luo J. Delineating the molecular events underlying development of prostate cancer variants with neuroendocrine/small cell carcinoma characteristics. Int J Mol Sci. 2021;22(23):12742.
47. Abdulfatah E, Fine SW, Lotan TL, Mehra R. De novo neuroendocrine features in prostate cancer. Hum Pathol. 2022;127:112–22.
48. Alabi BR, Liu S, Stoyanova T. Current and emerging therapies for neuroendocrine prostate cancer. Pharmacol Ther. 2022;238:108255. https://doi.org/10.1016/j.pharmthera.2022.108255.
49. Liauw SL, Son CH, Shergill A, Shogan BD. Circulating tumor-tissue modified HPV DNA analysis for molecular disease monitoring after chemoradiation for anal squamous cell carcinoma: a case report. J Gastrointest Oncol. 2021;12(6):3155–62. https://doi.org/10.21037/jgo-21-300.
50. Antonov P, Raycheva G. A rare case of a patient with primary urothelial carcinoma of the prostate urethra - multidisciplinary approach. Urol Case Rep. 2021;38:101643. https://doi.org/10.1016/j.eucr.2021.101643.
51. Cackowski FC, Heath EI. Prostate cancer dormancy and recurrence. Cancer Lett. 2022;524:103–8. https://doi.org/10.1016/j.canlet.2021.09.037.
52. Jakstas T, et al. The association of TP53, BCL2, BAX and NOXA SNPs and laryngeal squamous cell carcinoma development. Int J Mol Sci. 2024;25(21):11849. https://doi.org/10.3390/ijms252111849.
53. Liu Y, Lijun F, Liu W. High SQLE expression and gene amplification correlates with poor prognosis in head and neck squamous cell carcinoma. Cancer Manag Res. 2021;13:4709–23. https://doi.org/10.2147/CMAR.S305719.
54. Xu H, et al. Development and validation of a nomogram for predicting prostatic urethral involvement in bladder cancer. Sci Rep. 2025;15(1):10431. https://doi.org/10.1038/s41598-025-95684-6.
55. Packeiser E-M, Engels L, Nolte I, Goericke-Pesch S, Murua Escobar H. MDR1 inhibition reverses doxorubicin-resistance in six doxorubicin-resistant canine prostate and bladder cancer cell lines. Int J Mol Sci. 2023;24(9):8136. https://doi.org/10.3390/ijms24098136.
56. Park J, et al. Label-free optical redox ratio from urinary extracellular vesicles as a screening biomarker for bladder cancer. Am J Cancer Res. 2022;12(5):2068–83.
57. Croce S, et al. Uterine sarcomas and rare uterine mesenchymal tumors with malignant potential. Diagnostic guidelines of the French Sarcoma Group and the Rare Gynecological Tumors Group. Gynecol Oncol. 2022;167(2):373–89. https://doi.org/10.1016/j.ygyno.2022.07.031.

58. Trinidad CM, Wangsiricharoen S, Prieto VG, Aung PP. Rare variants of dermatofibrosarcoma protuberans: clinical, histologic, and molecular features and diagnostic pitfalls. Dermatopathology. 2023; https://doi.org/10.3390/dermatopathology10010008.
59. Schipper LJ, et al. Clinical impact of prospective whole genome sequencing in sarcoma patients. Cancers. 2022; https://doi.org/10.3390/cancers14020436.
60. Takahashi T. Prostate cancer screening and Gleason score: empirical clinical practice. Virchows Arch. 2024; https://doi.org/10.1007/s00428-024-03900-x.
61. Montironi R, et al. Narrative review of prostate cancer grading systems: will the Gleason scores be replaced by the Grade Groups? Transl Androl Urol. 2021;10(3):1530–40. https://doi.org/10.21037/tau-20-853.
62. Saunders EJ, Kote-Jarai Z, Eeles RA. Identification of germline genetic variants that increase prostate cancer risk and influence development of aggressive disease. Cancers (Basel). 2021;13(4):760. https://doi.org/10.3390/cancers13040760.
63. Boehm BE, York ME, Petrovics G, Kohaar I, Chesnut GT. Biomarkers of aggressive prostate cancer at diagnosis. Int J Mol Sci. 2023;24(3):2185. https://doi.org/10.3390/ijms24032185.
64. Shah N, Ioffe V, Chang JC. Increasing aggressive prostate cancer. Can J Urol. 2022;29(6):11384–90.
65. Sun BL, et al. A humanized monoclonal antibody targeting extracellular nicotinamide phosphoribosyltransferase prevents aggressive prostate cancer progression. Pharmaceuticals. 2021;14(12):1322. https://doi.org/10.3390/ph14121322.
66. Shah RB, et al. Genitourinary Pathology Society and International Society of Urological Pathology White Paper on defining indolent prostate cancer: call for a multidisciplinary approach. Eur Urol. 2025; https://doi.org/10.1016/j.eururo.2025.02.029.
67. Georgiou LA, Scarbrough BE. PSA screening for prostate cancer in the United States: 30 years of controversy. J Public Health Policy. 2024;45(3):552–61. https://doi.org/10.1057/s41271-024-00502-4.
68. Bhattacharya I, et al. Selective identification and localization of indolent and aggressive prostate cancers via CorrSigNIA: an MRI-pathology correlation and deep learning framework. Med Image Anal. 2022;75:102288. https://doi.org/10.1016/j.media.2021.102288.
69. Okpua NC, Okekpa SI, Njaka S, Emeh AN. Clinical diagnosis of prostate cancer using digital rectal examination and prostate-specific antigen tests: a systematic review and meta-analysis of sensitivity and specificity. Afr J Urol. 2021;27(1):32. https://doi.org/10.1186/s12301-021-00129-x.
70. Bergengren O, et al. 2022 update on prostate cancer epidemiology and risk factors—a systematic review. Eur Urol. 2023;84(2):191–206. https://doi.org/10.1016/j.eururo.2023.04.021.
71. Rivera-Izquierdo M, et al. Obesity as a risk factor for prostate cancer mortality: a systematic review and dose-response meta-analysis of 280,199 patients. Cancers (Basel). 2021;13(16):4169. https://doi.org/10.3390/cancers13164169.
72. Oczkowski M, Dziendzikowska K, Pasternak-Winiarska A, Włodarek D, Gromadzka-Ostrowska J. Dietary factors and prostate cancer development, progression, and reduction. Nutrients. 2021;13(2):496. https://doi.org/10.3390/nu13020496.
73. Greco L, Auricchio R. Chapter 3 – Genetic predisposition. In: Corazza GR, Troncone R, Lenti MV, Silano M, editors. Pediatric and adult celiac disease. Academic Press; 2024. p. 25–40. https://doi.org/10.1016/B978-0-443-13359-6.00020-0.
74. Song SH, Byun SS. Polygenic risk score for genetic evaluation of prostate cancer risk in Asian populations: a narrative review. Investig Clin Urol. 2021;62(3):256–66. https://doi.org/10.4111/icu.20210124.
75. Wu Y, Sarkissyan M, Vadgama JV. Epigenetics in breast and prostate cancer. Methods Mol Biol. 2015;1238:425–66. https://doi.org/10.1007/978-1-4939-1804-1_23.
76. Pardo JC, Ruiz de Porras V, Gil J, Font A, Puig-Domingo M, Jordà M. Lipid metabolism and epigenetics crosstalk in prostate cancer. Nutrients. 2022;14(4):851. https://doi.org/10.3390/nu14040851.
77. Liu M, et al. Gene polymorphism-related differences in the outcomes of abiraterone for prostate cancer: a systematic overview. Am J Cancer Res. 2021;11(5):1873–94.

78. Johnson E, Nussenzveig R, Agarwal N, Swami U. Germline variants and response to systemic therapy in advanced prostate cancer. Pharmacogenomics. 2020;21(1):75–81. https://doi.org/10.2217/pgs-2019-0125.
79. Abida W, et al. Genomic correlates of clinical outcome in advanced prostate cancer. Proc Natl Acad Sci USA. 2019;116(23):11428–36. https://doi.org/10.1073/pnas.1902651116.
80. Borque-Fernando A, et al. Genetic counseling in prostate cancer: how to implement it in daily clinical practice? Actas Urol Esp. 2021;45(1):8–20. https://doi.org/10.1016/j.acuro.2020.08.009.
81. Ornish D, et al. Changes in prostate gene expression in men undergoing an intensive nutrition and lifestyle intervention. Proc Natl Acad Sci USA. 2008;105(24):8369–74. https://doi.org/10.1073/pnas.0803080105.
82. Tan K, Naylor MJ. The influence of modifiable factors on breast and prostate cancer risk and disease progression. Front Physiol. 2022;13:840826. https://doi.org/10.3389/fphys.2022.840826.
83. Xu X, et al. The landscape of N(6)-methyladenosine in localized primary prostate cancer. Nat Genet. 2025;57(4):934–48. https://doi.org/10.1038/s41588-025-02128-y.
84. Sener TE, et al. Resveratrol treatment may preserve the erectile function after radiotherapy by restoring antioxidant defence mechanisms, SIRT1 and NOS protein expressions. Int J Impot Res. 2018;30(4):179–88. https://doi.org/10.1038/s41443-018-0042-6.
85. Porter CM, Shrestha E, Peiffer LB, Sfanos KS. The microbiome in prostate inflammation and prostate cancer. Prostate Cancer Prostatic Dis. 2018;21(3):345–54. https://doi.org/10.1038/s41391-018-0041-1.
86. Hoyt MA, Bower JE, Irwin MR, Weierich MR, Stanton AL. Sleep quality and depressive symptoms after prostate cancer: the mechanistic role of cortisol. Behav Neurosci. 2016;130(3):351–6. https://doi.org/10.1037/bne0000107.
87. Global burden and strength of evidence for 88 risk factors in 204 countries and 811 subnational locations, 1990-2021: a systematic analysis for the Global Burden of Disease Study 2021. Lancet (London, England). 2024;403(10440):2162–203. https://doi.org/10.1016/S0140-6736(24)00933-4.
88. Youogo LM-AK, Parent M-E, Hystad P, Villeneuve PJ. Ambient air pollution and prostate cancer risk in a population-based Canadian case-control study. Environment Epidemiol (Philadelphia, Pa.). 2022;6(4):e219. https://doi.org/10.1097/EE9.0000000000000219.
89. Li H, et al. Cancer incidence in a Swedish cohort with high exposure to perfluoroalkyl substances in drinking water. Environ Res. 2022;204(Pt C):112217. https://doi.org/10.1016/j.envres.2021.112217.
90. Gore AC, et al. EDC-2: the Endocrine Society's second scientific statement on endocrine-disrupting chemicals. Endocr Rev. 2015;36(6):E1–E150. https://doi.org/10.1210/er.2015-1010.
91. Leiker AJ, Desai NB, Folkert MR. Rectal radiation dose-reduction techniques in prostate cancer: a focus on the rectal spacer. Future Oncol. 2018;14(26):2773–88. https://doi.org/10.2217/fon-2018-0286.
92. McDermott N, et al. Fractionated radiation exposure amplifies the radioresistant nature of prostate cancer cells. Sci Rep. 2016;6:34796. https://doi.org/10.1038/srep34796.
93. Fanshawe JB, et al. Decision regret in patients with localised prostate cancer: a systematic review and meta-analysis. Eur Urol Oncol. 2023;6(5):456–66. https://doi.org/10.1016/j.euo.2023.02.005.
94. Schover LR. Sexual healing in patients with prostate cancer on hormone therapy. Am Soc Clin Oncol Educ Book. 2015:e562–6. https://doi.org/10.14694/EdBook_AM.2015.35.e562.
95. Raj S, Piang LK, Nair KS, Tiwari VK, Kaur H, Singh B. Awareness regarding risk factors, symptoms and treatment facilities for cancer in selected states of India. Asian Pac J Cancer Prev. 2012;13(8):4057–62. https://doi.org/10.7314/apjcp.2012.13.8.4057.
96. De Langhe S, et al. Acute radiation-induced nocturia in prostate cancer patients is associated with pretreatment symptoms, radical prostatectomy, and genetic markers in the TGFβ1 gene. Int J Radiat Oncol Biol Phys. 2013;85(2):393–9. https://doi.org/10.1016/j.ijrobp.2012.02.061.

97. Kalra S, Dhingra A, Kapoor N. Adrenal asthenia. J Pak Med Assoc. 2025;75(3):498–500. https://doi.org/10.47391/JPMA.25-18.
98. Janardanan S, Nigam A, Moschonas D, Perry M, Patil K. Urinary bladder diverticulum: a single-center experience in the management of refractory lower urinary symptoms using a robotic platform. Cureus. 2023;15(7):e42354. https://doi.org/10.7759/cureus.42354.
99. Oh JH, et al. Predicting the germline dependence of hematuria risk in prostate cancer radiotherapy patients. Radiother Oncol J Eur Soc Ther Radiol Oncol. 2023;185:109723. https://doi.org/10.1016/j.radonc.2023.109723.
100. Muermann MM, Wassersug RJ. Prostate cancer from a sex and gender perspective: a review. Sex Med Rev. 2022;10(1):142–54. https://doi.org/10.1016/j.sxmr.2021.03.001.
101. Amarasekera C, Wong V, Yura E, Manjunath A, Schaeffer E, Kundu S. Prostate cancer in sexual minorities and the influence of HIV status. Nat Rev Urol. 2019;16(7):404–21. https://doi.org/10.1038/s41585-019-0194-2.
102. Hoyt MA, Carpenter KM. Sexual self-schema and depressive symptoms after prostate cancer. Psychooncology. 2015;24(4):395–401. https://doi.org/10.1002/pon.3601.
103. Kotb AF, Beltagy A, Ismail AM, Hashad MM. Sexual activity and the risk of prostate cancer: review article. Arch Ital di Urol Androl organo Uff [di] Soc Ital di Ecogr Urol e Nefrol. 2015;87(3):214–5. https://doi.org/10.4081/aiua.2015.3.214.
104. Turner CJ, Edwards CM. The role of the microenvironment in prostate cancer-associated bone disease. Curr Osteoporos Rep. 2016;14(5):170–7. https://doi.org/10.1007/s11914-016-0323-2.
105. Humphrey PA, Andriole GL. Prostate cancer diagnosis. Mo Med. 2010;107(2):107–12.
106. Cao Y, Giovannucci E. Obesity and Prostate Cancer. Recent Results Cancer Res. 2016;208:137–53. https://doi.org/10.1007/978-3-319-42542-9_8.
107. Khan FM. Predicting advanced prostate cancer from modeling early indications in biopsy and prostatectomy samples via transductive semi-supervised survival analysis. Biomed Res Int. 2018;2018:2178645. https://doi.org/10.1155/2018/2178645.
108. Mesci A, et al. RSPO3 is a prognostic biomarker and mediator of invasiveness in prostate cancer. J Transl Med. 2019;17(1):125. https://doi.org/10.1186/s12967-019-1878-3.
109. Willems RAL, Winckers K, Biesmans C, de Vos-Geelen J, Ten Cate H. Evolving data on cardiovascular complications in cancer. Thromb Res. 2022;213(Suppl):S87–94. https://doi.org/10.1016/j.thromres.2022.01.003.
110. Goodwin BC, et al. Cancer-related help-seeking in cancer survivors living in regional and remote Australia. Psychooncology. 2021;30(7):1068–76. https://doi.org/10.1002/pon.5643.
111. Gnanapragasam VJ, Greenberg D, Burnet N. Urinary symptoms and prostate cancer—the misconception that may be preventing earlier presentation and better survival outcomes. BMC Med. 2022;20(1):264. https://doi.org/10.1186/s12916-022-02453-7.
112. Zanvit P, et al. Antitumor activity of AZD0754, a dnTGFβRII-armored, STEAP2-targeted CAR-T cell therapy, in prostate cancer. J Clin Invest. 2023;133(22). https://doi.org/10.1172/JCI169655.
113. Hakam N, et al. Hematospermia is rarely associated with urologic malignancy: analysis of United States claims data. Andrology. 2022;10(5):919–25. https://doi.org/10.1111/andr.13189.
114. Pizzol D, Trott M, Grabovac I, Yang L, Barnett Y, Parris C, et al. Ejaculation disorders in male patients with cancer: a systematic review and meta-analysis of prevalence. J Urol. 2021;206(6):1361–72.
115. Lane JA, et al. Functional and quality of life outcomes of localised prostate cancer treatments (Prostate Testing for Cancer and Treatment [ProtecT] study). BJU Int. 2022;130(3):370–80. https://doi.org/10.1111/bju.15739.
116. Lillard JW Jr, Moses KA, Mahal BA, George DJ. Racial disparities in Black men with prostate cancer: a literature review. Cancer. 2022;128(21):3787–95. https://doi.org/10.1002/cncr.34433.
117. King-Okoye M, Arber A, Faithfull S. Routes to diagnosis for men with prostate cancer: men's cultural beliefs about how changes to their bodies and symptoms influence help-seeking

actions. A narrative review of the literature. Eur J Oncol Nurs. 2017;30:48–58. https://doi.org/10.1016/j.ejon.2017.06.005.
118. Williams IS, et al. Modern paradigms for prostate cancer detection and management. Med J Aust. 2022;217(8):424–33. https://doi.org/10.5694/mja2.51722.
119. Wollersheim BM, et al. Type of treatment, symptoms and patient satisfaction play an important role in primary care contact during prostate cancer follow-up: results from the population-based PROFILES registry. BMC Fam Pract. 2021;22(1):218. https://doi.org/10.1186/s12875-021-01567-w.
120. Tichanek F, Försti A, Hemminki A, Hemminki O, Hemminki K. Long-term periodic and conditional survival trends in prostate, testicular, and penile cancers in the Nordic countries, marking timing of improvements. Cancers (Basel). 2023;15(17):4261. https://doi.org/10.3390/cancers15174261.
121. Ilic D, et al. Prostate cancer screening with prostate-specific antigen (PSA) test: a systematic review and meta-analysis. BMJ. 2018;362:k3519. https://doi.org/10.1136/bmj.k3519.
122. Nguyen-Nielsen M, Borre M. Diagnostic and therapeutic strategies for prostate cancer. Semin Nucl Med. 2016;46(6):484–90. https://doi.org/10.1053/j.semnuclmed.2016.07.002.
123. Wei JT, et al. Early detection of prostate cancer: AUA/SUO guideline part I: prostate cancer screening. J Urol. 2023;210(1):46–53. https://doi.org/10.1097/JU.0000000000003491.
124. Scattoni V, Russo A, Di Trapani E, Capitanio U, La Croce G, Montorsi F. Repeated biopsy in the detection of prostate cancer: when and how many cores. Arch Ital Urol Androl. 2014;86(4):311–3. https://doi.org/10.4081/aiua.2014.4.311.
125. Wei JT, et al. Early detection of prostate cancer: AUA/SUO guideline part II: considerations for a prostate biopsy. J Urol. 2023;210(1):54–63. https://doi.org/10.1097/JU.0000000000003492.
126. Gibney GT, Weiner LM, Atkins MB. Predictive biomarkers for checkpoint inhibitor-based immunotherapy. Lancet Oncol. 2016;17(12):e542–51. https://doi.org/10.1016/S1470-2045(16)30406-5.
127. Mizuno K, Beltran H. Future directions for precision oncology in prostate cancer. Prostate. 2022;82 Suppl 1(Suppl 1):S86–96. https://doi.org/10.1002/pros.24354.
128. Duffy MJ. Biomarkers for prostate cancer: prostate-specific antigen and beyond. Clin Chem Lab Med. 2020;58(3):326–39. https://doi.org/10.1515/cclm-2019-0693.
129. Bi WL, et al. Artificial intelligence in cancer imaging: clinical challenges and applications. CA Cancer J Clin. 2019;69(2):127–57.
130. Ström P, Kartasalo K, Olsson H, Solorzano L, Delahunt B, Berney DM, et al. Artificial intelligence for diagnosis and grading of prostate cancer in biopsies: a population-based, diagnostic. Lancet Oncol. 2020;21(2):222–32. https://doi.org/10.1016/S1470-2045(19)30738-7.
131. Saha A, et al. Artificial intelligence and radiologists in prostate cancer detection on MRI (PI-CAI): an international, paired, non-inferiority, confirmatory study. Lancet Oncol. 2024;25(7):879–87. https://doi.org/10.1016/S1470-2045(24)00220-1.
132. Suarez-Ibarrola R, et al. Artificial intelligence in magnetic resonance imaging-based prostate cancer diagnosis: where do we stand in 2021? Eur Urol Focus. 2022;8(2):409–17. https://doi.org/10.1016/j.euf.2021.03.020.
133. Zhu M, et al. Artificial intelligence in pathologic diagnosis, prognosis and prediction of prostate cancer. Am J Clin Exp Urol. 2024;12(4):200–15. https://doi.org/10.62347/JSAE9732.
134. Zhang K-X, Yu Z-P, Shen T-Y, Tang H. Application of artificial intelligence in the diagnosis of prostate cancer. Zhonghua Nan Ke Xue. 2023;29(12):1043–7.
135. Zopf EM, et al. Effects of a 15-month supervised exercise program on physical and psychological outcomes in prostate cancer patients following prostatectomy: the ProRehab study. Integr Cancer Ther. 2015;14(5):409–18. https://doi.org/10.1177/1534735415583552.
136. Burbridge C, et al. Understanding symptomatic experience, impact, and emotional response in recently diagnosed metastatic castration-resistant prostate cancer: a qualitative study. Support Care Cancer. 2020;28(7):3093–101. https://doi.org/10.1007/s00520-019-05079-3.
137. Spratt DE, Shore N, Sartor O, Rathkopf D, Olivier K. Treating the patient and not just the cancer: therapeutic burden in prostate cancer. Prostate Cancer Prostatic Dis. 2021;24(3):647–61.

138. Donachie K, et al. What interventions affect the psychosocial burden experienced by prostate cancer patients undergoing active surveillance? A scoping review. Support Care Cancer. 2022;30(6):4699–709. https://doi.org/10.1007/s00520-022-06830-z.
139. Johansen S, Cvancarova M, Ruland C. The effect of cancer patients' and their family caregivers' physical and emotional symptoms on caregiver burden. Cancer Nurs. 2018;41(2):91–9. https://doi.org/10.1097/NCC.0000000000000493.
140. Potosky AL, et al. Demographic and clinical factors associated with health-related quality-of-life profiles among prostate cancer survivors. JCO Oncol Pract. 2024;20(7):921–31. https://doi.org/10.1200/OP.24.00076.
141. Yamada Y, Beltran H. The treatment landscape of metastatic prostate cancer. Cancer Lett. 2021;519:20–9. https://doi.org/10.1016/j.canlet.2021.06.010.
142. Yang B, Wang J. Effects of exercise on cancer-related fatigue and quality of life in prostate cancer patients undergoing androgen deprivation therapy: a meta-analysis of randomized clinical trials. Chinese Med Sci J = Chung-kuo i hsueh k'o hsueh tsa chih. 2017;32(1):13–21. https://doi.org/10.24920/j1001-9242.2007.002.
143. Thompson D, et al. Long-term health-related quality of life in patients on active surveillance for prostate cancer: a systematic review. Eur Urol Oncol. 2023;6(1):4–15. https://doi.org/10.1016/j.euo.2022.09.001.
144. Rafikova G, Gilyazova I, Enikeeva K, Pavlov V, Kzhyshkowska J. Prostate cancer: genetics, epigenetics and the need for immunological biomarkers. Int J Mol Sci. 2023;24(16):12797. https://doi.org/10.3390/ijms241612797.
145. Launer BM, Lloyd GL. Sociodemographic index and global trends in prostate cancer: 1990-2017. Prostate. 2021;81(12):825–31. https://doi.org/10.1002/pros.24178.
146. Venkateswaran V, Klotz LH. Diet and prostate cancer: mechanisms of action and implications for chemoprevention. Nat Rev Urol. 2010;7(8):442–53. https://doi.org/10.1038/nrurol.2010.102.
147. Mahal BA, et al. Travel distance and stereotactic body radiotherapy for localized prostate cancer. Cancer. 2018;124(6):1141–9. https://doi.org/10.1002/cncr.31190.
148. Brown LC, et al. Clinical outcomes in patients with metastatic renal cell carcinoma and brain metastasis treated with ipilimumab and nivolumab. J Immunother Cancer. 2021;9(9):e003281. https://doi.org/10.1136/jitc-2021-003281.
149. Suman S, et al. Therapeutic efficacy, prognostic variables and clinical outcome of (177) Lu-PSMA-617 PRLT in progressive mCRPC following multiple lines of treatment: prognostic implications of high FDG uptake on dual tracer PET-CT vis-à-vis Gleason score in such cohort. Br J Radiol. 2019;92(1104):20190380. https://doi.org/10.1259/bjr.20190380.
150. Schiano C, Soricelli A, De Nigris F, Napoli C. New challenges in integrated diagnosis by imaging and osteo-immunology in bone lesions. Expert Rev Clin Immunol. 2019;15(3):289–301. https://doi.org/10.1080/1744666X.2019.1561283.
151. Akhoundova D, Feng FY, Pritchard CC, Rubin MA. Molecular genetics of prostate cancer and role of genomic testing. Surg Pathol Clin. 2022;15(4):617–28. https://doi.org/10.1016/j.path.2022.08.002.
152. Vietri MT, et al. Hereditary prostate cancer: genes related, target therapy and prevention. Int J Mol Sci. 2021;22(7):3753. https://doi.org/10.3390/ijms22073753.
153. Ballon-Landa E, Parsons JK. Nutrition, physical activity, and lifestyle factors in prostate cancer prevention. Curr Opin Urol. 2018;28(1):55–61. https://doi.org/10.1097/MOU.0000000000000460.
154. Hussain Y, et al. Quercetin and its nano-scale delivery systems in prostate cancer therapy: paving the way for cancer elimination and reversing chemoresistance. Cancers (Basel). 2021;13(7):1602. https://doi.org/10.3390/cancers13071602.
155. Burden of disease scenarios by state in the USA, 2022–50: a forecasting analysis for the Global Burden of Disease Study 2021. Lancet (London, England). 2024;404(10469):2341–70. https://doi.org/10.1016/S0140-6736(24)02246-3.

The Role of Biomarkers in Prostate Cancer Diagnosis

2

Rahul Kumar, Vaishali Bhagwani, Rakesh Sahu, and Ankita Kabi

Abbreviations

PSA	prostate-specific antigen
DRE	digital rectal examination
PCA3	prostate cancer antigen 3
CTCs	circulating tumor cells
miRNA	microRNA
DNA	deoxyribonucleic acid
RNA	ribonucleic acid
PSAD	PSA density
PSAV	PSA velocity
EPI	ExoDx Prostate IntelliScore
HOXC6	homeobox C6 gene
DLX1	distal-less homeobox 1 gene
TMPRSS2	transmembrane protease, serine 2
ERG	ETS-related gene
cfDNA	cell-free DNA

R. Kumar
Faculty of Pharmacy, Vidya University, Meerut, Uttar Pradesh, India

V. Bhagwani
Department of Pharmacy, K.P Singh Memorial Institute of Pharmacy, Siapur, Uttar Pradesh, India

R. Sahu
School of Pharmacy, Sharda University, Knowledge Park III, Greater Noida, Uttar Pradesh, India

A. Kabi (✉)
Department of Anaesthesiology, Pain Medicine and Critical Care, AIIMS Gorakhpur, Gorakhpur, Uttar Pradesh, India

S. Srivastava et al. (eds.), *Biosensor Technologies for Prostate Cancer*, https://doi.org/10.1007/978-981-95-8644-8_2

2.1 Introduction

The diagnosis of prostate cancer requires immediate attention because it represents a prominent worldwide health matter that requires effective early-stage detection to boost patient outcomes [1]. The heterogeneous nature of the disease presents difficulties in identifying it because disease forms display both slow-growing and fast-moving characteristics [2]. Standard diagnostic methods, including prostate-specific antigen (PSA) testing and digital rectal examinations (DREs), are used to provide care; however, they often fail to deliver optimal results [3]. PSA produces too many false signals because it lacks precision, while DRE fails to detect substantial numbers of the disease. The failure to properly differentiate between important and non-significant cancers leads to medical procedures being performed on both types of cancers. Research has concentrated on prostate cancer biomarkers in an attempt to resolve the existing challenges [4]. The availability of biological fluid-based measurements represents a significant step toward enhanced disease detection, as these indicators provide specific and informative information about the disease state through improved sensitivity levels, risk assessment capabilities, and non-invasive test capabilities [5].

2.1.1 Burden of Prostate Cancer and the Need for Improved Diagnosis

Prostate cancer exists as a major healthcare problem globally because it maintains its position among the principal cancers that affect male populations worldwide, while generating significant mortality rates due to cancer [6]. Effective diagnostic strategies remain essential for medical practice due to the vast scope of this disease. Detecting prostate cancer in its early stages, together with precise diagnosis, becomes essential for obtaining prompt treatment along with better clinical results, which leads to improved patient prognosis [7]. The diagnosis of prostate cancer becomes challenging because this condition exists across several distinct disease categories, from harmless yet low risk to advanced and rapidly growing tumor types [8]. Due to the variations in prostate cancer characteristics, professionals need complex instruments that detect cancer and tell significant from insignificant cases [9]. Medical practice requires proactive innovations in diagnostic systems, which need to eliminate present evaluation techniques to deliver doctors better, specific, detailed patient disease analysis and risk assessment results [10].

2.1.2 Limitations of Traditional Diagnostic Methods (PSA, DRE)

Health professionals have used prostate-specific antigen (PSA) screening and digital rectal examination (DRE) as the primary methods for detecting prostate cancer since the 1970s [11]. Table 2.1 presents a comparative analysis of

Table 2.1 Comparing biomarker-based and conventional diagnostic techniques for the detection of prostate cancer

Aspect	Traditional methods (PSA, DRE)	Biomarker-based approaches	References
Specificity	Low PSA is elevated in many non-cancerous conditions	Higher biomarkers are more specific to prostate cancer pathology	[14, 15]
Sensitivity	Variable may miss tumor, especially small or anterior-located ones with DRE	Improved more precisely finds aggressive and early-stage types	[11, 16]
Risk stratification	Limited cannot distinguish between indolent and aggressive cancers	Provides detailed risk profiles, aiding in targeted patient management	[17, 18]
Invasiveness	PSA is non-invasive; DRE is mildly invasive and uncomfortable	Mostly non-invasive (e.g., blood or urine-based biomarker)	[19, 20]
False positives/ negatives	High rate leads to unnecessary biopsies or missed diagnosis	Reduced Biomarkers help avoid overtreatment and missed aggressive cancer	[21, 22]
Clinical utility	Widely available, easy to use but with limited diagnostic value	Still emerging, requires validation, but shows strong potential for enhancing clinical care	[23, 24]
Patient-centric approach	Generic, less tailored to individual patient risk	Enables personalized diagnostics and treatment strategies	[18, 25]

conventional diagnostic methods, such as PSA and DRE, against new biomarker-based approaches, highlighting the drawbacks of traditional tools and the potential benefits of biomarkers in terms of specificity, sensitivity, risk stratification, and patient experience [12]. PSA testing has produced early identification outcomes in select men, yet it faces important performance barriers. The prostate-specific antigen PSA gets elevated in levels beyond typical ranges from benign prostatic hyperplasia (BPH), together with prostatitis and physical exercise [13]. The nonspecific nature of these tests results in numerous false-positive outcomes, therefore initiating avoidable and uncomfortable biopsies that endanger patient health. PSA screening has received criticism because it fails to properly distinguish between aggressive cancers and indolent ones, which results in the medical intervention of non-significant diseases [14].

Digital rectal examination (DRE) performs physical prostate gland evaluations, but these assessments rely strictly on feelings that affect sensitivity, especially for both small tumors and tumors located in the gland's front section [26]. A DRE works best to identify cancer through the experience of examiners and the tumor dimensions and position. The diagnostic field shows deficiencies when using PSA and DRE alone because this practice leads to doctors missing dangerous cancers, as well as identifying non-threatening conditions [16].

2.1.3 The Promise of Biomarkers in Enhancing Diagnostic Accuracy

This interest in new prostate cancer diagnostic biomarkers reflects dissatisfaction with PSA and DRE in detection [27]. Defined as quantifiable signs of a biological state or condition, prostate cancer is an imaging disturbance from biomarkers. Because they provide more precise information on the existence, aggressiveness, and possible behavior of prostate cancer, such molecular markers, detectable (for example) in biological fluids, including blood, urine, or tissue, offer the prospect of enhanced diagnostic accuracy [28]. Figure 2.1 illustrates the transition from conventional prostate cancer diagnostic tools to biomarker-driven approaches, highlighting the disease burden, the limitations of current techniques, and the role biomarkers play in enhancing diagnostic accuracy through non-invasive and targeted approaches [23]. The study of the biomarkers will help to address the main drawbacks of the conventional approaches [29]: *Improvement of specificity*: Finding indicators more specifically connected to prostate cancer and less likely to be described by other diseases using prostate biopsy helps to reduce false positives and the necessity for pointless biopsies [30]. Finding indicators that can identify cancer

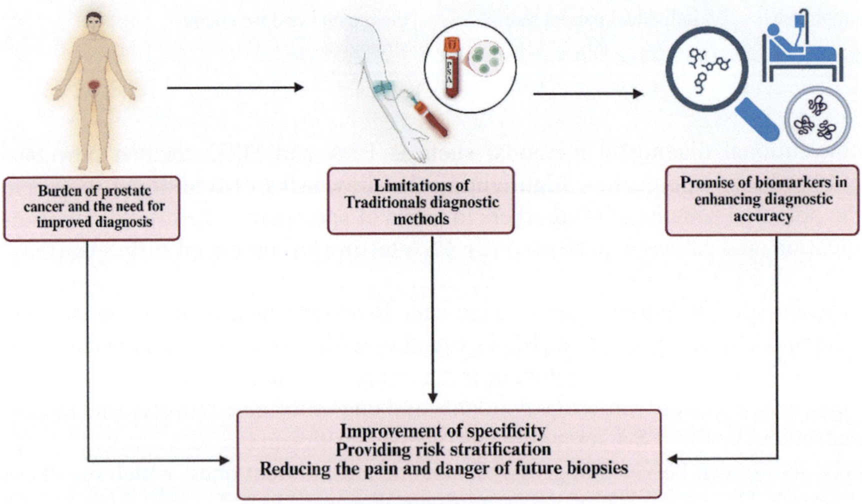

Fig. 2.1 The progression of prostate cancer diagnosis from disease burden and limitations of traditional methods to biomarker-based approaches that improve diagnostic specificity, enable risk stratification, and reduce unnecessary biopsies

sooner than previously and even more possibilities of being treated early helps to make cancer more sensitive. *Providing risk stratification*: Indicators that forecast certain individuals at risk for acquiring high-grade illness as opposed to low-grade disease so that more targeted management methods and maybe lowering the danger of excessive treatment of indolent malignancies may be offered [31]. *Reducing the pain and danger of future biopsies*: Non-invasive or minimally invasive detection is the capacity to create blood or urine-detectable biomarkers with the goal of lowering pain and danger of future biopsies [19].

2.2 Understanding Biomarkers: A Fundamental Overview

A biomarker's fundamental quality is a quantifiable material, next to traits that serve as signs of biological states and situations [32]. Among the imaging findings, markers employed for disease diagnosis and monitoring in prostate cancer patients include proteins, nucleic acids (such as DNA and RNA), metabolites, and circulating tumor cells. The key feature of a biomarker is the identification of biological disease processes ignored by conventional medical diagnostics [33]. Biomarkers are classified according to three primary categories: molecular composition, clinical goal, and detection site. Correctly classifying biomarkers allows for their proper application in clinical practice and data interpretation [34]. Two main points of view help one identify biomarkers by means of categories, including the nature of biomarkers, which are constituted of proteins such as PSA and PCA3, nucleic acids like TMPRSS2-ERG fusion and microRNAs, and metabolites like sarcosine, together with cells like circulating tumor cells [35]. The biomarkers indicate their origin as either serum biomarkers in blood serum or urine biomarkers in urine samples, or as tissue biomarkers taken from prostate tissue biopsies and surgical operations, or imaging biomarkers obtained via medical imaging techniques [15]. Among all clinical biomarker categories of prostate cancer, the system that defines functional use in disease treatment is the most relevant [36].

2.2.1 Type of Biomarkers in Prostate Cancer (Diagnostic, Prognostic, Predictive)

The medical profession employs three separate clinical categories of prostate cancer biomarkers for different objectives (Fig. 2.2) [37]. Throughout medical testing, these indicators help to identify prostate cancer. Their basic goal is to find disease presence in patients as opposed to those without prostate cancer [38].

Diagnostic Biomarker An ideal diagnostic biomarker must show high sensitivity to properly detect cancer cases and high specificity to properly categorize those without cancer, hence lowering both false-positive and false-negative results [39]. The case studies examined in this chapter focus on PCA3 and urine-based testing, aiming to enhance the accuracy of PSA tests and reduce the number of unnecessary treatments

Fig. 2.2 Clinical classification of biomarkers in prostate cancer

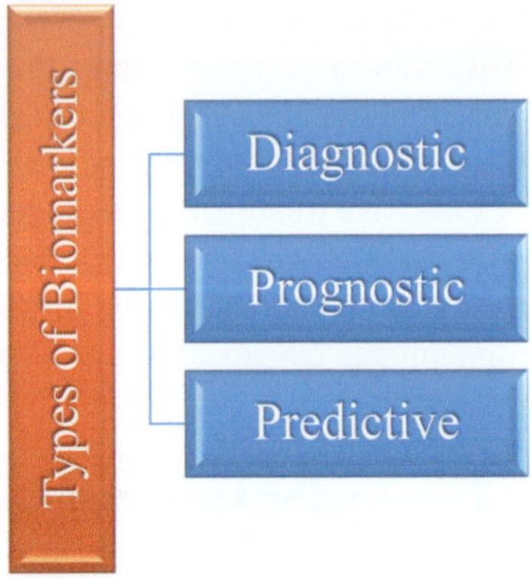

resulting from elevated PSA levels [40]. *Prognostic biomarker*: Regardless of their treatment choice, such indicators assist in forecasting how prostate cancer will progress in people with a diagnosis. The biomarkers provide useful information that helps to create forecasts about the future progression of illness and occurrences of cancer recurrence or death from prostate cancer [41]. By identifying patients with aggressive disease potential for more aggressive therapies and those with less aggressive disease features for active monitoring programs, the use of prognostic biomarkers allows doctors to conduct precise risk categorization. Researcher-created genetic risk scores based on prostate tissue biopsy data serve to determine patient likelihoods for disease recurrence after radical prostatectomy operations [42].

Predictive Biomarker The predictive character of biomarkers enables doctors to forecast therapy response probabilities with their patients [43]. Predictive biomarkers reflect treatment outcomes; hence, their relevance relies on whether a patient receives or does not receive a specific therapy [18]. A predictive biomarker enables doctors to identify patients who will derive the most benefit from treatment approaches, such as radiation therapy and androgen deprivation therapy, as well as those who will not respond to them. Such biomarkers allow healthcare professionals to create individualized treatment plans that increase efficacy and lower unnecessary toxicities from therapeutic drugs [44]. The study of specific genetic alterations in tumor tissue provides an illustration to evaluate treatment sensitivity or drug resistance for systemic drugs. It is crucial to note that some biomarkers can exhibit characteristics of more than one category. For instance, a biomarker might have diagnostic utility in detecting the presence of cancer and also provide prognostic information about its potential aggressiveness [45].

2.2.2 Biological Sources of Biomarkers (Serum, Urine, Tissue)

Several biological sources provide prostate cancer biomarkers that offer distinct qualities in terms of sample availability, coupled with invasive collection techniques, and their capacity to deliver particular disease data [46]. Figure 2.3 shows

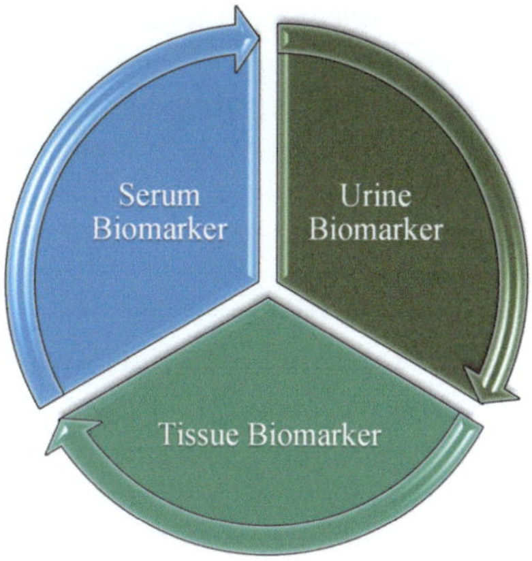

Fig. 2.3 Classification of biomarkers used in prostate cancer diagnosis. Biomarkers are generally grouped based on the type of biological sample analyzed, such as serum, urine, or tissue, each providing distinct diagnostic, prognostic, and predictive significance

the classification of biomarkers used in prostate cancer diagnosis, including serum, urine, and tissue biomarkers [47].

Serum Biomarker Biomarkers are found in the blood serum after blood clots. Tests using blood serum as their origin are relatively non-invasive, allowing them to follow patients over time and screen populations [20]. The best-known blood biomarker now available for prostate cancer is PSA. Currently undergoing scientific study are many serum-based indicators that might improve diagnostic tools for prostate cancer and strategies for predicting disease progression. Because their direct connection to prostate tumor molecular activity is not always present, systemic factors tend to influence serum biomarkers [48].

Urine Biomarker Since it requires only urine samples, urine provides biomarkers via a simple, non-invasive technique. Cells and chemicals from the prostate are let go into urine via the urinary system, which enables their detection [49]. Because evaluating this biological fluid enables the investigation of prostate tissues using non-invasive techniques, the study of biomarkers discovered in urine shows great promise for both early-stage diagnosis and risk assessment of prostate disorders [50]. Urine-based biomarkers include PCA3, as well as more recent urine markers assessing specific prostate cancer-related mRNA and protein profiles in samples collected during digital rectal exams.

Tissue Biomarker Medical practitioners employ tissue biomarkers obtained from surgical resections and prostate gland biopsies [51]. Through tissue-based biomarkers, doctors obtain unambiguous information about tumors, including their genetic data, protein alterations, and gene expression patterns. For both diagnostic confirmation and Gleason score evaluation, as well as identification of significant indicators guiding treatment decisions, tissue biomarkers are of fundamental importance [52]. The TMPRSS2-ERG gene fusion is one example of genomic testing used in prostate tissue acquired during biopsy operations. Although it offers useful knowledge, the collection of tissue biomarkers requires invasive medical treatments [53]. Prostate cancer diagnosis and medical management benefit from understanding biomarker definitions, alongside their biological origins and various types [54]. The following sections analyze biomarkers that are already available and those under development within different categories to provide solutions to prostate cancer's diagnostic obstacles.

2.2.3 Established Biomarkers in Prostate Cancer Diagnosis

2.2.3.1 PSA and Its Refinements: Utility and Limitations

Measured mostly as total PSA in serum, prostate-specific antigen (PSA) is still a basic biomarker in prostate cancer detection [55]. Examining its isoforms, free PSA (% fPSA), and complexed PSA (cPSA) sharpens risk assessment, especially in the diagnostic "gray zone." Lower % fPSA and maybe greater cPSA ratios might raise suspicion for cancer, hence better directing biopsy choices [56]. Beyond raw numbers, PSA density (PSAD), which takes into account prostate size, enhances specificity by considering benign prostatic enlargement. For a particular PSA level, Higher PSAD indicates a higher cancer probability. Cancer may also be indicated by PSA velocity (PSAV), the rate of PSA changes over time. Fast rises cause worry even within normal levels [57]. These improvements aim to enhance PSA's accuracy in detecting clinically relevant illnesses. Still, there are significant drawbacks and ongoing debates regarding the interpretation of PSA screening. Its lack of selectivity causes regular false positives and needless biopsies of benign diseases. Without obvious survival advantages, over-detection of an indolent tumor may lead to over-treatment and its related adverse effects (e.g., erectile dysfunction, urine incontinence) [58]. Moreover, PSA's sensitivity for aggressive illness is not total, which can result in false negatives. Age and race also affect PSA levels, which complicates the use of consistent threshold values [21]. The effect on death of population-based PSA screening remains controversial, as it weighs any advantages against the drawbacks of overdiagnosis [59]. Current recommendations thus support a more tailored, risk-adapted strategy for PSA testing, emphasizing joint decision-making and considering patient-specific factors [60]. Although OSA and its modifications provide useful information, their inherent limitations underscore the crucial need for ongoing research and the incorporation of new, more specific biomarkers to improve prostate cancer detection and management.

2.2.3.2 PCA3: A Urine-Based Biomarker Enhancing Prostate Cancer Risk Assessment

Prostate cancer tissue exhibits significantly higher overexpression of prostate cancer antigen 3 (PCA3), as shown in Fig. 2.4, a non-protein-coding mRNA, compared to normal prostatic tissue [61]. While its role in cancer is still under investigation, its overexpression in normal tissue makes it a useful urine biomarker. Quantifying the PCA3 mRNA level relative to PSA mRNA on a post-digital rectal

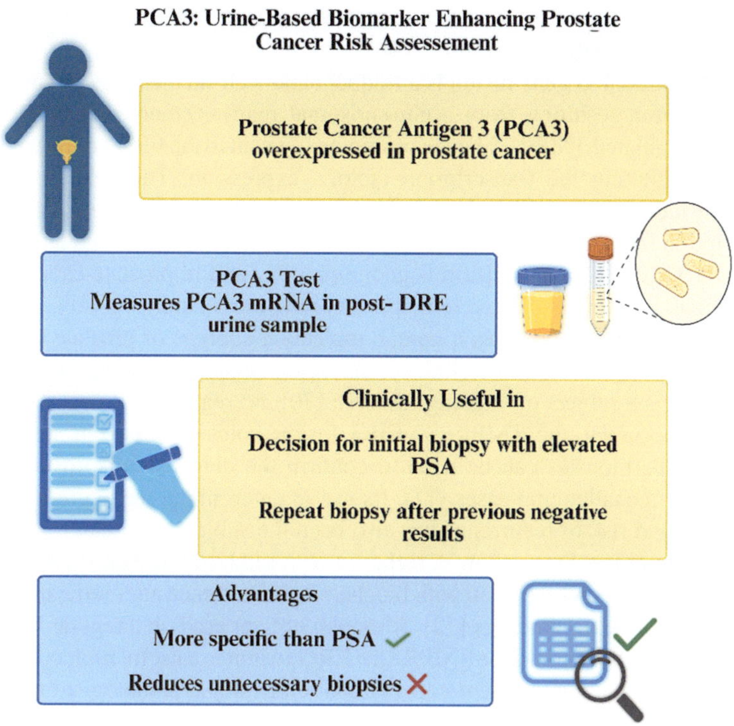

Fig. 2.4 The PCA3 urine-based biomarker plays a role in assessing prostate cancer risk: it is overexpressed in prostate cancer and used in post-DRE urine testing to guide initial or repeat biopsies, improving specificity over PSA and reducing unnecessary biopsies

examination (DRE) urine sample, which is prostate cell-enriched, the PCA3 test results in a PCA3 score that reflects the probability of finding prostate cancer on future biopsy [62]. Clinically, PCA3 has been helpful in various situations. Most importantly, it helps men with increased PSA, especially those in the "gray zone," make the decision about the issue of the first biopsy. A low PCA3 score can be an indicator of a lower risk of cancer, thus preventing some men from undergoing unnecessary urgent biopsy [63]. Second, PCA3 can be helpful in men with persistently increased PSA and previous negative biopsies undergoing repeat biopsies. In this scenario, a high PCA3 score elevates the risk of cancer and can be an indicator to proceed further [64]. PCA3 has several advantages over PSA. Its overexpression in cancer makes it more specific, thus reducing the false-positive rate of benign prostatic disease [65]. Following a DRE, a urine test is less vulnerable to factors that potentially influence serum PSA [66]. PCA3, however, has some drawbacks. For the detection of cancer during screening, its sensitivity is not necessarily superior to that of PSA; its predictive value may depend on the level of PSA and a history of previous biopsy [67].

2.2.3.3 TMPRSS2-ERG Gene Fusion: A Molecular Marker for Prostate Cancer Subtyping and Risk

The TMPRSS2-ERG gene fusion is a frequent and well-defined genetic mutation in prostate cancer, resulting from a chromosomal rearrangement that positions the androgen-regulated TMPRSS2 gene promoter adjacent to the ERG coding sequence, thereby facilitating the transcription factor's expression. This leads to ectopic, androgen-induced overexpression of the ERG protein, an ETS family member of transcription factors involved in cell proliferation, differentiation, and angiogenesis [69]. The TMPRSS2-ERG fusion is geographically and in prostate cancer cohorts heterogeneous, but is estimated to be present in approximately 40–60% of prostate cancers. Its occurrence defines a unique molecular subtype of prostate cancer and has been associated with some clinicopathological features, although its prognostic significance is a subject of ongoing research [70]. As regards risk stratification and diagnostic accuracy, the TMPRSS2-ERG fusion holds promise. Its detection in prostate tissue biopsies can be used to confirm the diagnosis of prostate cancer, particularly in challenging cases [71]. Its use in determining the aggressiveness of the disease and risk of recurrence has also been the subject of research, albeit with conflicting findings. Some show correlation with reduced Gleason scores, whereas others examine their correlation with biochemical recurrence after radical prostatectomy, with conflicting findings [72]. Although not yet used on a regular basis as an isolated diagnostic marker, the TMPRSS2-ERG fusion is a useful molecular marker that can be used to complement conventional clinical and pathological parameters [73]. Its use in multi-marker panels and risk prediction models is being explored to improve patient stratification for active surveillance or aggressive treatment protocols. Additional studies are required to more fully define its prognostic and predictive value in various stages of disease and treatment regimens [74].

2.2.3.4 Genomic Biomarkers: Multi-gene Assays for Personalized Prostate Cancer Risk Assessment

Genomic biomarkers, in the form of multi-gene expression tests, are a valuable innovation in prostate cancer risk stratification [75]. These commercially available tests, such as Oncotype DX Prostate and Decipher, quantify the expression of a panel of genes in prostate tissue samples obtained from biopsies. These panels of genes are chosen with care to reflect various biological pathways of tumor growth, development, and response to treatment [76]. The major use of these assays is the prediction of the aggressiveness of prostate cancer in men with localized disease. By measuring the expression of these sets of genes, the tests provide an accompanying risk score that predicts the risk of adverse pathological features (e.g., high Gleason grade, extracapsular extension) and the risk of biochemical recurrence after radical prostatectomy [77]. This information is highly valuable to both patients and clinicians in making informed decisions about disease treatment and in distinguishing between those who can be safely managed through active surveillance and those who require more aggressive treatment [78]. Although most widely applied after diagnosis to enhance risk stratification and direct treatment, the possibility of genomic biomarkers directing initial biopsy choice is also being investigated [79].

By selecting men at a greater underlying risk of aggressive cancer using pre-biopsy characteristics and possibly incorporating genomic markers from initial limited biopsies, they have the potential to enhance patient selection into more extensive diagnostic testing [80]. Additional evaluation is required to further establish their place in the pre-biopsy context. Genomic biomarkers are an individualized approach to defining the biological features of a man's prostate cancer, resulting in more individualized and effective care [81].

2.2.4 Emerging Biomarkers with Diagnostic Potential

2.2.4.1 Urine Biomarkers in Prostate Cancer: Clinically Available Innovations and Emerging Candidates

Although existing biomarkers, such as PSA and PCA3, have aided in the identification of prostate cancer, the pursuit of more precise and specific non-invasive technologies is driving research on new diagnostic biomarkers [82]. These new markers, discovered in various biological matrices, hold great potential to overcome the limitations of current methods and enhance early detection and risk classification. This section examines several of the most promising new biomarkers in the sector [83]. Due to its non-invasive collection and direct interaction with the prostate gland, urine offers an especially appealing source of biomarkers [84]. Many encouraging urine indicators indicate possibilities for enhancing prostate cancer detection and lowering the need for pointless biopsies. *SelectMDx*: A urine-based molecular diagnostic tool called SelectMDx tracks the urinary mRNA levels of two genes, i.e., HOXC6 and DLX1, linked to high-grade prostate cancer [85]. Particularly in males with higher PSA levels, studies have shown its capacity to forecast the probability of discovering clinically relevant cancer on biopsy. SelectMDx may assist in saving unnecessary biopsies by identifying those with a low risk of aggressive illness [86]. *ExoDx*: Another commercially available urine test is ExoDx Prostate IntelliScore (EPI), which examines exosomal RNA from three genes: ERG, PCA3, and SPDEF. This test has demonstrated use in men with raised PSA or abnormal DRE and offers a risk score for the existence of high-grade prostate cancer (Gleason score ≥ 7), hence guiding the choice to have a biopsy [87]. Its non-invasive character and capacity to provide risk stratification make it a useful instrument in the diagnostic process. Many other urine biomarkers are under active research beyond these accepted assays, among them are the following [88]: *TMPRSS2-ERG fusion*: Detection of this gene fusion product in urine samples provides a non-invasive technique to detect a molecular subtype of prostate cancer. *Specific protein markers*: Studies are looking at the use of certain proteins lost into the urine that are particularly elevated or changed in prostate cancer. *Metabolomic profiles*: Examining the unique chemical fingerprint in urine samples might highlight trends suggesting prostate cancer. *Cell-free DNA (cfDNA)*: Detecting and examining tumor-derived DNA fragments in urine offers promise for non-invasive cancer screening and surveillance. Ongoing studies in urine biomarkers seek to find very specialized and

Table 2.2 Advanced technologies for characterization and detection of CTCs

Advanced technologies	Characterization and detection of CTCs	References
Genomic analysis	Finding genetic changes and mutations in CTCs	[90, 92]
Transcriptomic analysis	Examining the gene expression patterns of CTCs to determine their metastatic potential and treatment susceptibility	[91, 92]
Proteomic analysis	Examining the proteins CTCs express to find possible treatment targets constitutes a proteomic study	[83, 93]

sensitive indicators that may precisely diagnose prostate cancer, especially aggressive types, without requiring intrusive treatments [89].

2.2.4.2 Circulating Tumor Cells in Prostate Cancer: Technological Advances and Emerging Roles in Detection and Monitoring

Cancer cells that have detached from the main tumor and entered the circulation are called circulating tumor cells (CTCs). Their identification and characterization constitute a "liquid biopsy" method that may provide insightful analysis of the condition without requiring a tissue sample [90]. Isolating and examining CTCs is technically difficult since they are uncommon in the blood. Significant developments in detection technologies, including microfluidic devices and antibody-based capture techniques, have helped us to find and count these cells; nevertheless, challenges remain [91]. Moreover, Table 2.2 shows that advanced methods are being created to describe CTCs at the molecular level.

Although CTCs are more well-known in the context of metastatic disease surveillance, their possible use in early detection is being vigorously investigated [92]. Even a small percentage of CTCs with certain traits might suggest early-stage malignancy. Studies are focusing on developing highly sensitive CTC detection techniques that can identify CTCs in males with localized illness, finding CTC subtypes or molecular characteristics unique to early-stage or high-risk prostate cancer, and predicting disease progression and guiding initial therapy choices using CTC enumeration and characterization. Although there are still difficulties in converting CTC detection into standard early diagnostic practice, continuous studies offer hope for their future relevance in this context [94].

2.2.4.3 Exosomes and microRNAs in Prostate Cancer: Encapsulated Biomarkers and Molecular Regulators in Diagnosis

Small extracellular vesicles, known as exosomes, are released by cells, including cancer cells, and contain a variety of biomolecules, including proteins, lipids, nucleic acids, and microRNAs [93]. Small non-coding RNA molecules, known as microRNAs (miRNAs), regulate gene expression and play a crucial role in cancer formation and progression [95]. Exosomes produced by prostate cancer cells convey a molecular payload that reflects the features of the source tumor [96]. Examining the contents of exosomes extracted from blood, urine, and other physiological fluids provides a non-invasive view into the tumor microenvironment.

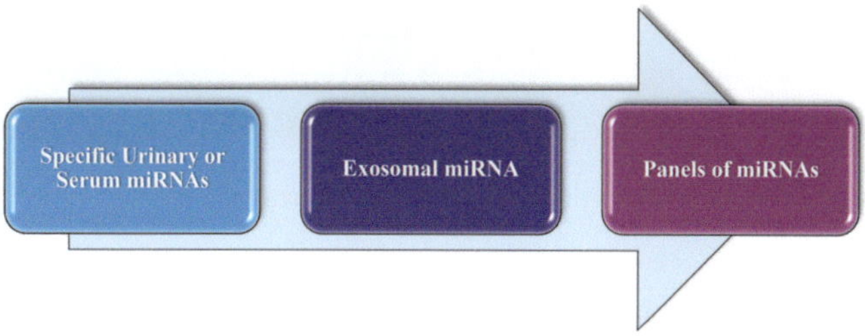

Fig. 2.5 Role of microRNA in detection and development of prostate cancer

Studies are concentrating on findings [97]: particular proteins abundant in exosomes from prostate cancer; distinct lipid profiles of exosomes produced from cancer; DNA and RNA signals characteristic of exosomes; and unique lipid profiles of cancer-derived exosomes. Relatively stable and shielded from degradation, exosomal RNA, particularly mRNA and miRNA, is a potential source of diagnostic indicators. Key biological processes linked to prostate cancer, including cell proliferation, apoptosis, and metastasis, are significantly regulated by microRNAs [25]. Figure 2.5 illustrates that prostate cancer tissues and body fluids exhibit consistently aberrant expression patterns of certain miRNAs. Research is currently looking into the possibilities of [98]. Non-invasive diagnostic indicators for prostate cancer identification include certain urine or serum miRNAs. Panels of miRNAs can distinguish between low-risk and high-risk illnesses, as well as benign prostatic problems and prostate cancer. Exosomal miRNAs are highly stable and serve as useful diagnostic markers.

Certain miRNAs' stability and disease specificity make them appealing candidates for clinical translation as diagnostic tools [99].

2.2.4.4 Epigenetic Markers in Prostate Cancer: Aberrant DNA Methylation as a Molecular Signature for Non-invasive Diagnosis

Heritable changes in gene expression, excluding changes to the underlying DNA sequence, include epigenetic modifications such as DNA methylation [100]. A hallmark of cancer, particularly prostate cancer, aberrant DNA methylation patterns may cause the silencing or activation of important genes implicated in the formation and progression of tumors. Certain genes show regular and notable changes in their methylation state in prostate cancer relative to normal prostate tissue. Different biological samples include the following [101]: *prostate tissue*—finding methylation markers that could help with diagnosis and forecast disease aggressiveness; *plasma and serum*—finding circulating methylated DNA fragments from cancer cells in serum and plasma; *urine*—examining methylation DNA lost from the prostate into the urinary system. Prostate cancer diagnosis shows great potential from the discovery of abnormal DNA methylation patterns in non-invasively gathered samples, including serum and urine [102]. The benefits of using DNA methylation as a biomarker are as follows [103]: Some methylation changes are quite particular to

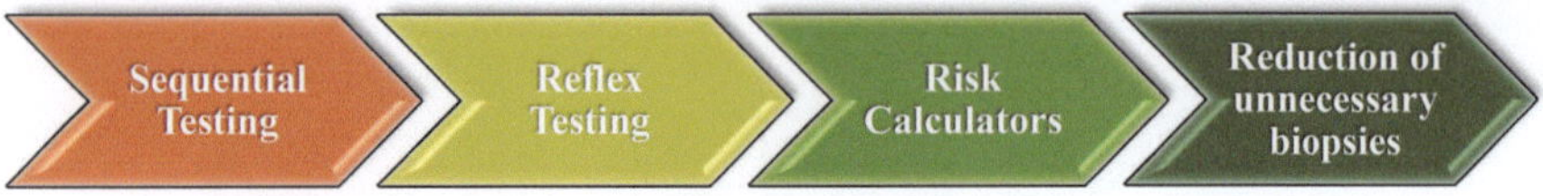
Sequential Testing
Reflex Testing
Risk Calculators
Reduction of unnecessary biopsies

Fig. 2.6 Integration of biomarkers in the diagnosis of prostate cancer

malignancy; methylated DNA is quite stable in bodily fluids; early detection potential, as abnormal methylation may happen early in carcinogenesis. Current studies aim to identify robust, clinically relevant methylation markers that can be consistently detected in liquid samples for early prostate cancer diagnosis and risk stratification [104].

2.2.5 Integrating Biomarkers into Diagnostic Algorithms

When properly included in diagnostic algorithms, prostate cancer biomarkers' actual clinical use becomes clear [105]. Instead of being utilized alone, biomarkers may be deliberately used at different points throughout the diagnostic journey to fine-tune risk assessment, direct decisions, and finally enhance patient outcomes [106]. Figure 2.6 represents the key techniques for integrating biomarkers, which are discussed in this part.

2.2.5.1 Sequential and Reflex Testing Strategies

Sequential testing is one efficient way to include biomarkers. This approach calls for a first, generally less intrusive test, such as a PSA [107]. A supplementary, more particular biomarker test is then used to further stratify the patient's risk if the result suggests an intermediate risk or falls inside a predetermined "gray zone" [108]. Aiming to increase the specificity of the diagnostic procedure, this sequential strategy reduces the number of men who undergo biopsy solely based on a moderately elevated PSA [109]. Reflex testing, which automatically runs a specific biomarker test based on the initial test's findings, is another comparable concept [110]. For instance, a reflex test for free PSA or PCA3 may be automatically requested if a patient's total PSA falls within a certain range, thereby providing more information and assisting in assessing the probability of a clinically relevant malignancy [111]. The advantages of sequential and reflex testing strategies include the following: *Improved specificity*: Using a second-line biomarker in a chosen group of men at intermediate risk helps to lower the proportion of false-positive PSA values, causing needless biopsies [112]. *Cost-effectiveness*: A small proportion of patients should be targeted for more costly or specialized biomarker testing to maximize resource use. *Personalized risk assessment*: Based on many lines of evidence, sequential testing offers a more sophisticated and personalized evaluation of risk. Free PSA percentage, PSA density, PSA velocity, and PCA3 are among the biomarkers often employed in sequential or reflex testing [113]. Clinical guidelines and local practices influence the algorithms and cutoffs used.

2.2.5.2 Risk Calculators Incorporating Biomarkers

Including biomarkers in risk calculators is one more effective way to combine them [114]. Particularly for clinically relevant illnesses, these techniques provide a more precise estimation of an individual's chance of developing prostate cancer by combining biomarker findings with many clinical criteria, like age, family history, DRE results, and PSA level. By offering a numerical chance of a positive biopsy, risk calculators help patients and doctors to decide more wisely whether or not to go on with a prostate biopsy [115]. These calculators may increase the accuracy of risk prediction by including the extra value of biomarkers, therefore enhancing models based just on conventional risk elements [116]. Among the biomarkers included in prostate cancer risk calculators are the following [117]: *PCA3*: Its incorporation has been proven to increase the predicted accuracy of risk calculators, especially in males with past negative biopsies. *TMPRSS2-ERG fusion*: Especially for aggressive illness, this molecular marker helps to improve risk projections. *Urine-based biomarkers*: These more recent urine-based biomarkers, including SelectMDx and ExoDx Prostate IntelliScore, are being included more and more into risk calculators to improve their capacity to forecast the existence of high-grade malignancy. *Genomic risk scores*: Although usually employed after a positive biopsy for prognosis, several genetic markers are being investigated for their possible ability to enhance first risk assessment in biopsy-naive males.

2.2.5.3 Impact on Reducing Unnecessary Biopsies

Reducing the amount of pointless prostate biopsies is a main objective of including biomarkers into diagnostic algorithms [118]. Relying mostly on PSA has resulted in a notable number of biopsies in men who are finally discovered to have benign diseases or low-risk, clinically inconsequential prostate cancer [119]. These biopsies are intrusive, may cause problems, and add to patient anxiety and medical expenditures. Integrating Biomarkers into Prostate Cancer Diagnostic Algorithms [120]. Table 2.2 key techniques for employing biomarkers within clinical workflows—including sequential and reflex testing, integration into risk calculators, and their combined function in lowering unneeded biopsies—are summarized in this table. It also emphasizes frequently utilized biomarkers and their related clinical advantages [121]. Strategically adding more particular biomarkers into the diagnostic route will help us to [122]: *Identify men at really greater risk*: Better selection of people who are more likely to have clinically relevant cancer is possible using biomarkers with enhanced specificity, hence raising the positive predictive value of biopsy. *Reassure men at low risk*: Findings suggesting a low likelihood of aggressive cancer should let some men with moderately raised PSA skip initial biopsy and think about other options, including active monitoring or repeat PSA testing. *Improve biopsy indications*: By providing a more objective evaluation of biopsy need, risk calculators using biomarkers may help to employ this invasive technique more wisely (Table 2.3).

Table 2.3 Clinical integration of biomarkers in prostate cancer diagnostic pathways

Integration strategy	Description	Common biomarkers used	Benefits	References
Sequential testing	Initial screening (e.g., PSA) followed by a more specific biomarker test in intermediate or uncertain cases	Free PSA, PSA density, PCA3	Improves specificity Reduces unnecessary biopsies Personalized assessment	[67]
Reflex testing	Automatic secondary biomarker testing triggered by certain PSA results	Free PSA, PCA3	Streamlined process Adds predictive value to borderline PSA results	[107]
Risk calculators	Biomarkers combined with clinical parameters (e.g., age, DRE, family history) to predict cancer risk more accurately	PCA3, TMPRSS2-ERG, SelectMDx, ExoDx, genomic scores	Objective decision-making Improved prediction of clinically significant cancers	[39]
Reduction of unnecessary biopsies	Biomarker use helps distinguish between aggressive and indolent cancers, reducing patient burden from unneeded procedures	PSA, PCA3, genomic risk scores	Fewer invasive biopsies Lower patient anxiety Cost-effective use of medical resources	[112]

2.2.6 Challenges and Future Directions in Biomarker Research

Researchers in prostate cancer biomarkers confront multiple vital barriers before clinical biomarkers can transform discovered data into effective diagnostic tools [123]. The complete execution of biomarkers depends on overcoming these essential obstacles for improved diagnosis and patient outcomes. Technological progress and increased knowledge about prostate cancer biology create new promising directions within the field at the same time [124].

2.2.6.1 Validation and Standardization of Biomarkers

An important hurdle in biomarker studies consists of performing comprehensive validation on potential biomarkers [125]. Many initial findings regarding promising biomarkers do not show stable performance across large independent patient populations. Numerous causes lead to the lack of reproducibility, including [126]: *Small sample sizes*: The insufficient number of patients enrolled in first-stage research makes it difficult to show disease heterogeneity accurately. *Lack of independent validation*: The results must receive confirmation through separate, well-designed studies for general-purpose validity and strength assessment. *Methodological variability*: Various techniques for sample collection, as well as differences in processing methods and analytical procedures between studies, result in irregular outcomes. *Confounding factors*: Medical investigators must handle patient-specific factors, including age, along with comorbidities and medications, to prevent their influence on biomarker measurement levels. Widespread clinical adoption of biomarkers becomes challenging because of the absence of standardization in their measuring procedures [127]. Different laboratories tend to employ inconsistent reagents and definitions of protocols, which must use diverse instruments, resulting in divergent measurement outcomes, thus blocking proper results comparison [128]. For reliable clinical biomarker data, several key measures must be created, including standardized tests with clear performance characteristics and quality control systems and reference standard materials [129]. Academic institutions, in collaboration with industry partners and regulatory agencies, must work together to establish these standards.

It is doubtful that a single biomarker can provide the whole picture or the full truth of prostate cancer due to its complexity and heterogeneity [130]. Often, using only one marker renders it unsuitable either particularly or sensitively. This has resulted in a solid agreement that a multi-marker panel with multi-marker information should be created to improve diagnosis accuracy, risk stratification, and prediction of treatment response [131]. These panels enable the combination of biomarkers from multiple biological sources (e.g., serum and urine), various molecular types (e.g., protein and genomic markers), or biomarkers that reflect distinct biological pathways associated with prostate cancer development and progression. Multi-marker strategies have numerous motivations [132]: *Increased sensitivity and specificity*: Markers that are independently linked to cancer may raise the overall specificity and/or sensitivity of cancer detection. *Improved risk stratification*: A more informative image of disease aggressiveness may be produced by integrating tumor biology prognostic indicators, which represent different features of disease aggressiveness. *Enhanced prediction of treatment response*: Combined predictive indicators aimed at various therapeutic pathways may clarify patient selection for certain therapies to improve treatment response prediction [133]. Selecting and validating the panel of biomarkers in the shape of a panel using advanced statistical and computational techniques that support the identification of the best panel of biomarkers and the creation of strong algorithms for data integration and interpretation [134].

2.2.6.2 Personalized Approaches to Prostate Cancer Diagnosis

A heterogeneous bag of tumor biology notably highlights the importance of taking a personalized approach to diagnosis, owing to the knowledge that prostate cancer is not a single disease, but one with a wide range of clinical behaviors [135]. This is exactly where (bio)markers are crucial because they enable us to understand the molecular characteristics present in each disease of an individual patient [136]. Personalized diagnosis is an approach whereby the diagnostic pathway could be tailored depending on an individual's risk, biomarker profiles, and additional clinical information. This may involve the following [137]: *risk-adapted screening*—targeting identification of men at increased risk using biomarkers who may derive greater benefit from screening and considering de-intensifying screening in men at lower risk; *customizing biopsy decisions*—using biomarkers to identify which men should undergo prostate biopsy, decreasing unnecessary procedures among men at low risk based on biomarker profiles; *reassessment of individual risk*—using prognostic biomarkers to better stratify a patient's risk for disease progression, informing treatment vs active surveillance decision-making. For personalized diagnostic strategies to be developed and implemented, we need a better understanding of the molecular heterogeneity of prostate cancer and markers that will stratify patients into clinically relevant groups [138]. This approach should also be combined with clinical data, imaging data, and patient preferences to make the vision of personalized management of prostate cancer a reality [139].

2.2.6.3 Technological Advancements in Biomarker Discovery and Detection

Rapid technological developments are driving the discovery of new biomarkers and allowing more sensitive and effective detection techniques [17]. These technical developments are crucial for overcoming current constraints and expanding the range of clinically relevant biomarkers. The important areas of development are the following [140]: *High-throughput omics technologies*: By enabling the simultaneous examination of hundreds of molecules, genomics, transcriptomics, proteomics, and metabolomics, they help to identify new biomarkers and fully map the molecular landscape of prostate cancer [141]. *Liquid biopsy technologies*: Advances in the identification and analysis of circulating tumor cells (CTCs), circulating tumor DNA (ctDNA), and exosomes in blood and urine provide less invasive methods for diagnosis, monitoring, and predicting therapy response [142]. These technologies provide great promise for serial monitoring and real-time knowledge of disease development. *Advanced imaging techniques*: Non-invasive visualization of tumor features and assistance in diagnosis and staging may be achieved by combining molecular imaging with new tracers aimed at certain biomarkers [143]. *Microfluidics and nanotechnology*: They might help to create very sensitive and particular point-of-care devices for biomarker identification, hence enabling fast and easily available diagnostic testing. *Artificial intelligence and machine learning*: AI and ML are being used to examine massive, complicated biomarker databases, find new trends and connections, and create prediction models for diagnosis, prognosis, and therapy response. Accelerating the identification and translation of significant prostate cancer biomarkers into clinical practice will depend on ongoing investment and innovation in these technology domains [144].

2.2.7 Conclusion: The Evolving Role of Biomarkers in Precision Diagnosis

The research examined prostate cancer detection, considering both the shortcomings of traditional approaches and the significant potential advantages of biomarkers. Starting with a look at the worldwide prostate cancer incidence, our study advocates better diagnosis methods, lowering patient invasiveness. The combination of PSA and DRE diagnostic errors, which exhibit poor sensitivity and specificity, makes precision highly essential. Examining biomarkers involves determining their basic meaning, as well as their diagnostic, prognostic, and predictive classification, and biological source identification in serum, urine, and tissue. A solid knowledge base on biomarkers allowed researchers to thoroughly investigate established biomarkers, including PSA with its many variations, as well as PCA3 and TMPRSS2-ERG fusion, and separate genetic risk assessment methodologies. The diagnostic developments of these markers draw attention to the requirement for more precise responses, as they all have different drawbacks. The following section emphasized exciting changes in biomarker generation by means of urine-based diagnostic assays and cancer cell tracking, as well as exosomal and microRNA analysis and DNA methylation studies. These new diagnostic technologies could provide patients with additional detection possibilities and better risk assessment, together with milder diagnostic approaches. Using biomarkers, strategies for clinical practice evaluation included diagnostic algorithm systems, sequential testing methods, and risk assessment calculators. These strategies will help physicians make better clinical decisions and reduce biopsies. For the study on biomarkers to be useful, it needs thorough validation and standardization, as well as the creation of integrated multi-marker panels. Prostate cancer testing direction is tailored to strategies motivated by modern technology, aiming to provide new indicators indicating exact care-focused knowledge about patients. Modern medical research is increasing the diagnostic power of biomarkers for prostate cancer assessment quickly. Accurate prostate cancer diagnosis calls for conventional techniques to connect with biomarkers, providing higher accuracy. This development plan aims to remove current diagnostic limitations so that clinicians may find important prostate cancer cases sooner and guarantee accurate tumor classification and lower surgery costs associated with slow-growing tumors, hence improving outcomes for patients. Medical research initiatives to confirm fresh biomarkers drive the development of more individualized prostate cancer treatment for patients.

2.3 Summary

The changing field of biomarkers for prostate cancer diagnosis is examined in this chapter. It highlights the urgent need for more precise, sensitive, and non-invasive techniques by starting with the shortcomings of conventional diagnostic techniques like PSA and DRE. Following a classification of biomarkers by type (diagnostic, prognostic, predictive) and source (serum, urine, tissue), in-depth discussions of well-known markers such as PSA, PCA3, TMPRSS2-ERG fusion, and genomic assays are presented. The diagnostic potential of emerging biomarkers, such as circulating tumor cells (CTCs), exosomal and microRNAs, urinary assays (SelectMDx, ExoDx), and epigenetic markers (DNA methylation), is assessed. To demonstrate how biomarkers can decrease needless biopsies and promote individualized diagnosis, integration strategies are provided, including risk calculators and sequential testing. Future directions are discussed in the chapter's conclusion, with a focus on precision medicine techniques, multi-marker panels, validation, and technology developments.

Glossary

Biomarker a measurable indicator of a biological condition or disease

PSA (prostate-specific antigen) a protein produced by the prostate gland; used as a traditional biomarker for prostate cancer

PCA3 a prostate cancer-associated non-coding RNA overexpressed in malignant tissue

TMPRSS2-ERG fusion a gene fusion common in prostate cancer that helps define molecular subtypes

Genomic assays tests analyzing multiple gene expressions to stratify prostate cancer risk

CTCs (circulating tumor cells) tumor cells that have entered the bloodstream, used in liquid biopsy

Exosomes small extracellular vesicles containing RNA, DNA, and proteins, used in biomarker discovery

MicroRNAs (miRNAs) small, non-coding RNA molecules involved in gene regulation and cancer development

DNA methylation an epigenetic modification where methyl groups are added to DNA, influencing gene expression

References

1. Nevo A, Navaratnam A, Andrews P. Prostate cancer and the role of biomarkers. Abdom Radiol. 2020;45:2120–32.
2. Porzycki P, Ciszkowicz E. Modern biomarkers in prostate cancer diagnosis. Cent Eur J Urol. 2020;73(3):300.
3. Cozar JM, Robles-Fernandez I, Rodriguez-Martinez A, Puche-Sanz I, Vazquez-Alonso F, Lorente JA, et al. The role of miRNAs as biomarkers in prostate cancer. Mutat Res Mutat Res. 2019;781:165–74.
4. Salciccia S, Capriotti AL, Laganà A, Fais S, Logozzi M, De Berardinis E, et al. Biomarkers in prostate cancer diagnosis: from current knowledge to the role of metabolomics and exosomes. Int J Mol Sci. 2021;22(9):4367.
5. Chistiakov DA, Myasoedova VA, Grechko AV, Melnichenko AA, Orekhov AN. New biomarkers for diagnosis and prognosis of localized prostate cancer. Semin Cancer Biol. Elsevier. 2018:9–16.
6. Kelly SP, Anderson WF, Rosenberg PS, Cook MB. Past, current, and future incidence rates and burden of metastatic prostate cancer in the United States. Eur Urol Focus. 2018;4(1):121–7.
7. Spratt DE, Shore N, Sartor O, Rathkopf D, Olivier K. Treating the patient and not just the cancer: therapeutic burden in prostate cancer. Prostate Cancer Prostatic Dis. 2021;24(3):647–61.
8. Smith-Palmer J, Takizawa C, Valentine W. Literature review of the burden of prostate cancer in Germany, France, the United Kingdom and Canada. BMC Urol. 2019;19:1–16.

9. Gustavsen G, Gullet L, Cole D, Lewine N, Bishoff JT. Economic burden of illness associated with localized prostate cancer in the United States. Future Oncol. 2019;16(1):4265–77.
10. Ngcamphalala C, Östensson E, Ginindza TG. The economic burden of prostate cancer in Eswatini. BMC Health Serv Res. 2022;22(1):483.
11. Matsukawa A, Yanagisawa T, Bekku K, Parizi MK, Laukhtina E, Klemm J, et al. Comparing the performance of digital rectal examination and prostate-specific antigen as a screening test for prostate cancer: a systematic review and meta-analysis. Eur Urol Oncol. 2024;7(4):697–704.
12. Ji WT, Wang YK, Han ZY, Wang SQ, Wang Y. Construction of a clinically significant prostate cancer risk prediction model based on traditional diagnostic methods. Front Oncol. 2024;14:1474891.
13. Descotes JL. Diagnosis of prostate cancer. Asian J Urol. 2019;6(2):129–36.
14. Sharma S, Zapatero-Rodriguez J, O'Kennedy R. Prostate cancer diagnostics: clinical challenges and the ongoing need for disruptive and effective diagnostic tools. Biotechnol Adv. 2017;35(2):135–49.
15. Filella X, Foj L. Prostate cancer detection and prognosis: from prostate specific antigen (PSA) to exosomal biomarkers. Int J Mol Sci. 2016;17(11):1784.
16. Gurwin A, Kowalczyk K, Knecht-Gurwin K, Stelmach P, Nowak Ł, Krajewski W, et al. Alternatives for MRI in prostate cancer diagnostics—review of current ultrasound-based techniques. Cancers (Basel). 2022;14(8):1859.
17. Wu Y, Wang Y, Huang Z, Liu Q. Recent advances in analysis technology for detection of prostate cancer biomarkers. Microchem J [Internet]. 2023;190:108740. Available from: https://www.sciencedirect.com/science/article/pii/S0026265X23003582.
18. Saxby H, Mikropoulos C, Boussios S. An update on the prognostic and predictive serum biomarkers in metastatic prostate cancer. Diagnostics. 2020;10(8):549.
19. Mbita Z, Miya TV, Ramagoma RB, Jeyapalan JN, Brzozowski L, Dlamini Z. Diagnostic Advances: innovative techniques and biomarkers for prostate cancer diagnosis. In: Transforming prostate cancer care: advancing cancer treatment with insights from Africa. Springer; 2024. p. 47–78.
20. Nguyen LT, Sharma AR, Chakraborty C, Saibaba B, Ahn ME, Lee SS. Review of prospects of biological fluid biomarkers in osteoarthritis. Int J Mol Sci. 2017;18(3):601.
21. Merriel SWD, Pocock L, Gilbert E, Creavin S, Walter FM, Spencer A, et al. Systematic review and meta-analysis of the diagnostic accuracy of prostate-specific antigen (PSA) for the detection of prostate cancer in symptomatic patients. BMC Med [Internet]. 2022;20(1):54. Available from: https://doi.org/10.1186/s12916-021-02230-y.
22. Eskra JN, Rabizadeh D, Pavlovich CP, Catalona WJ, Luo J. Approaches to urinary detection of prostate cancer. Prostate Cancer Prostatic Dis [Internet]. 2019;22(3):362–81. Available from: https://doi.org/10.1038/s41391-019-0127-4.
23. Kretschmer A, Tilki D. Biomarkers in prostate cancer–current clinical utility and future perspectives. Crit Rev Oncol Hematol. 2017;120:180–93.
24. Meehan J, Gray M, Martínez-Pérez C, Kay C, McLaren D, Turnbull AK. Tissue-and liquid-based biomarkers in prostate cancer precision medicine. J Pers Med. 2021;11(7):664.
25. Hussen BM, Ahmadi G, Marzban H, Azar MEF, Sorayyayi S, Karampour R, et al. The role of HPV gene expression and selected cellular MiRNAs in lung cancer development. Microb Pathog. 2021;150:104692.
26. Ying Y, He W, Xiong Q, Wang Z, Wang M, Chen Q, et al. Value of digital rectal examination in patients with suspected prostate cancer: a prospective cohort analysis study. Transl Androl Urol. 2023;12(11):1666.
27. Koo KM, Mainwaring PN, Tomlins SA, Trau M. Merging new-age biomarkers and nanodiagnostics for precision prostate cancer management. Nat Rev Urol. 2019;16(5):302–17.
28. Madu CO, Lu Y. Novel diagnostic biomarkers for prostate cancer. J Cancer. 2010;1:150.
29. Brönimann S, Pradere B, Karakiewicz P, Abufaraj M, Briganti A, Shariat SF. An overview of current and emerging diagnostic, staging and prognostic markers for prostate cancer. Expert Rev Mol Diagn. 2020;20(8):841–50.

30. Agbetuyi-Tayo P, Gbadebo M, Rotimi OA, Rotimi SO. Advancements in biomarkers of prostate cancer: a review. Technol Cancer Res Treat. 2024;23:15330338241290028.
31. Mohammed AA. Biomarkers in prostate cancer: new era and prospective. Med Oncol. 2014;31:1–6.
32. Velonas VM, Woo HH, dos Remedios CG, Assinder SJ. Current status of biomarkers for prostate cancer. Int J Mol Sci. 2013;14(6):11034–60.
33. Chen JY, Wang PY, Liu MZ, Lyu F, Ma MW, Ren XY, et al. Biomarkers for prostate cancer: from diagnosis to treatment. Diagnostics. 2023;13(21):3350.
34. Sopyllo K, Erickson AM, Mirtti T. Grading evolution and contemporary prognostic biomarkers of clinically significant prostate cancer. Cancers (Basel). 2021;13(4):628.
35. Gadzinski AJ, Cooperberg MR. Prostate cancer markers. In: Genitourin Cancers; 2018. p. 55–86.
36. Kohaar I, Petrovics G, Srivastava S. A rich array of prostate cancer molecular biomarkers: opportunities and challenges. Int J Mol Sci. 2019;20(8):1813.
37. Kontos CK, Adamopoulos PG, Scorilas A. Prognostic and predictive biomarkers in prostate cancer. Expert Rev Mol Diagn. 2015;15(12):1567–76.
38. Fujita K, Nonomura N. Urinary biomarkers of prostate cancer. Int J Urol. 2018;25(9):770–9.
39. Visser WCH, de Jong H, Melchers WJG, Mulders PFA, Schalken JA. Commercialized blood-, urinary-and tissue-based biomarker tests for prostate cancer diagnosis and prognosis. Cancers (Basel). 2020;12(12):3790.
40. Das S, Dey MK, Devireddy R, Gartia MR. Biomarkers in cancer detection, diagnosis, and prognosis. Sensors. 2023;24(1):37.
41. Balázs K, Antal L, Sáfrány G, Lumniczky K. Blood-derived biomarkers of diagnosis, prognosis and therapy response in prostate cancer patients. J Pers Med. 2021;11(4):296.
42. Yan Y, Yeon SY, Qian C, You S, Yang W. On the road to accurate protein biomarkers in prostate cancer diagnosis and prognosis: current status and future advances. Int J Mol Sci. 2021;22(24):13537.
43. Montironi R, Cimadamore A, Lopez-Beltran A, Cheng L, Scarpelli M. Update on prostate cancer diagnosis, prognosis, and prediction to response to therapy. Vol. 10, Cells. MDPI; 2020. p. 20.
44. Kdadra M, Höckner S, Leung H, Kremer W, Schiffer E. Metabolomics biomarkers of prostate cancer: a systematic review. Diagnostics. 2019;9(1):21.
45. McNally CJ, Ruddock MW, Moore T, McKenna DJ. Biomarkers that differentiate benign prostatic hyperplasia from prostate cancer: a literature review. Cancer Manag Res. 2020;12:5225–41.
46. Celec P, Vlková B, Lauková L, Bábíčková J, Boor P. Cell-free DNA: the role in pathophysiology and as a biomarker in kidney diseases. Expert Rev Mol Med. 2018;20:e1.
47. Xue C, Yang B, Fu L, Hou H, Qiang J, Zhou C, et al. Urine biomarkers can outperform serum biomarkers in certain diseases. Urine. 2023;5:57–64.
48. Balhara N, Devi M, Balda A, Phour M, Giri A. Urine; a new promising biological fluid to act as a non-invasive biomarker for different human diseases. Urine. 2023;5:40–52.
49. Larsen LK, Lind GE, Guldberg P, Dahl C. DNA-methylation-based detection of urological cancer in urine: overview of biomarkers and considerations on biomarker design, source of DNA, and detection technologies. Int J Mol Sci. 2019;20(11):2657.
50. Lima T, Henrique R, Vitorino R, Fardilha M. Bioinformatic analysis of dysregulated proteins in prostate cancer patients reveals putative urinary biomarkers and key biological pathways. Med Oncol. 2021;38(1):9.
51. Zhang M, Shao C, Sun H, Zhang B, Guo Z, Sun J, et al. Blood-and urine-based liquid biopsy for early-stage cancer investigation: taken clear renal cell carcinoma as a model. Mol Cell Proteomics. 2023;22(8)
52. Navajas R, Corrales F, Paradela A. Quantitative proteomics-based analyses performed on pre-eclampsia samples in the 2004–2020 period: a systematic review. Clin Proteomics. 2021;18:1–12.

53. Chao MR, Evans MD, Hu CW, Ji Y, Møller P, Rossner P, et al. Biomarkers of nucleic acid oxidation–a summary state-of-the-art. Redox Biol. 2021;42:101872.
54. Legg KM, Powell R, Reisdorph N, Reisdorph R, Danielson PB. Verification of protein biomarker specificity for the identification of biological stains by quadrupole time-of-flight mass spectrometry. Electrophoresis. 2017;38(6):833–45.
55. Sundaresan VM, Smani S, Rajwa P, Renzulli J, Sprenkle PC, Kim IY, et al. Prostate-specific antigen screening for prostate cancer: diagnostic performance, clinical thresholds, and strategies for refinement. Urol Oncol Semin Orig Investig [Internet]. 2025;43(1):41–8. Available from: https://www.sciencedirect.com/science/article/pii/S1078143924005052.
56. Eldred-Evans D, Tam H, Sokhi H, Padhani AR, Winkler M, Ahmed HU. Rethinking prostate cancer screening: could MRI be an alternative screening test? Nat Rev Urol [Internet]. 2020;17(9):526–39. Available from: https://doi.org/10.1038/s41585-020-0356-2.
57. Leapman MS, Wang R, Park H, Yu JB, Sprenkle PC, Cooperberg MR, et al. Changes in Prostate-specific antigen testing relative to the revised US preventive services task force recommendation on Prostate Cancer screening. JAMA Oncol [Internet]. 2022;8(1):41–7. Available from: https://doi.org/10.1001/jamaoncol.2021.5143.
58. French WW, Wallen EM. Advances in the diagnostic options for prostate cancer. Postgrad Med [Internet]. 2020;132(sup4):52–62. Available from: https://doi.org/10.1080/00325481.2020.1822067.
59. Kim JH, Hong SK. Clinical utility of current biomarkers for prostate cancer detection. Investig Clin Urol. 2021;62(1):1–13.
60. Stabile A, Giganti F, Rosenkrantz AB, Taneja SS, Villeirs G, Gill IS, et al. Multiparametric MRI for prostate cancer diagnosis: current status and future directions. Nat Rev Urol [Internet]. 2020;17(1):41–61. Available from: https://doi.org/10.1038/s41585-019-0212-4.
61. Lemos AEG, Matos A d R, Ferreira LB, Gimba ERP. The long non-coding RNA PCA3: an update of its functions and clinical applications as a biomarker in prostate cancer. Oncotarget. 2019;10(61):6589–603.
62. Akinloye O, Kareem OI, Popoola OA, Samuel TA, Adaramoye O. Diagnostic potential value of circulating PCA3 mRNA in plasma and urine of prostate cancer patients. Sci African [Internet]. 2022;17:e01343. Available from: https://www.sciencedirect.com/science/article/pii/S2468227622002502.
63. Raja N, Russell CM, George AK. Urinary markers aiding in the detection and risk stratification of prostate cancer. Transl Androl Urol. 2018;7(Suppl 4):S436–42.
64. Lima AR, Pinto J, Azevedo AI, Barros-Silva D, Jerónimo C, Henrique R, et al. Identification of a biomarker panel for improvement of prostate cancer diagnosis by volatile metabolic profiling of urine. Br J Cancer [Internet]. 2019;121(10):857–68. Available from: https://doi.org/10.1038/s41416-019-0585-4.
65. Sequeira JP, Salta S, Freitas R, López-López R, Díaz-Lagares Á, Henrique R, et al. Biomarkers for pre-treatment risk stratification of prostate cancer patients: a systematic review. Cancers (Basel) [Internet]. 2024;16(7). Available from: https://www.mdpi.com/2072-6694/16/7/1363
66. Gunelli R, Fragalà E, Fiori M. PCA3 in prostate cancer. In: Salvi S, Casadio V, editors. Urinary biomarkers: methods and protocols [Internet]. New York: Springer US; 2021. p. 105–13. Available from: https://doi.org/10.1007/978-1-0716-1354-2_9.
67. Chang EK, Gadzinski AJ, Nyame YA. Blood and urine biomarkers in prostate cancer: are we ready for reflex testing in men with an elevated prostate-specific antigen? Asian J Urol [Internet]. 2021;8(4):343–53. Available from: https://www.sciencedirect.com/science/article/pii/S2214388221000540.
68. Rodon N, Trias I, Verdú M, Calvo M, Banus JM, Puig X. Correlation of mRNA-PCA3 urine levels with the new grading system in prostate cancer. Rev Española Patol [Internet]. 2019;52(1):20–6. Available from: https://www.sciencedirect.com/science/article/pii/S1699885518300382.
69. Kohaar I, Li Q, Chen Y, Ravindranath L, Young D, Ali A, et al. Association of germline genetic variants with TMPRSS2-ERG fusion status in prostate cancer. Oncotarget. 2020 Apr;11(15):1321–33.

70. Song C, Chen H. Predictive significance of TMRPSS2-ERG fusion in prostate cancer: a meta-analysis. Cancer Cell Int [Internet]. 2018;18(1):177. Available from: https://doi.org/10.1186/s12935-018-0672-2.
71. Chalmers ZR, Burns MC, Ebot EM, Frampton GM, Ross JS, Hussain MHA, et al. Early-onset metastatic and clinically advanced prostate cancer is a distinct clinical and molecular entity characterized by increased TMPRSS2–ERG fusions. Prostate Cancer Prostatic Dis [Internet]. 2021;24(2):558–66. Available from: https://doi.org/10.1038/s41391-020-00314-z.
72. Kobelyatskaya AA, Pudova EA, Snezhkina AV, Fedorova MS, Pavlov VS, Guvatova ZG, et al. Impact TMPRSS2–ERG molecular subtype on prostate cancer recurrence. Life [Internet]. 2021;11(6). Available from: https://www.mdpi.com/2075-1729/11/6/588.
73. Bugoye FC, Torrorey-Sawe R, Biegon R, Dharsee N, Mafumiko F, Kibona H, et al. Exploring therapeutic applications of PTEN, TMPRSS2:ERG fusion, and tumour molecular subtypes in prostate cancer management. Front Oncol. 2025;15:1521204.
74. Xu C, Luo J, Wang M, Wang Y, Chen Z, Cao Y, et al. Detection of tmprss2-erg and tmprss2-egr1 gene fusion in prostate cancer from a Chinese population. Egypt J Med Hum Genet [Internet]. 2020;21(1):53. Available from: https://doi.org/10.1186/s43042-020-00092-2.
75. Iacobas S, Iacobas DA. A personalized genomics approach of the Prostate Cancer. Cells [Internet]. 2021;10(7). Available from: https://www.mdpi.com/2073-4409/10/7/1644
76. Alarcón-Zendejas AP, Scavuzzo A, Jiménez-Ríos MA, Álvarez-Gómez RM, Montiel-Manríquez R, Castro-Hernández C, et al. The promising role of new molecular biomarkers in prostate cancer: from coding and non-coding genes to artificial intelligence approaches. Prostate Cancer Prostatic Dis [Internet]. 2022;25(3):431–43. Available from: https://doi.org/10.1038/s41391-022-00537-2.
77. Abu Hijlih R, Sharaf B, Salah S, Bani Hani H, Nielsen SM, Heald B, et al. Patterns and frequency of pathogenic germline variants among prostate cancer patients utilizing multi-gene panel genetic testing. World J Oncol. 2024;15(5):801–8.
78. Zhu W, Wu J, Lai W, Li F, Zeng H, Li X, et al. Harnessing machine learning and multi-omics to explore tumor evolutionary characteristics and the role of AMOTL1 in prostate cancer. Int J Biol Macromol [Internet]. 2025;286:138402. Available from: https://www.sciencedirect.com/science/article/pii/S0141813024092134.
79. Dameri M, Ferrando L, Cirmena G, Vernieri C, Pruneri G, Ballestrero A, et al. Multi-gene testing overview with a clinical perspective in metastatic triple-negative breast Cancer. Int J Mol Sci [Internet]. 2021;22(13). Available from: https://www.mdpi.com/1422-0067/22/13/7154
80. Cragun D, Beckstead J, Farmer M, Hooker G, Dean M, Matloff E, et al. IMProving care after inherited Cancer testing (IMPACT) study: protocol of a randomized trial evaluating the efficacy of two interventions designed to improve cancer risk management and family communication of genetic test results. BMC Cancer [Internet]. 2021;21(1):1099. Available from: https://doi.org/10.1186/s12885-021-08822-4.
81. Kwon DHM, Borno HT, Cheng HH, Zhou AY, Small EJ. Ethnic disparities among men with prostate cancer undergoing germline testing. Urol Oncol Semin Orig Investig [Internet]. 2020;38(3):80.e1–7. Available from: https://www.sciencedirect.com/science/article/pii/S1078143919303618.
82. Condrat CE, Thompson DC, Barbu MG, Bugnar OL, Boboc A, Cretoiu D, et al. miRNAs as biomarkers in disease: latest findings regarding their role in diagnosis and prognosis. Cells [Internet]. 2020;9(2). Available from: https://www.mdpi.com/2073-4409/9/2/276
83. Khoo A, Liu LY, Nyalwidhe JO, Semmes OJ, Vesprini D, Downes MR, et al. Proteomic discovery of non-invasive biomarkers of localized prostate cancer using mass spectrometry. Nat Rev Urol [Internet]. 2021;18(12):707–24. Available from: https://doi.org/10.1038/s41585-021-00500-1.
84. Jedinak A, Loughlin KR, Moses MA. Approaches to the discovery of non-invasive urinary biomarkers of prostate cancer. Oncotarget. 2018;9(65):32534–50.
85. Liu Y, Hatano K, Nonomura N. Liquid biomarkers in prostate cancer diagnosis: current status and emerging prospects. World J Mens Health. 2025;43(1):8–27.

86. Olson P, Wagner J. Established and emerging liquid biomarkers for prostate cancer detection: a review. Urol Oncol Semin Orig Investig [Internet]. 2025;43(1):3–14. Available from: https://www.sciencedirect.com/science/article/pii/S1078143924004861.
87. Tutrone R, Donovan MJ, Torkler P, Tadigotla V, McLain T, Noerholm M, et al. Clinical utility of the exosome based ExoDx Prostate(IntelliScore) EPI test in men presenting for initial biopsy with a PSA 2–10 ng/mL. Prostate Cancer Prostatic Dis [Internet]. 2020;23(4):607–14. Available from: https://doi.org/10.1038/s41391-020-0237-z.
88. Linscott JA, Meeks JJ, Dyrskjøt L, Li R. The elusive horizon: biomarkers in urothelial carcinoma. Eur Urol [Internet]. 2024;85(4):317–9. Available from: https://www.sciencedirect.com/science/article/pii/S030228382400006X.
89. Dinges SS, Hohm A, Vandergrift LA, Nowak J, Habbel P, Kaltashov IA, et al. Cancer metabolomic markers in urine: evidence, techniques and recommendations. Nat Rev Urol [Internet]. 2019;16(6):339–62. Available from: https://doi.org/10.1038/s41585-019-0185-3.
90. Vidlarova M, Rehulkova A, Stejskal P, Prokopova A, Slavik H, Hajduch M, et al. Recent Advances in methods for circulating tumor cell detection. Int J Mol Sci [Internet]. 2023;24(4). Available from: https://www.mdpi.com/1422-0067/24/4/3902
91. Kumar J, Basak S, Kalkal A, Packirisamy G. Recent advances in nanotechnology and microfluidic-based approaches for isolation and detection of circulating tumor cells (CTCs). Nano-Struct Nano-Objects [Internet]. 2022;31:100886. Available from: https://www.sciencedirect.com/science/article/pii/S2352507X22000294
92. Habli Z, AlChamaa W, Saab R, Kadara H, Khraiche ML. Circulating tumor cell detection technologies and clinical utility: challenges and opportunities. Cancers (Basel) [Internet]. 2020;12(7). Available from: https://www.mdpi.com/2072-6694/12/7/1930
93. Bhome R, Del Vecchio F, Lee GH, Bullock MD, Primrose JN, Sayan AE, et al. Exosomal microRNAs (exomiRs): small molecules with a big role in cancer. Cancer Lett. 2018;420:228–35.
94. Ju S, Chen C, Zhang J, Xu L, Zhang X, Li Z, et al. Detection of circulating tumor cells: opportunities and challenges. Biomark Res [Internet]. 2022;10(1):58. Available from: https://doi.org/10.1186/s40364-022-00403-2.
95. Masaoutis C, Korkolopoulou P, Theocharis S. Exosomes in sarcomas: tiny messengers with broad implications in diagnosis, surveillance, prognosis and treatment. Cancer Lett. 2019;449:172–7.
96. Ingenito F, Roscigno G, Affinito A, Nuzzo S, Scognamiglio I, Quintavalle C, et al. The role of exo-miRNAs in cancer: a focus on therapeutic and diagnostic applications. Int J Mol Sci. 2019;20(19):4687.
97. Li X, Han Y, Meng Y, Yin L. Small RNA-big impact: exosomal miRNAs in mitochondrial dysfunction in various diseases. RNA Biol. 2024;21(1):236–55.
98. Chen F, Xiao M, Hu S, Wang M. Keap1 Nrf2 pathway: a key mechanism in the occurrence and development of cancer. Front Oncol. 2024;14:1381467.
99. Panta P, Manavathi B, Nagini S. Genetics and molecular mechanisms in oral cancer progression. In: Oral Cancer Detect Nov Strateg Clin Impact; 2019. p. 29–80.
100. Ko A, Liao C. Based colorimetric sensors for point-of-care testing. Anal Methods. 2023;15(35):4377–404.
101. Habeshian TS, Cannavale KL, Slezak JM, Shu YH, Chien GW, Chen X, et al. DNA methylation markers for risk of metastasis in a cohort of men with localized prostate cancer. Epigenetics. 2024;19(1):2308920.
102. Rendek T, Pos O, Duranova T, Saade R, Budis J, Repiska V, et al. Current challenges of methylation-based liquid biopsies in cancer diagnostics. Cancers (Basel). 2024;16(11):2001.
103. Chen K, Sun J, Zhao H, Jiang R, Zheng J, Li Z, et al. Non-invasive lung cancer diagnosis and prognosis based on multi-analyte liquid biopsy. Mol Cancer. 2021;20:1–7.
104. Zhao SG, Chen WS, Li H, Foye A, Zhang M, Sjöström M, et al. The DNA methylation landscape of advanced prostate cancer. Nat Genet. 2020;52(8):778–89.
105. Pellacani D, Droop AP, Frame FM, Simms MS, Mann VM, Collins AT, et al. Phenotype-independent DNA methylation changes in prostate cancer. Br J Cancer. 2018;119(9):1133–43.

106. Liu Q, Reed M, Zhu H, Cheng Y, Almeida J, Fruhbeck G, et al. Epigenome-wide DNA methylation and transcriptome profiling of localized and locally advanced prostate cancer: uncovering new molecular markers. Genomics. 2022;114(5):110474.
107. Zhou S, Sikorski D, Xu H, Zubarev A, Chergui M, Lagacé F, et al. Defining the criteria for reflex testing for BRAF mutations in cutaneous melanoma patients. Cancers (Basel). 2021;13(9):2282.
108. Truong H, Breen K, Nandakumar S, Sjoberg DD, Kemel Y, Mehta N, et al. Gene-based confirmatory germline testing following tumor-only sequencing of prostate cancer. Eur Urol. 2023;83(1):29–38.
109. Roy S, Grimes S, Morgan SC, Eapen L, Malone J, Craig J, et al. Patient-reported outcomes from a phase 3 randomized controlled trial exploring optimal sequencing of short-term androgen deprivation therapy with prostate radiation therapy in localized prostate cancer. Int J Radiat Oncol Biol Phys. 2021;110(4):1101–13.
110. Zacharias M, Konjic S, Kratochwill N, Absenger G, Terbuch A, Jost PJ, et al. Expanding broad molecular reflex testing in non-small cell lung cancer to squamous histology. Cancers (Basel). 2024;16(5):903.
111. Russo J, Giri VN. Germline testing and genetic counselling in prostate cancer. Nat Rev Urol. 2022;19(6):331–43.
112. Van Poppel H, Albreht T, Basu P, Hogenhout R, Collen S, Roobol M. Serum PSA-based early detection of prostate cancer in Europe and globally: past, present and future. Nat Rev Urol. 2022;19(9):562–72.
113. Braxton DR, Huang Y, Darabi S, Chavez F, Das PM, Bowen TJ. Pathology molecular reflex testing improves turn-around-time and overall molecular testing rates in NSCLC. Wolters Kluwer Health; 2021.
114. Osses DF, Roobol MJ, Schoots IG. Prediction medicine: biomarkers, risk calculators and magnetic resonance imaging as risk stratification tools in prostate cancer diagnosis. Int J Mol Sci. 2019;20(7):1637.
115. Denijs FB, van Harten MJ, Meenderink JJL, Leenen RCA, Remmers S, Venderbos LDF, et al. Risk calculators for the detection of prostate cancer: a systematic review. Prostate Cancer Prostatic Dis. 2024;27(3):544–57.
116. Jalali A, Kitching M, Martin K, Richardson C, Murphy TB, FitzGerald SP, et al. Integrating inflammatory serum biomarkers into a risk calculator for prostate cancer detection. Sci Rep. 2021;11(1):2525.
117. Ankerst DP, Goros M, Tomlins SA, Patil D, Feng Z, Wei JT, et al. Incorporation of urinary prostate cancer antigen 3 and TMPRSS2: ERG into prostate cancer prevention trial risk calculator. Eur Urol Focus. 2019;5(1):54–61.
118. Donato P, Morton A, Yaxley J, Teloken PE, Coughlin G, Esler R, et al. Improved detection and reduced biopsies: the effect of a multiparametric magnetic resonance imaging-based triage prostate cancer pathway in a public teaching hospital. World J Urol. 2020;38:371–9.
119. Ahlering T, Huynh LM, Kaler KS, Williams S, Osann K, Joseph J, et al. Unintended consequences of decreased PSA-based prostate cancer screening. World J Urol. 2019;37:489–96.
120. Drost FJH, Osses D, Nieboer D, Bangma CH, Steyerberg EW, Roobol MJ, et al. Prostate magnetic resonance imaging, with or without magnetic resonance imaging-targeted biopsy, and systematic biopsy for detecting prostate cancer: a Cochrane systematic review and meta-analysis. Eur Urol [Internet]. 2020;77(1):78–94. Available from: https://www.sciencedirect.com/science/article/pii/S0302283819305135.
121. Pilatz A, Veeratterapillay R, Köves B, Cai T, Bartoletti R, Wagenlehner F, et al. Update on strategies to reduce infectious complications after prostate biopsy. Eur Urol Focus [Internet]. 2019;5(1):20–8. Available from: https://www.sciencedirect.com/science/article/pii/S2405456918303651.
122. Lomas DJ, Ahmed HU. All change in the prostate cancer diagnostic pathway. Nat Rev Clin Oncol [Internet]. 2020;17(6):372–81. Available from: https://doi.org/10.1038/s41571-020-0332-z.

123. Swami U, McFarland TR, Nussenzveig R, Agarwal N. Advanced prostate cancer: treatment advances and future directions. Trends in Cancer [Internet]. 2020;6(8):702–15. Available from: https://doi.org/10.1016/j.trecan.2020.04.010.
124. Lima AR, Pinto J, Amaro F, Bastos M d L, Carvalho M, de Pinho P. Advances and perspectives in prostate cancer biomarker discovery in the last 5 years through tissue and urine metabolomics. Metabolites [Internet]. 2021;11(3). Available from: https://www.mdpi.com/2218-1989/11/3/181.
125. Narayan VM. A critical appraisal of biomarkers in prostate cancer. World J Urol [Internet]. 2020;38(3):547–54. Available from: https://doi.org/10.1007/s00345-019-02759-x.
126. McKiernan J, Donovan MJ, Margolis E, Partin A, Carter B, Brown G, et al. A prospective adaptive utility trial to validate performance of a novel urine exosome gene expression assay to predict high-grade prostate cancer in patients with prostate-specific antigen 2–10ng/ml at initial biopsy. Eur Urol [Internet]. 2018;74(6):731–8. Available from: https://www.sciencedirect.com/science/article/pii/S0302283818306043.
127. Yekula A, Muralidharan K, Kang KM, Wang L, Balaj L, Carter BS. From laboratory to clinic: Translation of extracellular vesicle-based cancer biomarkers. Methods [Internet]. 2020;177:58–66. Available from: https://www.sciencedirect.com/science/article/pii/S1046202319303135.
128. Wang A, Shen J, Rodriguez AA, Saunders EJ, Chen F, Janivara R, et al. Characterizing prostate cancer risk through multi-ancestry genome-wide discovery of 187 novel risk variants. Nat Genet. 2023;55(12):2065–74.
129. Kiebish MA, Cullen J, Mishra P, Ali A, Milliman E, Rodrigues LO, et al. Multi-omic serum biomarkers for prognosis of disease progression in prostate cancer. J Transl Med [Internet]. 2020;18(1):10. Available from: https://doi.org/10.1186/s12967-019-02185-y.
130. Cucchiara V, Cooperberg MR, Dall'Era M, Lin DW, Montorsi F, Schalken JA, et al. Genomic markers in prostate cancer decision making. Eur Urol. 2018;73(4):572–82.
131. Filella X, Fernandez-Galan E, Fernandez Bonifacio R, Foj L. Emerging biomarkers in the diagnosis of prostate cancer. Pharmgenomics Pers Med. 2018;11:83–94.
132. Kim H, Park S, Jeong IG, Song SH, Jeong Y, Kim CS, et al. Noninvasive precision screening of prostate cancer by urinary multimarker sensor and artificial intelligence analysis. ACS Nano. 2020;15(3):4054–65.
133. Van den Broeck T, van den Bergh RCN, Briers E, Cornford P, Cumberbatch M, Tilki D, et al. Biochemical recurrence in prostate cancer: the European Association of Urology prostate cancer guidelines panel recommendations. Eur Urol Focus. 2020;6(2):231–4.
134. Pang B, Zhu Y, Ni J, Thompson J, Malouf D, Bucci J, et al. Extracellular vesicles: the next generation of biomarkers for liquid biopsy-based prostate cancer diagnosis. Theranostics. 2020;10(5):2309.
135. Spohn SKB, Bettermann AS, Bamberg F, Benndorf M, Mix M, Nicolay NH, et al. Radiomics in prostate cancer imaging for a personalized treatment approach – current aspects of methodology and a systematic review on validated studies. Theranostics. 2021;11(16):8027–42.
136. Sekhoacha M, Riet K, Motloung P, Gumenku L, Adegoke A, Mashele S. Prostate cancer review: genetics, diagnosis, treatment options, and alternative approaches. Molecules [Internet]. 2022;27(17). Available from: https://www.mdpi.com/1420-3049/27/17/5730
137. Arita Y, Roest C, Kwee TC, Paudyal R, Lema-Dopico A, Fransen S, et al. Advancements in artificial intelligence for prostate cancer: optimizing diagnosis, treatment, and prognostic assessment. Asian J Urol [Internet]. 2025; Available from: https://www.sciencedirect.com/science/article/pii/S2214388225000074
138. Kucera R, Pecen L, Topolcan O, Dahal AR, Costigliola V, Giordano FA, et al. Prostate cancer management: long-term beliefs, epidemic developments in the early twenty-first century and 3PM dimensional solutions. EPMA J [Internet]. 2020;11(3):399–418. Available from: https://doi.org/10.1007/s13167-020-00214-1.
139. Bax C, Taverna G, Eusebio L, Sironi S, Grizzi F, Guazzoni G, et al. Innovative diagnostic methods for early prostate cancer detection through urine analysis: a review. Cancers (Basel) [Internet]. 2018;10(4). Available from: https://www.mdpi.com/2072-6694/10/4/123.

140. Chai K, Xu C, Man J, Deng Y, Yang L. Evolving paradigms in prostate cancer screening: a decade of bibliometric insights and technological advancements. Front Oncol. 2025;15:1511880.
141. Kumar RR, Kumar A, Chuang CH, Shaikh MO. Recent advances and emerging trends in cancer biomarker detection technologies. Ind Eng Chem Res [Internet]. 2023;62(14):5691–713. Available from: https://doi.org/10.1021/acs.iecr.2c04097.
142. Das S, Dey MK, Devireddy R, Gartia MR. Biomarkers in cancer detection, diagnosis, and prognosis. Sensors [Internet]. 2024;24(1). Available from: https://www.mdpi.com/1424-8220/24/1/37.
143. Khan T, Altamimi MA, Hussain A, Ramzan M, Ashique S, Alhuzani MR, et al. Understanding of PSA biology, factors affecting PSA detection, challenges, various biomarkers, methods, and future perspective of prostate cancer detection and diagnosis. Adv Cancer Biol Metastasis [Internet]. 2022;5:100059. Available from: https://www.sciencedirect.com/science/article/pii/S2667394022000338.
144. Tenchov R, Sapra AK, Sasso J, Ralhan K, Tummala A, Azoulay N, et al. Biomarkers for early cancer detection: a landscape view of recent advancements, spotlighting pancreatic and liver cancers. ACS Pharmacol Transl Sci [Internet]. 2024;7(3):586–613. Available from: https://doi.org/10.1021/acsptsci.3c00346.

Fundamentals of Biosensors

3

Sakshi Patel, Gulam Muheyuddeen, Preeti Singh, and Shashank Shekhar

Abbreviations

DNA	Deoxyribonucleic acid
EIS	Electrochemical impedance spectroscopy
LOD	Limit of detection
MIP	Molecularly imprinted polymer
pH	Potential of hydrogen (measure of acidity/alkalinity)
POCT	Point-of-care testing
PSA	Prostate-specific antigen
QCM	Quartz crystal microbalance
RNA	Ribonucleic acid
SPCE	Screen-printed carbon electrode
SPR	Surface plasmon resonance

S. Patel
Department of Pharmaceutical Technology, Meerut Institute of Engineering & Technology, Meerut, Uttar Pradesh, India

G. Muheyuddeen
Department of Pharmaceutical Chemistry, Faculty of Pharmacy, Jahangirabad Institute of Technology, Jahangirabad Fort, Jahangirabad, Barabanki, Uttar Pradesh, India

P. Singh
School of Pharmacy, Sharda University, Knowledge Park III, Greater Noida, Uttar Pradesh, India

S. Shekhar (✉)
Department of Radiotherapy, AIIMS Gorakhpur, Gorakhpur, Uttar Pradesh, India

S. Srivastava et al. (eds.), *Biosensor Technologies for Prostate Cancer*, https://doi.org/10.1007/978-981-95-8644-8_3

3.1 Introduction: Defining the Biosensor

Biology and technology have given us more than wonderful tools that can peep into the complicated molecular world concealed beneath life and the environment [1]. The most important of these technologies is probably the biosensor. A biosensor is an intricate analytical device that is employed to identify the presence and the concentration of specific chemical or biological molecules, known as analytes [2]. These instruments operate by transforming a biological recognition event, the extremely specific interaction of a biological element and the analyte of interest, into some measurable signal [3]. This synergy is often found in complex combinations, providing sensitive and selective detection that alters how we monitor our health, safeguard our environment, sustain the quality of our food, and advance scientific studies [4]. Starting with the diagnostics and extending far beyond, this chapter introduces the basic components of a biosensor and traces its indispensable role [5]. Due to the ability of biosensors to analyze biological or chemical substances rapidly, precisely, and often in real time, they are rapidly gaining importance as research and clinical instruments of the modern scientific and clinical environment. Their appearance is due to the interaction of high-tech physicochemical transducers and biological recognition systems, which enable more complex molecular interactions to be converted into a readable signal [6]. They are devices that apply selective biological components (such as enzymes, antibodies, nucleic acids, or whole cells) to detect certain analytes with a high degree of specificity, even in a complex mixture (such as blood, urine, or environmental samples) [7]. This helps bridge the gap between biology and engineering. Due to their special ability, biosensors have diverse applications, including defense, environmental monitoring, drug development, disease diagnostics, and food quality control [8]. Recent developments in materials science, nanotechnology, and microfluidics have further enhanced biosensor performance, improving sensitivity and portability while enabling field and point-of-care use [9]. The development of biosensors has become a crucial element of technological innovation, driven by the increasing demand for real-time monitoring, personalized medicine, and the detection of diseases at an early stage [10]. In the sections that follow, we will examine the fundamental components and operation of biosensors, as well as how their architecture can directly influence their functionality and potential use in areas such as prostate cancer diagnostics, where the early detection of a biomarker may significantly contribute to patient outcomes [11]. To gain a comprehensive understanding of how biosensors work and why they are successful, it is essential to start with their structural and functional foundations [12]. This involves an in-depth analysis of the biological recognition elements that offer selectivity, the transducers that convert biological events to measurable and quantifiable signals, and signal processing units that ensure the accuracy and usability of data [13]. The chapter will then discuss the cooperation of these factors in the detection process, explore the classification of the biosensors based on their principal working mechanisms, and evaluate key performance parameters such as sensitivity, specificity, and detection limits [14]. The chapter will end with examples of how the underlying concepts were applied in real-life practice, with a special focus on how the concepts have transformed the diagnosis of prostate cancer [15, 16]. With this understanding, readers will be prepared to advance to more complicated biosensor designs and applications, which will be discussed in the following chapters.

3.2 Core Components of a Biosensor

A functional biosensor is a complex structure that is characterized by the connection of several specific components into a single system [17]. All the elements together drive the process, which initially began with the identification of a targeted molecule, leading to the formation of useful data products. To understand the most crucial functionality of a biosensor, it is possible to consider its three main components, which include recognition components that specify detection, an analytical transducer that converts the biological signals, and the steps that have to be undertaken to process the data outputs [18]. A basic understanding of these key aspects drives appreciation for how biosensing technology operates, its adaptability, and its design concepts.

3.2.1 The Layer of Recognition: Bioreceptors (Such as Enzymes, Antibodies, and Nucleic Acids)

The bioreceptor is the biological component of biosensors that carries out molecular recognition and is the central component in all biosensor designs [19]. The selectivity and specificity properties of the biosensor depend primarily on this recognition layer because it enables the device to selectively detect its intended target molecule in complex biological and environmental samples [20]. The biochemical interaction between the bioreceptor and its corresponding analyte activates the detection basis of the biosensing system. Different bioreceptors exhibit varying dependencies on the target analyte, in conjunction with the selected sensing approach. Common types include the following [21]. *Enzymes:* Biological catalysts known as enzymes work with the analytical substrate to perform a particular chemical transformation. The detection process involves either measuring substance depletion (e.g., oxygen) or observing product formation (e.g., hydrogen peroxide, ions, electrons, and heat and light emission) [22]. Active sites on enzymes determine their high selectivity because they are shaped perfectly to suit their specific function, like the "lock-and-key" model explains [23]. Glucose sensors function with glucose oxidase (GOx) as their main component to measure glucose concentration through hydrogen peroxide generation after glucose oxidation occurs inside the device. *Immunoglobulins (Antibodies):* They represent fundamental Y-shaped proteins that form the basis of the adaptive immune system by specifically recognizing their matching antigens (acceptable measurement targets which include proteins, peptides, toxins, small molecules, and others) [24]. The detection method uses the antibody–antigen binding action or the detection of secondary antibody binding with a label [25]. Neutralization assays find widespread application in medical diagnosis across tests such as pregnancy tests that identify hCG hormone signals and viral antigen identification tests for infectious disease detection. The specificity and batch reliability of monoclonal antibodies outperform those of polyclonal antibodies. *Nucleic Acids (DNA/RNA):* Biosensor probes based on short DNA or RNA sequences (probes) exhibit hybridization selectivity for complementary targets, which follow the Watson–Crick base pairing rules (A–T, G–C) [26]. Through this method, biosensors achieve highly specific detection of genetic material from pathogens and disease-related mutations and gene expression markers (mRNA). Aptamers, which are single-stranded DNA and RNA aptamers identified through SELEX and related selection methods, form structured three-dimensional shapes that bind target molecules securely, much like antibodies do [27]. Aptamers offer numerous benefits, including improved manufacturing processes, increased durability, and straightforward modifications. *Cells or Microorganisms:* Entire living cells, together with microorganisms, function as bioreceptors because they serve as detection tools [28]. A change in the biological state (e.g., respiration rate, production of specific metabolites, and stress responses) of these biological receptors occurs upon exposure to an analyte (e.g., toxins, nutrients, and pollutants), which can be measured electrochemically or optically. The BOD sensor represents one among several applications where these devices prove valuable for identifying general toxic exposure and determining bioavailability levels. *Biomimetic Receptors:* The integration of biomimetic receptors into chemical receptors expands the types of detection systems by utilizing synthetic analogs, such as molecularly imprinted polymers (MIPs) and synthetic peptides, which demonstrate advantages in terms of stability and cost efficiency [29].

3.2.2 The Signal Generator: Transducer (e.g., Electrochemical, Optical, and Piezoelectric)

The transducer functions as an essential communication point to produce measurable physical output from biophysical or biochemical events at the bioreceptor surface [30]. Signal transduction enables the conversion of biological interaction data, which proves difficult to directly measure through the use of well-defined physical methods [31]. The nature of output signals and biosensor sensitivity, as well as measurement range, along with interferences, stems primarily from the choice of transducer type. Major classes of transducers include the following [32].

Electrochemical Transducers: The electrochemical transducer stands out because it provides high sensitivity alongside low cost, instrumental ease, and possible device miniaturization. Measurement of electrical variations occurs after bioreceptor interaction with the analyte. *Amperometric:* This detection method calculates the current output that arises when electroactive species evolve or vanish during the bioreceptor reaction (for example, detecting H_2O_2 from GOx action). *Potentiometric:* This technique tracks voltage changes on electrode surfaces because of modifications in ion concentration and charge accumulation, which can be accomplished by using ion-selective electrodes (ISEs) or field-effect transistors (FETs) modified with enzymes or antibodies. *Conductometric/ Impedimetric:* This technique detects modifications in electric conductivity or impedance of the electrolytic solution and electrode-solution junction, which result from enzymatic transformations that affect ionic mobility or surface characteristics modifications.

Optical Transducers: The bioreceptor–analyte interaction is influenced by light absorption, reflection, or changes in the emission and propagation characteristics of light. The devices have high detection capabilities and also have flexible functionality [33]. *Absorbance:* The absorbance method allows colorimetric detection by observing changes in light transmission, which are caused by enzymatic reactions and binding assays. *Fluorescence:* The detection methods involve fluorescence, which tracks the intensity, lifetime, or polarization changes of emitted light of fluorescent molecules utilized as fluorophores in the reaction pathway or binding process (read FRET-based sensors). *Luminescence (Chemi-/Bio-/):* The sensitivity of absorbance methods allows detection of light emission with high sensitivity through the minimal background, at a high level. *Surface Plasmon Resonance (SPR):* It is a label-free technique that measures changes in refractive indices that occur just under a layer of metals like gold to monitor interactions between analyte biomolecules with bioreceptors immobilized on the sensor surface. *Interferometry/Waveguides Technology:* It is a label-free technique that measures the change of light phase conditions and propagation properties that result from the interaction between biomolecules that occur through the binding of analyte biomolecules with bioreceptors immobilized on the sensor surface.

Piezoelectric (Mass-Sensitive) Transducers: They use piezoelectric materials that produce voltage output upon external stress, and resonance occurs upon voltage application [34]. *Quartz Crystal Microbalance (QCM):* It detects alterations in the resonant frequency of an oscillating quartz crystal through its measurement. A decrease in frequency becomes detectable after the analyte binds to the bioreceptor that was immobilized on the surface of the crystal. This is a label-free technique. *Surface Acoustic Wave (SAW):* The system records variations in acoustic wave properties that travel through a piezoelectric substrate when analyzing mass loading or changes that occur to surface properties from binding events. *Thermal (Calorimetric) Transducers:* They determine heat energy changes from biological reactions through calorimetric measurements during enzymatic catalysis or fragment-binding events. The detection system relies on heat change events, although precise instrumentation with thermal control remains crucial. The selection of transducers primarily depends on the chosen bioreceptor, as well as the application's necessary characteristics, including sensitivity levels, cost, and mobility needs for the device, as well as the requirement for unmodified detection methods [35].

3.2.3 Data Interpretation: Signal Processing and Readout

The signal output by the transducer has low strength, is accompanied by significant noise, and exhibits an imperfect relationship between the analyte concentration and the usable display format. Signal processing and readout electronics are needed as the final ultimate processing stage in such systems [35]. This system achieves signal amplification while also providing filtering, analysis, and conversion of signals, which converts simple transducer signals into information that should be presented to users. Amplification: The output signal of the transducer (in the form of picoampere currents and microvolt potentials or small frequency changes) is amplified without viewing port enhancement before further processing by electrical amplifiers [36]. Raw signals have noise that is caused by electronic noise and environmental interferences, as well as nonspecific interactions. *Filtering:* Signal noise is also reduced before measurement by the use of filtering technology at the analog level or digital level to increase levels of SNR to improve the accuracy and sensitivity of measurement [37]. *Signal Conditioning and Conversion:* Measurement devices convert continuous analog signals into digital form by using analog-to-digital converters (ADCs) to further process the information to microcontrollers or computers [38]. Normalization operations or baseline correction operations are performed at this stage. *Analysis and Calibration:* Before the processed digital signal is used, it must be connected directly to the actual concentration of the analyte. The sensor is calibrated using a curve that is produced, which accurately depicts its responses to known concentrations of analytes under similar conditions. Its device memory has the algorithms that utilize calibration data to convert signal intensity measurements to concentration values, represented as quantities such as mg/dL, μM, or ng/mL. *Readout/ Display:* The device displays the results as concentrations in either quantitative or positive /negative results using an interface that includes LCD displays alongside indicator lights and audible signals in addition to smartphone or computer connectivity to log the data [39]. The transducer feeds the signal processing unit with the electrical or optical signal, which filters through noise, amplifies the signal when needed, and translates the signal into a readable output, either quantitative or qualitative. This sequence of detecting an analyte between recognition and readout is illustrated in Fig. 3.1 at the molecular scale, showing the schematic interaction of a biosensor with an analyte of interest.

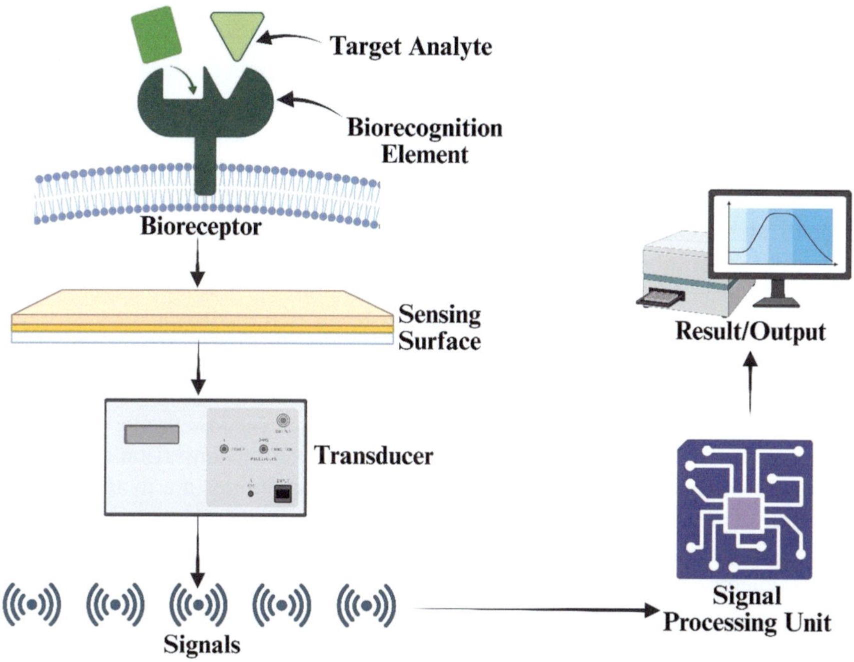

Fig. 3.1 Schematic representation of a biosensor mechanism

3.3 Detection Mechanism of Biosensors

The fundamental design is the result of the research on separate biosensor parts based on the description above [40]. A biosensor attains its remarkable function through a sophisticated method that activates the components to convert analyte detection into measurable signals. All biosensors perform two fundamental operational steps [41]. First, they allow precise molecular recognition through the bioreceptor, followed by a signal transduction step by the transducer. This section examines in detail the detection process, starting from specific molecule recognition through qualitative signal conversion, which enables detection to become possible [42].

3.3.1 The Biorecognition Event

Several bioreceptors recognize their targets through binding processes that utilize multiple non-covalent forces, such as hydrogen bonds, ionic interactions, van der Waals forces, and hydrophobic interactions [43]. The binding site union arises because bioreceptors have exact three-dimensional matching between their sites and analytes through lock-and-key or induced-fit models. *Binding-Based Recognition:* Bioreceptors achieve binding recognition by forming connections with their analytes through various non-covalent interactions, including hydrogen bonds, ionic bonds, van der Waals forces, and hydrophobic interactions. The bioreceptor achieves this level of accuracy thanks to just-right structural symmetry between its binding site and the analyte, which operates through mechanics that mirror lock-and-key mechanics or the precise induced-fit model, allowing both binding site and analyte to adapt their conformations [44]. For example, antibody–antigen binding, nucleic acid hybridization (probe-target DNA/RNA), aptamer–target binding, and lectin–carbohydrate interactions. The sensor surface development leads to the buildup of analyte matter at the location where bioreceptors remain fixed. The binding process brings about local change to the interfacial charge distribution, and dielectric properties and refractive index measurements at sensor interfaces, or causes a change in shape to the bioreceptors [45]. The strength degree of this affinal interaction is determined by its affinal constant along with its dissociation constant. *Catalysis-Based Recognition:* In catalysis-based bioreceptors, recognition occurs through catalase receptors that recognize their respective substrate (analyte) and catalyze the conversion of the substrate into more than one product. Its recognition capabilities are dictated by the multitude of properties, as well as the active site of the enzyme. For example, glucose oxidase accepts glucose as a substrate, which it chemically transforms into gluconic acid coupled with H_2O_2 formation [46].

The main effect emerges from chemical substrate breakdown. The substance analysis turns into chemical products such as H_2O_2 and H^+ ions alongside potential co-substrate usage (e.g., O_2) and produces heat discharge together with electron transfer (redox reactions) [47]. The reaction speed usually depends on the amount of analyte until the system becomes saturated. The biorecognition interaction between an analyte and its transducer surface results in a biochemical or biophysical change that occurs either at the transducer or in close proximity to it, regardless of binding or catalytic mechanism [48]. Successful analyte access to bioreceptors depends on their proper immobilization technique, in addition to maintaining the measurability of the biochemical or biophysical changes by the transducer. Achieving successful bioreceptor immobilization becomes challenging when preventing sample molecules from non-specifically binding with the sensor and maintaining bioreceptor stability over time.

3.3.2 Signal Transduction Principles

During signal transduction, the biochemical or biophysical results of biorecognition create alternative energy or signal formats, including optical, electrical, acoustic, or thermal signals that can be easily measured, enhanced, and processed for analytical needs [49]. The transducer serves as an interpreter that detects particular changes from bioreceptor–analyte interactions and creates output signals that should directly represent the analyte concentration. Different transducers use distinct conversion principles that determine their operation [50]. Table 3.1 provides a concise overview of the primary signal transduction strategies used in biosensors, highlighting their mechanisms and typical areas of application [51].

Table 3.1 Signal transduction principles in biosensors

Type of transduction	Method	Principle	Key measurement	Typical application	References
Electrochemical	Amperometry	Measures current from redox reactions at electrodes	Electron flow (current)	Glucose sensors (H_2O_2 detection)	[52]
	Potentiometry	Measures voltage between the sensing and reference electrodes with minimal current	Potential difference (voltage)	Ion-selective electrodes (pH sensors)	[53]
	Impedance spectroscopy (EIS)	Measures resistance and capacitance over AC frequency range	Impedance spectrum features	Antibody–antigen binding detection	[54]
Optical	Absorbance/fluorescence/luminescence	Measures changes in light absorbance, emission, or quenching	Light intensity, Wavelength, lifetime	Fluorescent immunoassays	[55]
	Surface plasmon resonance (SPR)/label-free	Detects refractive index changes on a metal surface	Resonance condition shifts	Real-time binding studies	[56]
Piezoelectric	Quartz crystal microbalance (QCM)	Measures mass change affecting crystal oscillation frequency	Frequency reduction	Biomolecules mass detection	[57]
Thermal	Thermal transduction	Measures heat from biochemical reactions	Temperature changes	Enzyme reaction monitoring	[58]

3.3.2.1 Electrochemical Transduction

These transduction methods measure electrical signal modifications in solutions [59]. *Amperometry:* The method of amperometry determines electron flow (current) that results from electrode surface-based redox (oxidation or reduction) reactions [60]. The reactions at the electrodes contain electroactive species (including H_2O_2 found in glucose sensors) whose redox states alter as the enzyme operates. The electrochemical reaction occurs while maintaining a particular voltage, and the produced current shows a direct relationship with the electroactive species levels to indicate the amount of analyte present. *Potentiometry:* This method measures the potential difference (voltage) between a sensing electrode and a reference electrode under near-zero current conditions [61]. The electrode interface accumulates charge that results in a potential shift because of analyte binding, enzymatic ion production, or consumption processes based on fundamental principles, including the Nernst equation. *Impedance Spectroscopy (EIS):* This method measures the resistance and capacitance (impedance) of the electrode–electrolyte interface over a range of AC frequencies [62]. The binding of an antibody–antigen pair or changes in ionic conditions caused by enzymatic processes at the interface modify its structural arrangement along with charge distribution, thus producing detectable impacts on impedance spectrum features.

3.3.2.2 Optical Transduction

The detection techniques based on optical transduction measure changes in light properties [63]. *Absorbance/Fluorescence/Luminescence:* The biorecognition process leads to chromophore formation and consumption through the production of fluorophores and luminophores, along with indicator-based optically modified properties (quenching and FRET included) [64]. Light absorbance or emission properties are measured while understanding their intensity and wavelength, as well as lifetime, through corresponding interpretations for analyte concentration. *Surface Plasmon Resonance (SPR)/Label-Free*: It measures how changes in the surface local refractive index affect the conditions needed to create surface plasmon resonance in a thin metal film, which contains immobilized bioreceptors [65]. Surface plasmon excitability depends on incident light conditions following changes in the metal film, which provide accurate and instant binding detection without relying on labels. The principle behind interferometry matches other label-free optical methods because they detect refractive index changes.

3.3.2.3 Piezoelectric Transduction

These methods depend on mass variation detection through the use of piezoelectric transduction [66]. *QCM:* The bioreceptor layer binding of analyte molecules to its surface on an oscillating quartz crystal causes a mass increase. Additional mass that attaches to the crystal makes its oscillation less efficient, which results in a detectable reduction in its resonant frequency [67]. The mass quantification of binding during the recognition process becomes possible through direct measurement of the frequency change using the Sauerbrey relationship for thin rigid films. *Thermal Transduction:* The detection system uses thermal transduction to measure heat generation or heat loss caused by biorecognition events that mainly include enzymatic reactions [68]. Near the bioreceptor layer, there exist thermistors or thermopiles that detect small temperature alterations to calculate both reaction velocity and analyte concentration levels.

3.4 Classification of Biosensors

The field of analytical technology places biosensors as its leading tools, which unite the study domains of biology with chemistry and engineering principles. The classification system helps scientists understand the different forms and usage methods of these devices [69]. Biosensors exist primarily in two classification groups, which distinguish them by their biorecognition elements or their transduction processes that convert biological signals to measurable outputs. Biosensor selection for analytical tasks finds support through these two framework methods. The selection of biosensors for analytics depends on these two structural frameworks. Table 3.2 presents a summary of fundamental biosensor categories according to their biorecognition elements, together with their transduction mechanisms [70].

Table 3.2 Classification of biosensors by biorecognition elements and transduction methods

Types of categorizations	Subtype	Recognition element/ mechanism	Applications	References
By biorecognition element	Enzyme-based	Enzymes (e.g., glucose oxidase); catalyze specific biochemical reactions	Blood glucose monitoring, clinical diagnostics	[52]
	Antibody-based (immunosensors)	Antibodies; highly specific antigen–antibody interactions	Pathogen detection, biomarker analysis, toxin detection	[71]
	Nucleic acid-based (geno sensors)	DNA/RNA probes; hybridize with complementary genetic sequences	Genetic diagnostics, mutation detection, pathogen identification	[72]
	Cell-based	Living cells; respond to environmental changes (pH, ion movement, oxygen levels)	Drug screening, cytotoxicity testing, environmental monitoring	[73]
	Aptamer-based	Synthetic oligonucleotides/ peptides; fold into 3D shapes to bind targets	Food safety testing, cancer diagnostics	[74]
	Molecularly imprinted polymers	Synthetic polymers with molecular recognition sites; mimic natural receptors	Harsh environment detection, reusable sensing	[75]

(continued)

Table 3.2 (continued)

Types of categorizations	Subtype	Recognition element/ mechanism	Applications	References
By transduction method	Electrochemical	Measures electric parameters (amperometric, potentiometric, impedimetric)	Personal glucose meters, point-of-care devices	[76]
	Optical	Detects changes in light properties (absorption, fluorescence, SPPR, luminescence)	Medical diagnostics, pharmaceutical research, environmental sensing	[56]
	Piezoelectric (acoustic)	Mass detection through changes in crystal vibration frequency	Label-free assays, low molecular weight compound detection	[57]
	Thermal (calorimetric)	Measures temperature changes from exothermic/ endothermic reactions	Label-free detection in non-standard conditions	[58]
	Magnetic	Tracks magnetic field changes due to the binding of magnetic particles	Multiplexed diagnostics, high-throughput testing, low-noise signal analysis	[77]

3.4.1 Classification by Biorecognition Element

The bioreceptor functions as the biorecognition element, which serves as the key component that enables selective analyte-recognition. The functional and specific properties of biosensors depend on their essential elements [78]. Figure 3.2 shows that the biosensor classification system depends on the type of biorecognition material [79].

Enzyme-Based Biosensors: These involve the use of enzymes as biological recognition components, as they are highly specific and have a catalytic activity. A typical example of a biosensor is the glucose biosensor that uses glucose oxidase [80]. The enzyme reaction is used to produce two products, including hydrogen peroxide, which are measurable substances. These biosensors are critical medical devices used frequently by research institutions to monitor the level of blood sugar in a clinical environment. *Antibody-Based (Immunosensors):* Immunosensors are used to detect specific antigens, the identification component of which is an antibody. The interaction of antibodies with antigens offers the highest level of specificity, with the selective attachment to yield excellent outcomes in pathogen detection, biomarker detection, and analysis of toxins [81]. The three analytical methods for

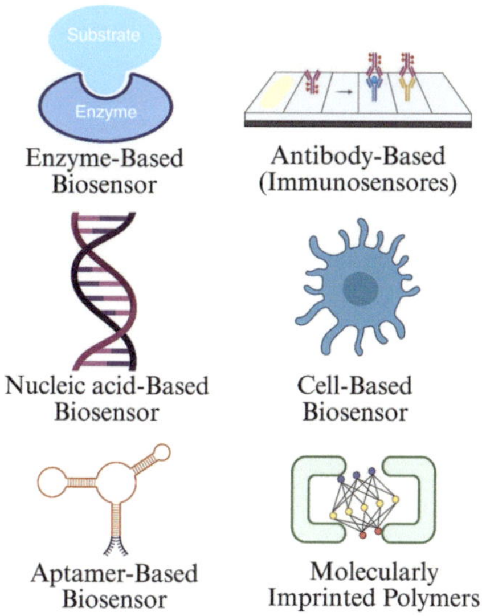

Fig. 3.2 Types of biosensors classified by biorecognition elements

biosensors are direct, sandwich, and competitive assays. *Nucleic Acid-Based Biosensors (Geno Sensors):* These biosensors detect specific DNA or RNA sequences through hybridization. These devices appear throughout genetic diagnostic procedures, pathogen identification protocols, and mutation analysis applications [82]. A binding interaction between probe and target occurs through either optical, electrochemical, or piezoelectric signals. *Cell-Based Biosensors:* The sensing elements in these biosensors consist of living cells that yield expanded biological feedback. Sensors of this kind serve researchers conducting cytotoxicity tests along with drug development work and environmental screening activities [83]. A cell detects changes in oxygen production and creates alterations in the acidity level and movement of ions. *Aptamer-Based Biosensors:* Aptamers consist of synthetic oligonucleotides and peptides, which develop specific three-dimensional shapes to recognize specific targets. Aptamers maintain high target recognition while being economically beneficial and durable at the same time as compared to antibody applications [74]. The development of biosensors based on aptamers continues for different applications within food safety and cancer detection fields; *Molecularly Imprinted Polymers (MIPs):* Though not biological, MIPs imitate natural recognition systems by creating polymer frameworks with holes complementary to the target molecule [84]. These are strong, reusable, and especially beneficial in severe settings where biomolecules may deteriorate.

3.4.2 Classification by Transduction Method

The biosensor takes measured biological signals through transduction to generate detectable signals. As shown in Fig. 3.3, the main types of biosensors exist based on

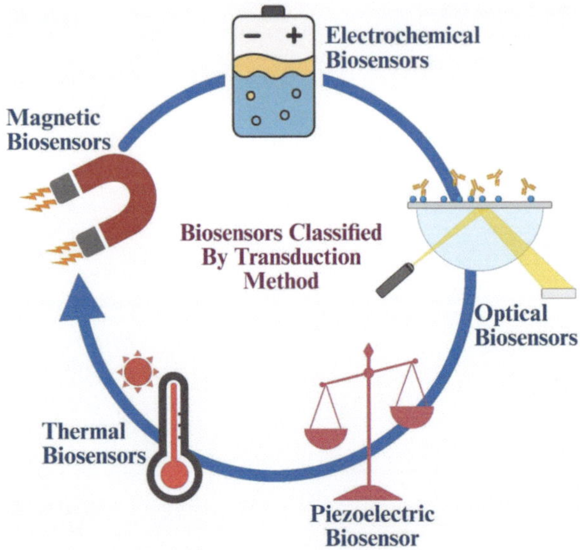

Fig. 3.3 Types of biosensors classified by transduction method

the transduction system mechanism as described below [85]. *Electrochemical Biosensors:* Biosensors of this type find wide acceptance because of their basic operation, along with effortless mobility and cost-effectiveness. Signal measurements can take the form of electrical parameters, including amperometric current, potentiometric potential, and impedance measurement (impedimetric). Glucose meters represent electrochemical biosensors, which currently serve patients widely throughout healthcare systems [86]. *Optical Biosensors:* The recognition event between biomolecules produces detectable changes in light properties, including absorption and fluorescence, together with luminescence and surface plasmon resonance (SPR) [87]. The sensors deliver high sensitivity detection, which medical diagnostics, together with environmental monitoring and pharmaceutical research, regularly apply. The SPR-based biosensor technology provides instant readout for biomolecular detection without requiring any labels.

Piezoelectric (Acoustic) Biosensors: The sensor detects surface mass changes, which make the piezoelectric crystal (usually quartz) frequency shift. A biomolecule binding to the sensor surface results in a change of the crystal's vibration frequency, which directly reveals its mass measurements [88]. These devices are used to perform label-free detection or identification of low molecular weight compounds and also label-free assays. *Thermal Biosensors (Calorimetric):* Temperature changes due to biological reactions, which could be endothermic or exothermic, are used as indicators of detection with these devices [89]. These detection mechanisms are not very common but can be used to make experiments that do not need labels or that cannot be used when the environment is incompatible with other operating systems. *Magnetic Biosensors:* The biosensors are based on magnetic particles that can be used to monitor changes in the magnetic field strength, which are caused by biorecognition interactions. Their application as diagnostic instruments in multiplexing tests and high-speed assessments attracts more attention due to weak background interference and the possibility of a small system size [90]. There are several categories of transduction systems that have disparate downsides and upsides between their sensitivity and operation speed, as well as integration capability and complexities. The selection procedure of transducers is a direct consequence of application specifications and needs, along with the detection precision requirements [91].

3.5 Gauging Performance: Key Biosensor Characteristics

The performance characteristics of any biosensor, especially in a complex area, such as the diagnostics of prostate cancer (PCa), are crucial to the clinical utility of the biosensor [92]. The parameters identified specify the reliability, accuracy, and applicability of the sensor to the diagnosis of diseases, future prognosis, and assessment of therapy outcomes.

Before biosensors can advance from laboratory to clinical use, it is crucial to make a thorough assessment of their performance characteristics [93]. As shown in Fig. 3.4, the essential characteristics of biosensors are key features such as

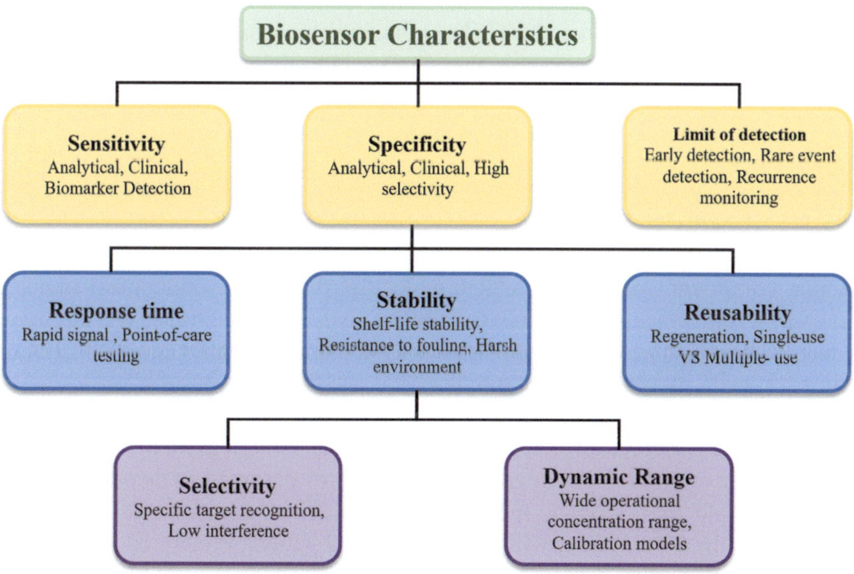

Fig. 3.4 Biosensors have several essential features, namely high sensitivity (analytical, clinical, and biomarker detection), high specificity, and low limit of detection, essential in detecting early and rare events. Other valuable characteristics include quick response time (point-of-care), stability over a wide range of conditions, regeneration, high selectivity with low interference, and a wide dynamic range ensured by stable calibration

sensitivity, specificity, limit of detection, response time, stability, reusability, selectivity, and dynamic range, all of which critically impact their performance in clinical and analytical settings [92].

3.5.1 Sensitivity, Specificity, and Limit of Detection (LOD)

The diagnostic performance of a biosensor depends on these three connected parameters since their application meets resistance from current biomarkers like prostate-specific antigen (PSA) [94]. Biosensor sensitivity within analytical settings means the change in sensor output signal per unit analyte concentration change, which displays as the slope value during the linear calibration range [95]. The translation of analytical sensitivity measurements into clinical sensitivity means the most for prostate cancer diagnosis. The clinical sensitivity of biosensors describes their capacity to correctly detect individuals who have prostate cancer (true positive rate). High clinical sensitivity is essential to detect prostate cancer at an early stage because patients need prompt treatment of their aggressive forms of disease [96]. The analysis of prostate cancer requires biomarker detection and the assessment of specific ratios regarding biomarker levels, including total PSA and free PSA as well as PCA3 and TMPRSS2 [97], ERG fusion transcripts, and multiple novel markers across specific microRNAs and extracellular vesicles currently under investigation. The main hurdle lies in making biosensors detectable for minimal yet crucial molecular disease alterations while preventing false detection of harmless cancer cells. Modern biosensors include several biomarker tests at once (p2PSA with other markers for PHI analysis) to improve the detection of aggressive prostate diseases.

3.5.1.1 Specificity

The ability of a biosensor to detect target analytes without interference from either similar compounds or other unrelated molecules that exist in biological samples (such as serum, plasma, and urine) constitutes analytical specificity. The ability of a test to identify those individuals correctly without prostate cancer constitutes clinical specificity regarding the true negative rate [98]. PSA tests create a significant problem due to their low clinical specificity because elevated PSA occurs in individuals with benign prostate conditions such as benign prostatic hyperplasia (BPH) and prostatitis. Current advanced biosensors designed to detect PCa need to demonstrate high clinical specificity so healthcare providers can minimize unnecessary biopsies, along with their associated patient anxiety and healthcare expenses. This is often achieved through [99]. The system utilizes biorecognition elements that exhibit high binding specificity toward their target using monoclonal antibodies and engineered aptamers. Detection of more cancer-specific biomarkers than total PSA (e.g., PCA3 in urine, specific glyco forms of PSA, and CTCs with specific phenotypes). Multiple biomarkers combined with algorithm analysis yield a malignancy signature that is more accurate than analysis of one marker only.

3.5.1.2 Limit of Detection (LOD)

The biosensor reaches its detection threshold (LOD) at the lowest concentration of target analyte that exceeds background signals or blank measurements, which typically follows statistical calculation methods through the addition of three standard deviations to the mean blank value [100]. The determination of the lower Limit of detection is crucial in various settings for PCa diagnosis. *Early Detection:* The detection of minimal amounts of biomarkers becomes possible through early-stage identification. Analysis of biochemical recurrence requires monitored prostate-specific antigen (PSA) levels to reach no-detectable status following prostatectomy and radiotherapy treatments [101]. The low level of PSA (above 0.1 ng/mL and above 0.2 ng/mL, depending on the definitions) may reflect a recurrence of disease; hence, sensitive testing techniques with detection limits of pg/mL are required. *Monitoring Biochemical Recurrence:* Biochemical recurrence requires unending monitoring, as adults who have had a radical prostatectomy or received radiation therapy should generate PSA results that cannot be detected [102]. Recurrence with PSA monitoring at low levels (over 0.1 or 0.2 ng/mL according to definitions) indicates that low concentrations of these exosomes demand highly sensitive assays working at the pg/mL level of detection. *Detection of Low-Incidence Substances:* Low-concentration biochemical substances, such as circulating tumor cells (CTCs) and individual exosomes, require detection assays since they hold valuable clinical information. Biosensors have signal amplification techniques with complicated amplification techniques (like enzyme reactions, beam-sensitive detection with nanoparticles, and nanoengineered transducers) to achieve clinically important detection limits [103].

3.5.2 Response Time, Stability, and Reusability

These working parameters determine the practicability in addition to the financial feasibility of the biosensor system [104]. Once a sample has been introduced into the biosensor system, a stable signal of some measurable value will then require time to appear. Biosensors that perform point-of-care testing (POCT) need to achieve response times that are faster than minutes, since this requirement is essential for clinical workflows [105]. The biosensor system enables clinicians to make decisions quickly, which can occur while meeting patients during their consultations. Laboratory assessments of PCa markers typically require extended periods, ranging from days to hours. Direct transduction biosensors functioning with electrochemical and optical mechanisms can detect signals quickly after sample introduction because they need minimal sample handling or incubation procedures [106]. Rapid results help speed up clinical diagnosis routines while enhancing patient care procedures.

3.5.2.1 Stability

The ability of a biosensor to preserve its performance traits (sensitivity, specificity, and baseline signal) throughout time spans storage periods and operational periods defines stability [107]. Sensor instability occurs due to three main factors: biological recognition element deterioration (antibody denaturation or enzyme inactivation), component leaching during sensor operation, non-specific sample matrix adsorption that damages the sensor surface, and transducer electronic component drift. Biosensors used to diagnose PCa require resistance to physical and environmental changes, such as temperature and humidity, as they will be employed across various clinical and resource-poor locations [108]. The stability of biosensors can be improved through better immobilization techniques and stronger bioreceptor choices, such as aptamers or nanobodies, along with the application of protective layers and effective surface anti-fouling methods, which are especially vital for complex matrix testing, such as blood or urine.

3.5.2.2 Reusability

A biosensor device demonstrates reusability when it performs dependable successive measurement operations with a single unit. The process of reusing biosensors involves an analytical removal procedure that returns the sensor surface to its original operating condition and preserves both the functionality of the bound bioreceptor and maintains signal stability [109]. The need to reduce laboratory testing expenses through test regeneration remains challenging because high-affinity systems face difficulties with effective regeneration and maintaining performance levels. Portable medical testing applications often require single-use sensors because they provide maximum performance alongside risk-free operation, although they might present a modest increase in test material expenses [110]. Organizations make their selection between reusable or single-use formats based on three main factors, which are specific application needs, along with performance requirements and operational complexity, as well as economic considerations [111].

3.5.3 Selectivity and Dynamic Range

The characteristics determine the exactness and measurement range of biological biosensors within real-life biological applications [112]. A sensor demonstrates selectivity when it can differentiate between its target substance and possible interferences that exist within the sample fluid. The measurement of biological fluids, including blood, serum, plasma, and urine, becomes problematic because these mixtures contain various proteins, salts, and lipids, as well as metabolites and cells [113]. The biomarkers used to detect PCa, such as PSA, experience interference from different kallikreins, including hK2, as well as high-abundance proteins and anticoagulants found in biological samples [114]. Selective sensors produce signals that originate entirely from the target analyte, which allows precise measurement of amounts. This is achieved through the following [115]: careful selection and engineering of the biorecognition element; optimization of assay conditions (pH, ionic strength, blocking agents); integration of sample pre-treatment steps (e.g., filtration and dilution); development of sensor interfaces that demonstrate resistance to nonspecific fouling.

3.5.3.1 Dynamic Range

The sensor produces quantitative results throughout its operational range, which starts from the lowest detectable concentration up to the analytical saturation point [116]. The measurement range of the biosensor system needs to extend from the lowest to the highest clinically important levels of the specific target biomarkers of PCa. The wide sequence of PCa biomarker concentration levels presents a strong challenge in biosensor detection applications. For instance [117], the concentration evaluation of total PSA extends from less than 0.1 ng/mL levels detected in prostatectomy patients to elevated amounts exceeding 100 ng/mL, which sometimes surpass 1000 ng/mL, in advanced metastatic conditions. The screening range for diagnosis usually spans from 0 to 10 ng/mL, while clinical practice uses 4 ng/mL and risk-adapted threshold values [118]. The relevant ranges of additional markers, such as PCA3 and CTCs, vary from one another. To function effectively in clinical settings, a biosensor needs an appropriate measurement range suitable for its intended use, which includes screening at low levels as well as diagnosis, therapy monitoring, and recurrence detection at very low levels altogether [119]. A wide linear dynamic range, which measures signal strength proportional to concentration, provides optimal calibration results, but non-linear responses can be calibrated through proper models. The achievement of appropriate dynamic range requires sufficient optimization of receptor content or transducer sensitivity and potentially involves sample dilution when dealing with highly concentrated samples [120].

3.6 Applications in Prostate Cancer Diagnostics

The specific use of biosensors in prostate cancer diagnosis, prognosis, and monitoring requires examination after a discussion of their main operating characteristics [121]. The existing diagnostic practices, which depend on PSA screening before performing invasive biopsies, show that more accurate diagnostic methods and less invasive procedures remain necessary. The unmet clinical needs find suitable solutions through biosensors, which present an attractive technological approach [122].

3.6.1 Medical Applications of Biosensors

The implementation of biosensors brings the most significant benefits to medical diagnostic procedures [123]. The detection capabilities of biosensors, which include rapidness, along with high sensitivity and specific biomarker identification, pathogen detection, and metabolite discovery, have transformed medical patient care [124].

Point-of-Care Testing (POCT): POCT enables clinical staff to perform laboratory-grade examinations at patient sites from bedsides to clinics and homes. Electrochemical glucose biosensors operate as a widespread medical example that diabetic patients use frequently for testing their blood sugar [136]. Rapid tests for detecting pregnancy, along with rapid infectious disease tests for Strep A and HIV,

Table 3.3 Application and roles of biosensors in diagnostics and beyond [125]

Application domain	Role of biosensor	Examples	References
Medical diagnostics	Enables rapid, sensitive, and specific detection of biomarkers and pathogens	Glucose monitoring (diabetes), HIV, HCG (pregnancy), Strep A tests, and coagulation monitoring	[126]
Point-of-care testing (POCT)	Brings lab-grade diagnostics to the bedside, clinics, and homes	Portable glucose meters, rapid infectious disease kits	[127]
Early disease detection	Detects low-level biomarkers to identify diseases at initial stages	Cancer markers, viral RNA/DNA, cardiac enzymes	[128]
Personalized medicine	Customizes treatments based on genetic and metabolic biosensor data	Pharmacogenomics, therapeutic monitoring	[129]
Environmental monitoring	Detects pollutants and monitors ecosystem health	Heavy metals, pesticides, air/water quality, endocrine disruptors	[130]
Food safety and quality control	Ensures food safety, detects spoilage, toxins, and verifies nutritional claims	Pathogen detection (*Salmonella*, *Listeria*), aflatoxins, allergens, and freshness sensors	[131]
Bioprocess monitoring	Real-time tracking of fermentation processes in biotech/pharma industries	Biomass, product yield, substrate concentration measurements	[132]
Drug discovery and development	Accelerates screening and interaction studies of pharmaceutical compounds	High-throughput assays, drug interaction testing	[133]
Agriculture	Monitors soil health, detects plant diseases, and optimizes crop management	Nutrient sensors, pathogen biosensors for crops	[134]
Defense and security	Detects chemical and biological threats	Biosensors for warfare agents, explosives, and narcotics	[135]

and rapid coagulation monitoring systems, make up additional well-known examples. The implementation of (Point-of-Care Testing) biosensors leads to enhanced patient care management through expedited clinical determination processes [137]. *Early Disease Detection*: It becomes possible with biosensors because they provide sensitive biomarker detection of extremely low concentrations, which helps medical professionals prevent diseases in their initial stages [138]. *Personalized Medicine:* Pharmacological vigilance and genetic marker evaluation for people can be achieved through smart biosensor systems designed according to patient requirements, as shown in Table 3.3. Biosensors provide value to multiple domains that go beyond healthcare facilities through their widespread usefulness to various scientific disciplines [139]. *Environmental Monitoring:* Biosensors serve environmental monitoring functions for detecting pollutants, which include pesticides, heavy metals, and endocrine disruptors, while assessing water and soil quality and monitoring air conditions as well as ecosystem health. *Food Safety and Quality Control*: The systems identify pathogens, including *Salmonella* and *Listeria*, while also detecting toxins like aflatoxins and allergens, in addition to spoilage indicators, as well as authenticating and determining the nutritional quality of products from end to end in the supply chain. *Bioprocess Monitoring:* Through bioprocess monitoring, pharmaceutical sectors and biotechnology facilities operate their fermentation systems in real time using substrate, product, and biomass detection methods. *Drug Discovery and Development:* During drug discovery, scientists perform fast screening of possible pharmaceutical substances, and they analyze drugs' reactions with each other. *Agriculture:* Soil conditions and plant diseases are monitored, as well as the delivery of optimal crop management through methods in agricultural contexts. *Defense and Security:* Biosensors are used for detecting biological and chemical warfare agents, explosives, and illicit drugs. Biosensors prove to be an effective analytical solution because they provide rapid detection of particular chemical or biological substances while maintaining excellent selectivity and sensitivity [140]. The disciplined progression of biosensors receives support through nanotechnology and materials science advances, as well as microfluidics and synthetic biology research, which will create more advanced sensing tools set to monitor physiological status automatically and survey environmental conditions across extended areas that strengthen their essential role in the workplace throughout our current era [141].

3.6.2 Suitability for Cancer Biomarker Detection

Biosensors show specific advantages for identifying cancer biomarkers from samples because of their detection capabilities [142]. Through superior biochemical detection, the following characteristics of biosensors fulfill the necessary criteria for better detection of prostate cancer. *High Sensitivity and Low Detection Limits:* Cancer biomarkers showing small concentrations of ng/mL to pg/mL or lower conditions, such as CTCs or specific nucleic acids, require biosensors because of their exceptional sensitivity and reduced detection thresholds [118]. Biosensors using advanced nanomaterials alongside enzymatic or nanoparticle-based amplification with electrochemical as well as plasmonic or photonic transducers meet the requirements for early PCa detection, together with post-treatment minimal residual disease monitoring because of their low detection limits [143]. *Specificity via Biorecognition:* Biosensor operation requires a specific biological recognition element for achieving its purpose. The development of biosensors depends on highly specific molecules, including PSA monoclonal antibodies for precise epitope targets as well as aptamers choosing PSMA for PCa antigens and probes targeting genetic sequences of PCA3 and TMPRSS2, ERG to select biomarkers indicating malignancy beyond total PSA [144]. Biosensors implementing biomarkers must exhibit greater analytical and clinical specificity for proper distinction between PCa and benign conditions such as BPH. *Rapid Analysis (Response Time):* Biosensor transduction methods give users instantaneous analysis capabilities by eliminating the time-consuming procedures normally found in traditional laboratory assays, including ELISA. Results from electrochemical and optical instruments and piezoelectric sensors become available within minutes [145]. The high rate of operation of biosensors enables point-of-care testing solutions, resulting in immediate clinical solutions and reducing the stress of waiting for patients. *Miniaturization and Portability:* With the help of microfabrication and microfluidic approaches, biosensor manufacturers are able to miniaturize the platform. The new manufacturing concepts create devices that are still portable or handheld and even benchtop machines to conduct testing outside the laboratory at clinics and doctor offices and eventually may be used directly by the patient in his or her home [146]. The downsizing of biosensors permits applications of smaller blood drops that are taken from fingers and smaller amounts of urine, along with decreased usage of reagents that enhance both the patient experience and potential cost savings of tests. *Multiplexing Capabilities:* The nonhomogeneous nature of prostate cancer requires the application of multiple biomarkers because of inadequate use alone to generate a precise medical determination [147]. Biosensor and microfluidic array-based biosensor applications can detect many biomarkers, such as total PSA, free PSA, and p2PSA for PHI determination, as well as PCA3, AMACR, TMPRSS2:ERG, and selected miRNAs and proteins of extracellular vesicles using small sample volumes. The evaluation has an augmented diagnostic and prognostic outcome by integrating numerous markers in a single test compared to standing-alone tests based on a single marker [148]. *Potential for Direct Detection in Complex Matrices:* Ongoing scientific research examines approaches to construct biosensor interfaces and methods of sample handling to analyze undisturbed or slightly processed complex biological samples (such as whole blood and urine). The workflow is made easier as an unnecessarily large setup of the laboratories is minimized to a bare minimum [149].

3.6.3 Linking Fundamentals to Application

The clinical value arising from the use of biosensors in the diagnostics of PCa is based on their simplistic operational capabilities, as stated in Sect. 3.5 of the paper, which satisfy the precise demands of the medical field [150]. *Sensitivity/LOD Early Recurrence Detection:* Biosensors are very sensitive with low pg/mL detection limits of PSA, which allows the appropriate recurrence monitoring following the prostatectomy and radiotherapy operation [151]. Timely identification of minimal changes in PSA (biochemical recurrence) using biosensors will allow providers to implement timely salvage therapy that may improve treatment outcomes. *Specificity/Selectivity Reducing Unnecessary Biopsies:* Experienced biosensors combine cancer-specific markers such as PCA3 and PHI components with current biomarkers and marker panels that generate high-level analytical selectivity to result in fewer unnecessary prostate biopsies [152]. Reduced incidences of false-positive test results would result in lowering the frequency of unnecessarily uncomfortable biopsies to the patient and would resolve one of the critical weaknesses of the current diagnosis techniques. *Response Time enabling Point-of-Care Risk Stratification:* A point-of-care test-based biosensor that provides risk assessment results in multiple biomarkers (enhanced PHI or novel panel) under 30 minutes would revolutionize patient assessment processes at the medical center [153]. The tool will allow medical practitioners to perform specialized risk management on their patients during the patient consultation time, in order to influence joint decisions regarding the use of the biopsy procedure and other similar investigations. *Stability and Reusability/Cost Impacting Accessibility:* A sensor's shelf life as well as its stability when in use will influence clinical accessibility by influencing its price and its capacity to be reused [154]. Technology access to healthcare systems is driven by the economic choice a healthcare system has between discarding cheap sensors to perform point-of-care testing and potentially low-priced reusable sensors to perform high-throughput environments. The availability of affordable biosensor systems that are stable offers opportunities to enrich the availability of advanced PCa diagnostic solutions at the widespread level [155]. *Dynamic Range to Comprehensive Disease Monitoring:* A biosensor provides comprehensive disease monitoring by having an extended dynamic range that can measure biomarkers at the proper level whether during screening or post-treatment level to advanced or metastatic disease levels with high concentration of biomarkers. This versatility gives a single platform a potential service ability in various stages of patient care [156]. *Multiplexing to Accurate Risk Stratification and Prognosis:* The most important strength of biosensor technology is the ability to combine PSA biomarker signals with PCA3/TMPRSS2: ERG genetic markers and protein/miRNA signals identified in exosomes on a single platform of detector [157]. The overall molecular testing method demonstrates its possible value in improving diagnostic accuracy and clinical risk assessment that would allow physicians to diagnose aggressive tumors that require immediate medical care compared to the less dangerous types of tumors that can be treated with active surveillance and, therefore, solve the problem of over-treating PCa [158].

3.7 Conclusion: Foundational Principles for Advanced Diagnostics

At the interface of biology, chemistry, and engineering, biosensors offer new methodologies for identifying and measuring biological markers. In analyzing its basic elements—the biorecognition component and the transducer—this chapter has developed a ground-level understanding of the biosensor technology and how the two parts work in combination to convert a given biological interaction into a measurable, typically electrical or optical signal. A look at the mechanism through which biosensors operate in detecting, transducing, and interpreting signals gives us an idea as to their accuracy and flexibility. The two-fold scheme of classification, which relies on either the type of bioreceptor or the methods of transduction, underscores the flexibility of the biosensor system that can be tailored to a great variety of analytical processes. The discussion about the key performance indicators, sensitivity, specificity, limit of detection (LOD), reaction time, and stability, particularly provides the requisite criteria to compare and contrast the performance of biosensors. These measures are of special concern, especially in a clinical setting where quick and accurate detection may have a direct effect on the patient. The significance of biosensors is even more evident when it comes to the diagnosis of prostate cancer. They are frequently absent in traditional diagnostics, particularly in their capacity to identify low-abundance biomarkers with high specificity, presenting a promising pathway for early diagnosis and monitoring. The flexibility of biosensor systems makes them a great fit to be incorporated into point-of-care devices, which will result in faster decision-making and more personalized healthcare solutions. After all, the concepts presented in this chapter offer the theoretical basis of understanding and developing next-generation biosensors. This primer shall be essential to the conception of the ways in which the biosensor technologies are transforming the future of diagnostics, especially the war on complex diseases such as prostate cancer, as we move to more advanced designs and uses in the chapters ahead.

3.8 Summary

Biosensors are an important technology at the interface of biology, chemistry, and engineering, which offer rapid, sensitive, and specific detection of diverse analytes. This chapter introduced the basics of biosensors, as well as described details of the key components of biosensors, such as biorecognition components, transducers, and signal processors, and their interactions to convert biological interactions into measurable signals. The various signal transduction mechanisms, including electrochemical, optical, piezoelectric, thermal, and magnetic, were also discussed along with the categorization of biosensors based on recognition elements. Performance attributes such as sensitivity, specificity, limit of detection, stability, reusability, and dynamic range were explored in regard to practical and clinical needs. This chapter also highlighted the use of biosensors in the diagnosis of prostate cancer, demonstrating their significance in actual biomedical contexts. Biosensors are set to become more and more important in environmental monitoring, personalized medicine, diagnostics, and more as materials science, nanotechnology, and data analytics continue to advance.

Glossary

Analyte A substance or chemical constituent that is being detected or measured.

Bioreceptor A biological molecule (e.g., enzyme, antibody, and nucleic acid) that specifically binds to the target analyte.

Limit of detection (LOD) The smallest concentration of an analyte that can be reliably detected.

Point-of-care testing Diagnostic testing performed near or at the site of patient care.

Quartz crystal microbalance (QCM) A piezoelectric sensor that detects mass changes on a surface.

Sensitivity The ability of a biosensor to detect small amounts of an analyte.

Signal processing unit Electronics/software that interprets and displays the output signal.

Specificity The ability to detect a specific analyte in the presence of others.

Surface plasmon resonance (SPR) A label-free optical detection method based on changes in refractive index.

Transducer A component that converts the biorecognition event into a measurable signal.

References

1. Kaya SI, Unal DN, Cetinkaya A, Uslu B, Ozkan SA. Overview of biosensors: definition, principles, and instrumentation. In: Biosensors. CRC Press; 2022. p. 3–23.
2. Baronas R, Ivanauskas F, Kulys J. Mathematical modeling of biosensors. Springer; 2021.
3. Carpenter AC, Paulsen IT, Williams TC. Blueprints for biosensors: design, limitations, and applications. Genes (Basel). 2018;9(8):375.
4. Morales MA, Halpern JM. Guide to selecting a biorecognition element for biosensors. Bioconjug Chem. 2018;29(10):3231–9.
5. Bollella P, Katz E. Biosensors—recent advances and future challenges. Sensors. 2020;20(22):6645.
6. Zhang X, Zhu Y, Wells M. A case study comparing lead-response in different bioreporters: what constitutes a good biosensor? Case Stud Chem Environ Eng. 2022;5:100192.
7. Mitra S, Cumming DRS. CMOS circuits for biological sensing and processing. Springer; 2018.
8. Kumar D, Prasad M, Mohan H. Biological recognition elements. In: Electrochemical sensors. Elsevier; 2022. p. 213–39.
9. Kozitsina AN, Svalova TS, Malysheva NN, Okhokhonin AV, Vidrevich MB, Brainina KZ. Sensors based on bio and biomimetic receptors in medical diagnostic, environment, and food analysis. Biosensors. 2018;8(2):35.
10. Saadati A, Hassanpour S, de la Guardia M, Mosafer J, Hashemzaei M, Mokhtarzadeh A, et al. Recent advances on application of peptide nucleic acids as a bioreceptor in biosensors development. TrAC Trends Anal Chem. 2019;114:56–68.
11. Mehrotra P. Biosensors and their applications–A review. Journal of oral biology and craniofacial research. 2016 May 1;6(2):153-9.
12. Zhang K, Gao G, Zhao C, Wang Y, Wang Y, Li J. Review of the design of power ultrasonic generator for piezoelectric transducer. Ultrason Sonochem. 2023;96:106438.
13. Zhang M, Zou CL, Jiang L. Quantum transduction with adaptive control. Phys Rev Lett. 2018;120(2):20502.
14. Polat EO, Cetin MM, Tabak AF, Bilget Güven E, Uysal BÖ, Arsan T, et al. Transducer technologies for biosensors and their wearable applications. Biosensors. 2022;12(6):385.
15. Wu A, He S, Ren Y, Wang N, Ho SCM, Song G. Design of a new stress wave-based pulse position modulation (PPM) communication system with piezoceramic transducers. Sensors. 2019;19(3):558.
16. Abdelbasset WK, Jasim SA, Bokov DO, Oleneva MS, Islamov A, Hammid AT, et al. RETRACTED ARTICLE: comparison and evaluation of the performance of graphene-based biosensors. Carbon Lett. 2022;32(4):927–51.
17. Tripathi MK, Nickhil C, Kate A, Srivastva RM, Mohapatra D, Jadam RS, et al. Biosensor: fundamentals, biomolecular component, and applications. In: Advances in biomedical polymers and composites. Elsevier; 2023. p. 617–33.

18. McLamore ES, Datta SPA. A connected world: system-level support through biosensors. Annu Rev Anal Chem. 2023;16(1):285–309.
19. Kumar A, Mahato K. Recent advancements in bioreceptors and materials for biosensors. In: Biosensors in precision medicine. Elsevier; 2024. p. 163–202.
20. Barreiros dos Santos M, Rodriguez-Lorenzo L, Queirós R, Espiña B. Fundamentals of biosensors and detection methods. In: Microfluidics and biosensors in cancer research: applications in cancer modeling and theranostics. Springer; 2022. p. 3–29.
21. Parmin NA, Hashim U, Gopinath SCB, Uda MNA. Biosensor recognizes the receptor molecules. In: Nanobiosensors for biomolecular targeting. Elsevier; 2019. p. 195–210.
22. Davis F, Altintas Z. General introduction to biosensors and recognition receptors. In: Biosensors and nanotechnology: applications in health care diagnostics. Wiley; 2018. p. 1–15.
23. Naresh V, Lee N. A review on biosensors and recent development of nanostructured materials-enabled biosensors. Sensors. 2021;21(4):1109.
24. Rodriguez OL, Safonova Y, Silver CA, Shields K, Gibson WS, Kos JT, et al. Genetic variation in the immunoglobulin heavy chain locus shapes the human antibody repertoire. Nat Commun. 2023;14(1):4419.
25. Subba D, Mete S, Haldar D, Saha S, Dolui BK. The solubility of four DNA-RNA bases in the aqueous calcium nitrate at nine temperatures and the insights into the solution thermodynamics. J Mol Liq. 2025;419:126729.
26. Bao L, Zhang X, Jin L, Tan ZJ. Flexibility of nucleic acids: from DNA to RNA. Chin Phys B. 2015;25(1):18703.
27. Huang CP, Hu WP, Yang W, Lee ZJ, Chen WY. In silico maturation of DNA aptamer against the prostate-specific antigen (PSA) and kinetic analysis. Biochem Biophys Res Commun [Internet]. 2025;759:151638. Available from: https://www.sciencedirect.com/science/article/pii/S0006291X25003523.
28. Shoaib M, Li H, Zareef M, Khan IM, Iqbal MW, Niazi S, et al. Recent Advances in food safety detection: split aptamer-based biosensors development and potential applications. J Agric Food Chem. 2025;73:4397.
29. Urbelienė N, Gasparavičiūtė R, Vaitekūnas J, Meškienė R, Valantinaitė U, Kruopis P, et al. A screening method for polyester films-degrading microorganisms and enzymes. J Hazard Mater. 2025;487:137177.
30. Niaki NM, Hatefnia F, Heidari MM, Tabean M, Mobed A. Alpha-Fetoprotein (AFP) biosensors. Clin Chim Acta. 2025;573:120293.
31. Mardanshahi A, Sreekumar A, Yang X, Barman SK, Chronopoulos D. Sensing techniques for structural health monitoring: a state-of-the-art review on performance criteria and new-generation technologies. Sensors. 2025;25(5):1424.
32. Srivastava BBL. Biosensor-signal transducers. In: Fundamentals of biosensors in healthcare. Elsevier; 2025. p. 71–85.
33. Pokale R, Rachana SP, Mukharya A, Colaco V, Naik GARR, Roy AA, et al. Core-shell nanoconstructs in cancer biosensing: techniques, applications, and fabrication strategies. In: Core-shell nano constructs for cancer theragnostic: current scenario, challenges and regulatory aspects. Springer; 2025. p. 137–77.
34. Rathee S, Saraf S, Raikwar S, Bidla PD, Jain SK. Biosensors for targeted therapeutics. In: Applications of biosensors in healthcare. Elsevier; 2025. p. 51–71.
35. Alaridhee ZAI, Alqaraguly MB, Formanova S, Kuryazov R, Mahdi MS, Taher WM, et al. Recent advances in microfluidic-based photoelectrochemical (PEC) sensing platforms for biomedical applications. Microchim Acta. 2025;192(5):297.
36. Yang H, Yan J, Tan J, Ren M, Li X, Wang S. High-precision readout circuits for portable biosensor devices—a review of IA. IEEE Sensors J. 2025;25:9233.
37. Li XQ, Yang HB, Ma XM, Zou CJ, Liu T, Zhou XC, et al. Readout electronics for the gamma detector of the HIRFL-CSR external target facility. Nucl Sci Tech. 2025;36(2):33.
38. Grinspoon SK, Zanni MV, Triant VA, Kantor A, Umbleja T, Diggs MR, et al. Performance of the pooled cohort equations and D: A: D risk scores among individuals with HIV

in a global cardiovascular disease prevention trial: a cohort study leveraging data from REPRIEVE. Lancet HIV. 2025;12(2):e118–29.

39. Garcia F, Amato A, Pfeiffer D, van Stenis M, Muller H, Oliveri E, et al. arXiv: The ultra-low material budget GEM based TPC for tracking with VMM3a readout. J Instrum. 2025;20(04):C04004.
40. Xu L, Lin Z, Tao H, Ye J, Fan M, Shen Y, et al. A dual-signal biosensor based on surface-enhanced Raman spectroscopy for high-sensitivity quantitative detection and imaging of circRNA in living cells. Biosens Bioelectron. 2025;268:116875.
41. Xiao H, Li M, Ohad N, Hao GF. Genetically encoded biosensors for spatiotemporal monitoring of plant proteins in growth and stress responses. Adv Agrochem. 2025;4:177.
42. Chen B, Yan Q, Li D, Xie J. Degradation mechanism and development of detection technologies of ATP-related compounds in aquatic products: recent advances and remaining challenges. Crit Rev Food Sci Nutr. 2025;65(1):101–22.
43. Yasri S, Wiwanitkit V. Biosensors in medical devices. In: Applications of biosensors in healthcare. Elsevier; 2025. p. 1–15.
44. Maher V, Martin D, Spetzler D, Zhao ZG, O'Neill H, Woodbury N. From randomness to recognition: modeling the evolution of DNA sequence information during SELEX. bioRxiv. 2025:2003–25.
45. Yang T, Yang B, Tian Z, Zhu G, Peng Y. Ratiometric, 3D Fluorescence Spectrum with abundant information for tetracyclines discrimination via dual biomolecules recognition and deep learning. Anal Chem [Internet]. 2025;97(12):6745–52. Available from: https://doi.org/10.1021/acs.analchem.4c07061.
46. Mirza S, Ateeq M, Fazil P, Zada A, Ahmad MS. Carbon-based nanoporous homochiral MOF as a highly efficient platform for chiral recognition and enantioselective electrooxidation. Cryst Growth Des [Internet]. 2025;25(4):903–11. Available from: https://doi.org/10.1021/acs.cgd.4c00674.
47. Yin Z, Liu X, Li S, Yuan R, Xiang Y. Highly sensitive β-amyloid1–42 oligomer aptamer-based assay via dual cyclic amplifications of three-way catalytic hairpin assembly and palindrome polymerase reaction. Sensors Actuators B Chem [Internet]. 2025;423:136750. Available from: https://www.sciencedirect.com/science/article/pii/S0925400524014801.
48. Yue MS, Luo N, Wang XD, Ao YF, Wang DX, Wang QQ. Cooperative anion–π catalysis with chiral molecular cages toward enantioselective desymmetrization of anhydrides. J Am Chem Soc [Internet]. 2025;147(3):2303–8. Available from: https://doi.org/10.1021/jacs.4c15978.
49. Sathish T, Ramasamy M, Kumar PS. Engineering a signal transduction mechanism for protein-based biosensors. In: Singh SK, Chandra P, editors. Protein biomarkers: discovery and applications in clinical diagnostics [Internet]. Singapore: Springer Nature Singapore; 2024. p. 351–68. Available from: https://doi.org/10.1007/978-981-97-5045-0_16.
50. Lin D, Shen Y, Liang T. Oncolytic virotherapy: basic principles, recent advances and future directions. Signal Transduct Target Ther [Internet]. 2023;8(1):156. Available from: https://doi.org/10.1038/s41392-023-01407-6.
51. Tetyana P, Shumbula PM, Njengele-Tetyana Z. Biosensors: design, development and applications. In: Ameen S, Akhtar MS, Shin HS, editors. Nanopores [Internet]. Rijeka: IntechOpen; 2021. Available from: https://doi.org/10.5772/intechopen.97576.
52. Wang J. Electrochemical Glucose Biosensors. Chem Rev [Internet]. 2008;108(2):814–25. Available from: https://doi.org/10.1021/cr068123a.
53. Bakker E, Pretsch E, Bühlmann P. Selectivity of potentiometric ion sensors. Anal Chem [Internet]. 2000;72(6):1127–33. Available from: https://doi.org/10.1021/ac991146n.
54. Magar HS, Hassan RYA, Mulchandani A. Electrochemical impedance spectroscopy (EIS): principles, construction, and biosensing applications. Sensors [Internet]. 2021;21(19). Available from: https://www.mdpi.com/1424-8220/21/19/6578.
55. Lakowicz JR. Instrumentation for fluorescence spectroscopy BT - principles of fluorescence spectroscopy. Boston, MA: Springer US; 2006. p. 27–61. Available from: https://doi.org/10.1007/978-0-387-46312-4_2.

56. Homola J. Surface plasmon resonance sensors for detection of chemical and biological species. Chem Rev [Internet]. 2008;108(2):462–93. Available from: https://doi.org/10.1021/cr068107d.
57. Marx KA. Quartz crystal microbalance: a useful tool for studying thin polymer films and complex biomolecular systems at the solution−surface interface. Biomacromolecules [Internet]. 2003;4(5):1099–120. Available from: https://doi.org/10.1021/bm020116i.
58. Yakovleva M, Bhand S, Danielsson B. The enzyme thermistor—a realistic biosensor concept. A critical review. Anal Chim Acta [Internet]. 2013;766:1–12. Available from: https://www.sciencedirect.com/science/article/pii/S0003267012017680.
59. Sakata T. Signal transduction interfaces for field-effect transistor-based biosensors. Commun Chem [Internet]. 2024;7(1):35. Available from: https://doi.org/10.1038/s42004-024-01121-6.
60. Fatima T, Bansal S, Husain S, Khanuja M. 1 – Biosensors. In: Maruccio G, Narang J, editors. Electrochemical sensors [Internet], Woodhead Publishing Series in Electronic and Optical Materials. Woodhead Publishing; 2022. p. 1–30. Available from: https://www.sciencedirect.com/science/article/pii/B9780128231487000015.
61. Yamani HZ, Safwat N, Mahmoud AM, Ayad MF, Abdel-Ghany MF, Gomaa MM. Point-of-care diagnostics for rapid determination of prostate cancer biomarker sarcosine: application of disposable potentiometric sensor based on oxide-conductive polymer nanocomposite. Anal Bioanal Chem [Internet]. 2023;415(22):5451–62. Available from: https://doi.org/10.1007/s00216-023-04818-0.
62. Simpkins LLC, Henriquez LA, Tran M, Adams TNG. Electrical impedance spectroscopy as a tool to detect the epithelial to mesenchymal transition in prostate cancer cells. Biosensors [Internet]. 2024;14(10). Available from: https://www.mdpi.com/2079-6374/14/10/503.
63. Kim J, Chun SH, Amornkitbamrung L, Song C, Yuk JS, Ahn SY, et al. Gold nanoparticle clusters for the investigation of therapeutic efficiency against prostate cancer under near-infrared irradiation. Nano Converg [Internet]. 2020;7(1):5. Available from: https://doi.org/10.1186/s40580-019-0216-z.
64. Kawatani M, Yamamoto K, Yamada D, Kamiya M, Miyakawa J, Miyama Y, et al. Fluorescence detection of prostate cancer by an activatable fluorescence probe for PSMA carboxypeptidase activity. J Am Chem Soc [Internet]. 2019;141(26):10409–16. Available from: https://doi.org/10.1021/jacs.9b04412.
65. Das S, Devireddy R, Gartia MR. Surface Plasmon Resonance (SPR) sensor for cancer biomarker detection. Biosensors [Internet]. 2023;13(3). Available from: https://www.mdpi.com/2079-6374/13/3/396.
66. Han Y, Liu C, Zhang D, Men H, Huo L, Geng Q, et al. Mechanosensitive ion channel Piezo1 promotes prostate cancer development through the activation of the Akt/mTOR pathway and acceleration of cell cycle. Int J Oncol [Internet]. 2019;55(3):629–44. Available from: https://doi.org/10.3892/ijo.2019.4839.
67. Sonklin T, Dhananjaya M, Sanong S, Pattanaphong J, Pojprapai S. Effect of surface modified quartz crystal microbalance (QCM) on detection sensitivity for prostate specific antigen (PSA). Integr Ferroelectr [Internet]. 2022;222(1):93–101. Available from: https://doi.org/10.1080/10584587.2021.1961519.
68. Sun F, Wu K, Yao Z, Mu X, Zheng Z, Sun M, et al. Long noncoding RNA LINC00963 induces NOP2 expression by sponging tumor suppressor miR-542-3p to promote metastasis in prostate cancer. Aging (Albany NY). 2020;12(12):11500–16.
69. Ayyad SM, Badawy MA, Shehata M, Alksas A, Mahmoud A, Abou El-Ghar M, et al. A new framework for precise identification of prostatic adenocarcinoma. Sensors [Internet]. 2022;22(5). Available from: https://www.mdpi.com/1424-8220/22/5/1848.
70. Rodrigues VC, Soares JC, Soares AC, Braz DC, Melendez ME, Ribas LC, et al. Electrochemical and optical detection and machine learning applied to images of genosensors for diagnosis of prostate cancer with the biomarker PCA3. Talanta [Internet]. 2021;222:121444. Available from: https://www.sciencedirect.com/science/article/pii/S0039914020307359.

71. Sun B, Qiao F, Chen L, Zhao Z, Yin H, Ai S. Effective signal-on photoelectrochemical immunoassay of subgroup J avian leukosis virus based on Bi2S3 nanorods as photosensitizer and in situ generated ascorbic acid for electron donating. Biosens Bioelectron [Internet]. 2014;54:237–43. Available from: https://www.sciencedirect.com/science/article/pii/S0956566313007999.
72. Sassolas A, Leca-Bouvier BD, Blum LJ. DNA biosensors and microarrays. Chem Rev [Internet]. 2008;108(1):109–39. Available from: https://doi.org/10.1021/cr0684467.
73. Su L, Jia W, Hou C, Lei Y. Microbial biosensors: a review. Biosens Bioelectron [Internet]. 2011;26(5):1788–99. Available from: https://www.sciencedirect.com/science/article/pii/S095656631000607X.
74. Campos-Fernández E, Oliveira Alqualo N, Moura Garcia LC, Coutinho Horácio Alves C, Ferreira Arantes Vieira TD, Caixeta Moreira D, et al. The use of aptamers in prostate cancer: a systematic review of theranostic applications. Clin Biochem [Internet]. 2021;93:9–25. Available from: https://www.sciencedirect.com/science/article/pii/S0009912021000837.
75. Zhang J, Cass AEG. Kinetic study of site directed and randomly immobilized his-tag alkaline phosphatase by flow injection chemiluminescence. J Mol Recognit [Internet]. 2006;19(3):243–6. Available from: https://onlinelibrary.wiley.com/doi/abs/10.1002/jmr.764.
76. Turner APF. Biosensors: sense and sensibility. Chem Soc Rev. 2013;42(8):3184–96.
77. Sahini MG, Malima NM. Chapter 14 – Multiferroic magnetoelectric-based biosensors in healthcare. In: Hasnain MS, Nayak AK, Aminabhavi TM, editors. Fundamentals of biosensors in healthcare [Internet]. Academic Press; 2025. p. 337–57. Available from: https://www.sciencedirect.com/science/article/pii/B9780443216589000255.
78. Li M, Jiang F, Xue L, Peng C, Shi Z, Zhang Z, et al. Recent progress in biosensors for detection of tumor biomarkers. Molecules [Internet]. 2022;27(21). Available from: https://www.mdpi.com/1420-3049/27/21/7327.
79. Zhu C, Li L, Wang Z, Irfan M, Qu F. Recent advances of aptasensors for exosomes detection. Biosens Bioelectron [Internet]. 2020;160:112213. Available from: https://www.sciencedirect.com/science/article/pii/S0956566320302104.
80. Chan KM, Gleadle JM, O'Callaghan M, Vasilev K, MacGregor M. Prostate cancer detection: a systematic review of urinary biosensors. Prostate Cancer Prostatic Dis [Internet]. 2022;25(1):39–46. Available from: https://doi.org/10.1038/s41391-021-00480-8.
81. Kumar P, Narwal V, Jaiwal R, Pundir CS. Construction and application of amperometric sarcosine biosensor based on SOxNPs/AuE for determination of prostate cancer. Biosens Bioelectron [Internet]. 2018;122:140–6. Available from: https://www.sciencedirect.com/science/article/pii/S0956566318306900.
82. Sánchez-Salcedo R, Miranda-Castro R, de-los-Santos-Álvarez N, Lobo-Castañón MJ. Dual electrochemical genosensor for early diagnosis of prostate cancer through lncRNAs detection. Biosens Bioelectron [Internet]. 2021;192:113520. Available from: https://www.sciencedirect.com/science/article/pii/S0956566321005571.
83. Sun S, Chen J. Recent advances in hydrogel-based biosensors for cancer detection. ACS Appl Mater Interfaces [Internet]. 2024;16(36):46988–7002. Available from: https://doi.org/10.1021/acsami.4c02317.
84. Fernández-Puig S, Lazo-Fraga AR, Korgel BA, Oza G, Dutt A, Vallejo-Becerra V, et al. Molecularly imprinted polymer-silica nanocomposite based potentiometric sensor for early prostate cancer detection. Mater Lett [Internet]. 2022;309:131324. Available from: https://www.sciencedirect.com/science/article/pii/S0167577X2102022X.
85. Saranyutanon S, Deshmukh SK, Dasgupta S, Pai S, Singh S, Singh AP. Cellular and molecular progression of prostate cancer: models for basic and preclinical research. Cancers (Basel) [Internet]. 2020;12(9). Available from: https://www.mdpi.com/2072-6694/12/9/2651.
86. Singh S, Gill AAS, Nlooto M, Karpoormath R. Prostate cancer biomarkers detection using nanoparticles based electrochemical biosensors. Biosens Bioelectron [Internet]. 2019;137:213–21. Available from: https://www.sciencedirect.com/science/article/pii/S0956566319302441.

87. Azab MY, Hameed MFO, Obayya SSA. Overview of optical biosensors for early cancer detection: fundamentals, applications and future perspectives. Biology (Basel) [Internet]. 2023;12(2). Available from: https://www.mdpi.com/2079-7737/12/2/232.
88. Sarkar S, Gogoi M, Mahato M, Joshi AB, Baruah AJ, Kodgire P, et al. Biosensors for detection of prostate cancer: a review. Biomed Microdevices [Internet]. 2022;24(4):32. Available from: https://doi.org/10.1007/s10544-022-00631-1.
89. Guliy OI, Staroverov SA, Karavaeva OA, Dykman LA. Heat shock proteins as biosensor instruments for cancer detection. In: Singh SK, Chandra P, editors. Protein biomarkers: discovery and applications in clinical diagnostics [Internet]. Singapore: Springer Nature Singapore; 2024. p. 209–44. Available from: https://doi.org/10.1007/978-981-97-5045-0_11.
90. Soares JC, Soares AC, Rodrigues VC, Melendez ME, Santos AC, Faria EF, et al. Detection of the prostate cancer biomarker PCA3 with electrochemical and impedance-based biosensors. ACS Appl Mater Interfaces [Internet]. 2019;11(50):46645–50. Available from: https://doi.org/10.1021/acsami.9b19180.
91. Takita S, Nabok A, Mussa M, Kitchen M, Lishchuk A, Smith D. Ultrasensitive prostate cancer marker PCA3 detection with impedimetric biosensor based on specific label-free aptamers. Biosens Bioelectron X [Internet]. 2024;18:100462. Available from: https://www.sciencedirect.com/science/article/pii/S2590137024000268.
92. Wang W, Liu J, Wu LA, Ko CN, Wang X, Lin C, et al. Nicking enzyme-free strand displacement amplification-assisted CRISPR-Cas-based colorimetric detection of prostate-specific antigen in serum samples. Anal Chim Acta [Internet]. 2022;1195:339479. Available from: https://www.sciencedirect.com/science/article/pii/S0003267022000502.
93. Yan L, Zhang C, Xi F. Disposable amperometric label-free immunosensor on chitosan–graphene-modified patterned ITO electrodes for prostate specific antigen. Molecules [Internet]. 2022;27(18). Available from: https://www.mdpi.com/1420-3049/27/18/5895.
94. Zhou L, Liu Y, Wang F, Jia Z, Zhou J, Jiang T, et al. Classification analyses for prostate cancer, benign prostate hyperplasia and healthy subjects by SERS-based immunoassay of multiple tumour markers. Talanta [Internet]. 2018;188:238–44. Available from: https://www.sciencedirect.com/science/article/pii/S0039914018305617.
95. Yazdani Z, Yadegari H, Heli H. A molecularly imprinted electrochemical nanobiosensor for prostate specific antigen determination. Anal Biochem [Internet]. 2019;566:116–25. Available from: https://www.sciencedirect.com/science/article/pii/S0003269718308856.
96. Phyo J Bin, Woo A, Yu HJ, Lim K, Cho BH, Jung HS, et al. Label-free SERS analysis of urine using a 3D-stacked AgNW-glass fiber filter sensor for the diagnosis of pancreatic cancer and prostate cancer. Anal Chem [Internet]. 2021;93(8):3778–85. Available from: https://doi.org/10.1021/acs.analchem.0c04200.
97. Han L, Wang D, Yan L, Petrenko VA, Liu A. Specific phages-based electrochemical impedimetric immunosensors for label-free and ultrasensitive detection of dual prostate-specific antigens. Sensors Actuators B Chem [Internet]. 2019;297:126727. Available from: https://www.sciencedirect.com/science/article/pii/S0925400519309281.
98. Felici E, González-Martínez C, Griñán TV, Gato-Zambrano S, Pereira SV, Fernández-Baldo MA, et al. Electrochemical immunoplatform for the quantification of epithelial extracellular vesicles applied to prostate cancer diagnosis. Talanta [Internet]. 2025;293:128130. Available from: https://www.sciencedirect.com/science/article/pii/S0039914025006204.
99. Hu Q, Gan S, Bao Y, Zhang Y, Han D, Niu L. Electrochemically controlled ATRP for cleavage-based electrochemical detection of the prostate-specific antigen at femtomolar level concentrations. Anal Chem [Internet]. 2020;92(24):15982–8. Available from: https://doi.org/10.1021/acs.analchem.0c03467.
100. Jamshidi A, Liu MC, Klein EA, Venn O, Hubbell E, Beausang JF, et al. Evaluation of cell-free DNA approaches for multi-cancer early detection. Cancer Cell [Internet]. 2022;40(12):1537–1549.e12. Available from: https://doi.org/10.1016/j.ccell.2022.10.022.
101. Liu S, Huo Y, Bai J, Ning B, Peng Y, Li S, et al. Rapid and sensitive detection of prostate-specific antigen via label-free frequency shift Raman of sensing graphene. Biosens Bioelectron

[Internet]. 2020;158:112184. Available from: https://www.sciencedirect.com/science/article/pii/S0956566320301810.
102. Deek MP, Van der Eecken K, Phillips R, Parikh NR, Isaacsson Velho P, Lotan TL, et al. The mutational landscape of metastatic castration-sensitive prostate cancer: the spectrum theory revisited. Eur Urol [Internet]. 2021;80(5):632–40. Available from: https://www.sciencedirect.com/science/article/pii/S0302283820310265.
103. Harmon SA, Tuncer S, Sanford T, Choyke PL, Türkbey B. Artificial intelligence at the intersection of pathology and radiology in prostate cancer. Diagn Interv Radiol. 2019;25(3):183–8.
104. Hu Q, Chen G, Han J, Wang L, Cui X, Wang P, et al. Determination of sarcosine based on magnetic cross-linked enzyme aggregates for diagnosis of prostate cancer. Biochem Eng J [Internet]. 2021;172:108039. Available from: https://www.sciencedirect.com/science/article/pii/S1369703X21001157.
105. Khumngern S, Thavarungkul P, Kanatharana P, Bejrananda T, Numnuam A. Molecularly imprinted electrochemical sensor based on poly(o-phenylenediamine-co-o-aminophenol) incorporated with poly(styrenesulfonate) doped poly(3,4-ethylenedioxythiophene) ferrocene composite modified screen-printed carbon electrode for highly sensitive and selective detection of prostate cancer biomarker. Microchem J [Internet]. 2022;177:107311. Available from: https://www.sciencedirect.com/science/article/pii/S0026265X22001394.
106. Mishra S, Kim ES, Sharma PK, Wang ZJ, Yang SH, Kaushik AK, et al. Tailored biofunctionalized biosensor for the label-free sensing of prostate-specific antigen. ACS Appl Bio Mater [Internet]. 2020;3(11):7821–30. Available from: https://doi.org/10.1021/acsabm.0c01002.
107. Kim H, Park S, Jeong IG, Song SH, Jeong Y, Kim CS, et al. Noninvasive precision screening of prostate cancer by urinary multimarker sensor and artificial intelligence analysis. ACS Nano. 2020;15(3):4054–65.
108. Shrestha S, Alsadoon A, Prasad PWC, Seher I, Alsadoon OH. A novel solution of using deep learning for prostate cancer segmentation: enhanced batch normalization. Multimed Tools Appl [Internet]. 2021;80(14):21293–313. Available from: https://doi.org/10.1007/s11042-021-10779-2.
109. Han L, Zhang X, Li D, Li M, Qin P, Tian S, et al. Fabrication of stable multivariate metal-organic frameworks with excellent adsorption performance toward bisphenols from environmental samples. Talanta [Internet]. 2021;235:122818. Available from: https://www.sciencedirect.com/science/article/pii/S0039914021007396.
110. Venkatesan M, Veeramuthu L, Liang FC, Chen WC, Cho CJ, Chen CW, et al. Evolution of electrospun nanofibers fluorescent and colorimetric sensors for environmental toxicants, pH, temperature, and cancer cells – a review with insights on applications Chem Eng J [Internet] 2020;397:125431. Available from: https://www.sciencedirect.com/science/article/pii/S1385894720314236.
111. Venkatesh K, Muthukutty B, Chen SM, Karuppiah C, Amanulla B, Yang CC, et al. Nanomolar level detection of non-steroidal antiandrogen drug flutamide based on ZnMn2O4 nanoparticles decorated porous reduced graphene oxide nanocomposite electrode. J Hazard Mater [Internet]. 2021;405:124096. Available from: https://www.sciencedirect.com/science/article/pii/S0304389420320860.
112. Babamiri B, Bahari D, Salimi A. Highly sensitive bioaffinity electrochemiluminescence sensors: recent advances and future directions. Biosens Bioelectron [Internet]. 2019;142:111530. Available from: https://www.sciencedirect.com/science/article/pii/S0956566319306098.
113. Sabahi A, Salahandish R, Ghaffarinejad A, Omidinia E. Electrochemical nano-genosensor for highly sensitive detection of miR-21 biomarker based on SWCNT-grafted dendritic au nanostructure for early detection of prostate cancer. Talanta [Internet]. 2020;209:120595. Available from: https://www.sciencedirect.com/science/article/pii/S0039914019312287.
114. Li X, Wei L, Pan L, Yi Z, Wang X, Ye Z, et al. Homogeneous immunosorbent assay based on single-particle enumeration using upconversion nanoparticles for the sensitive detection of cancer biomarkers. Anal Chem [Internet]. 2018;90(7):4807–14. Available from: https://doi.org/10.1021/acs.analchem.8b00251.

115. Yan R, Lu N, Han S, Lu Z, Xiao Y, Zhao Z, et al. Simultaneous detection of dual biomarkers using hierarchical MoS2 nanostructuring and nano-signal amplification-based electrochemical aptasensor toward accurate diagnosis of prostate cancer. Biosens Bioelectron [Internet]. 2022;197:113797. Available from: https://www.sciencedirect.com/science/article/pii/S0956566321008344.
116. Wei B, Mao K, Liu N, Zhang M, Yang Z. Graphene nanocomposites modified electrochemical aptamer sensor for rapid and highly sensitive detection of prostate specific antigen. Biosens Bioelectron [Internet]. 2018;121:41–6. Available from: https://www.sciencedirect.com/science/article/pii/S0956566318306730.
117. Wang Y, Ma S, Ruzzo WL. Spatial modeling of prostate cancer metabolic gene expression reveals extensive heterogeneity and selective vulnerabilities. Sci Rep [Internet]. 2020;10(1):3490. Available from: https://doi.org/10.1038/s41598-020-60384-w.
118. Kim WH, Lee JU, Jeon MJ, Park KH, Sim SJ. Three-dimensional hierarchical plasmonic nano-architecture based label-free surface-enhanced Raman spectroscopy detection of urinary exosomal miRNA for clinical diagnosis of prostate cancer. Biosens Bioelectron [Internet]. 2022;205:114116. Available from: https://www.sciencedirect.com/science/article/pii/S0956566322001567.
119. Hwang DJ, He Y, Ponnusamy S, Mohler ML, Thiyagarajan T, McEwan IJ, et al. New generation of selective androgen receptor degraders: our initial design, synthesis, and biological evaluation of new compounds with enzalutamide-resistant prostate cancer activity. J Med Chem [Internet]. 2019;62(2):491–511. Available from: https://doi.org/10.1021/acs.jmedchem.8b00973.
120. Ashrafizadeh M, Aghamiri S, Tan SC, Zarrabi A, Sharifi E, Rabiee N, et al. Nanotechnological approaches in prostate cancer therapy: integration of engineering and biology. Nano Today [Internet]. 2022;45:101532. Available from: https://www.sciencedirect.com/science/article/pii/S1748013222001591.
121. Boursier ME, Levin S, Zimmerman K, Machleidt T, Hurst R, Butler BL, et al. The luminescent HiBiT peptide enables selective quantitation of G protein–coupled receptor ligand engagement and internalization in living cells. J Biol Chem [Internet]. 2020;295(15):5124–35. Available from: https://www.sciencedirect.com/science/article/pii/S0021925817486030.
122. Datta A, Kim H, McGee L, Johnson AE, Talwar S, Marugan J, et al. High-throughput screening identified selective inhibitors of exosome biogenesis and secretion: a drug repurposing strategy for advanced cancer. Sci Rep [Internet]. 2018;8(1):8161. Available from: https://doi.org/10.1038/s41598-018-26411-7.
123. Haleem A, Javaid M, Singh RP, Suman R, Rab S. Biosensors applications in medical field: a brief review. Sensors Int. 2021;2:100100.
124. Prabowo BA, Cabral PD, Freitas P, Fernandes E. The challenges of developing biosensors for clinical assessment: a review. Chem. 2021;9(11):299.
125. Singh A, Sharma A, Ahmed A, Sundramoorthy AK, Furukawa H, Arya S, et al. Recent advances in electrochemical biosensors: applications, challenges, and future scope. Biosensors. 2021;11(9):336.
126. Fonseca WT, Parra Vello T, Lelis GC, Ferreira Deleigo AV, Takahira RK, Martinez DST, et al. Chemical sensors and biosensors for point-of-care testing of pets: opportunities for individualized diagnostics of companion animals. ACS Sensors [Internet]. 2025;10(5):3222–38. Available from: https://doi.org/10.1021/acssensors.4c03664.
127. Raj LV, Sasi S, Rajeswari P, Pushpa BR, Kulkarni AV, Biradar S. Design of FBG-based optical biosensor for the detection of malaria. J Opt [Internet]. 2025; Available from: https://doi.org/10.1007/s12596-025-02780-x.
128. Althobiti M, Nhung TTT, Verma S, Albugami RR, Kumar R. Artificial intelligence and biosensors: transforming cancer diagnostics. Med Nov Technol Devices [Internet]. 2025;27:100378. Available from: https://www.sciencedirect.com/science/article/pii/S2590093525000293.
129. Bhalla N, Pan Y, Yang Z, Payam AF. Opportunities and challenges for Biosensors and nanoscale analytical tools for pandemics: COVID-19. ACS Nano [Internet]. 2020;14(7):7783–807. Available from: https://doi.org/10.1021/acsnano.0c04421.

130. Anchidin-Norocel L, Iatcu OC, Lobiuc A, Covasa M. Heavy metal-gut microbiota interactions: probiotics modulation and biosensors detection. Biosensors. 2025;15(3):188.
131. Wang K, Lin X, Zhang M, Li Y, Luo C, Wu J. Review of electrochemical biosensors for food safety detection. Biosensors [Internet]. 2022;12(11). Available from: https://www.mdpi.com/2079-6374/12/11/959.
132. Rahmatnejad V, Wei Y, Rao G. In: Pörtner R, editor. Recent developments in bioprocess monitoring systems BT - biopharmaceutical manufacturing: progress, trends and challenges. Cham: Springer International Publishing; 2023. p. 39–66. Available from: https://doi.org/10.1007/978-3-031-45669-5_2.
133. Ramesh M, Janani R, Deepa C, Rajeshkumar L. Nanotechnology-enabled biosensors: a review of fundamentals, design principles, materials, and applications. Biosensors [Internet]. 2023;13(1). Available from: https://www.mdpi.com/2079-6374/13/1/40.
134. Patel N, Pathak P, Rai D, Chaudhary VK. Biosensors used for monitoring of environmental contaminants. In: Inamuddin, Asiri AM, editors. Nanosensor technologies for environmental monitoring. Cham: Springer International Publishing; 2020. p. 69–83. Available from: https://doi.org/10.1007/978-3-030-45116-5_4.
135. Moreira FTC, Sales MGF. Autonomous biosensing device merged with photovoltaic technology for cancer biomarker detection. J Electroanal Chem [Internet]. 2019;855:113611. Available from: https://www.sciencedirect.com/science/article/pii/S1572665719308793.
136. Kumar A, Parihar A, Panda U, Parihar DS. Microfluidics-based point-of-care testing (POCT) devices in dealing with waves of COVID-19 pandemic: the emerging solution. ACS Appl Bio Mater. 2022;5(5):2046–68.
137. Xu Z, Liu Z, Xiao M, Jiang L, Yi C. A smartphone-based quantitative point-of-care testing (POCT) system for simultaneous detection of multiple heavy metal ions. Chem Eng J. 2020;394:124966.
138. Ferentinos KP. Deep learning models for plant disease detection and diagnosis. Comput Electron Agric. 2018;145:311–8
139. Trivedi NK, Gautam V, Anand A, Aljahdali HM, Villar SG, Anand D, et al. Early detection and classification of tomato leaf disease using high-performance deep neural network. Sensors. 2021;21(23):7987.
140. Chowdhury MEH, Rahman T, Khandakar A, Ayari MA, Khan AU, Khan MS, et al. Automatic and reliable leaf disease detection using deep learning techniques. AgriEngineering. 2021;3(2):294–312.
141. Nandhini M, Kala KU, Thangadarshini M, Verma SM. Deep Learning model of sequential image classifier for crop disease detection in plantain tree cultivation. Comput Electron Agric. 2022;197:106915.
142. Bertok T, Bertokova A, Hroncekova S, Chocholova E, Svecova N, Lorencova L, et al. Novel prostate cancer biomarkers: aetiology, clinical performance and sensing applications. Chem Int. 2021;9(8). Available from: https://www.mdpi.com/2227-9040/9/8/205.
143. Yao J, Wang Y, Dai Y, Liu CC. Bioconjugated, single-use biosensor for the detection of biomarkers of prostate Cancer. ACS Omega [Internet]. 2018;3(6):6411–8. Available from: https://doi.org/10.1021/acsomega.8b00634.
144. Teng Y, Li W, Gunasekaran S. Biosensors based on single or multiple biomarkers for diagnosis of prostate cancer. Biosens Bioelectron X [Internet]. 2023;15:100418. Available from: https://www.sciencedirect.com/science/article/pii/S2590137023001152.
145. Damborský P, Damborská D, Belický Š, Tkáč J, Katrlík J. Sweet strategies in prostate cancer biomarker research: focus on a prostate specific antigen. Bionanoscience [Internet]. 2018;8(2):690–700. Available from: https://doi.org/10.1007/s12668-017-0397-z.
146. Sohrabi H, Bolandi N, Hemmati A, Eyvazi S, Ghasemzadeh S, Baradaran B, et al. State-of-the-art cancer biomarker detection by portable (Bio) sensing technology: a critical review. Microchem J [Internet] 2022;177:107248. Available from: https://www.sciencedirect.com/science/article/pii/S0026265X22000765.

147. Liu Y, Zhang N, Pan JB, Song J, Zhao W, Chen HY, et al. Bipolar electrode array for multiplexed detection of prostate cancer biomarkers. Anal Chem [Internet]. 2022;94(6):3005–12. Available from: https://doi.org/10.1021/acs.analchem.1c05383.
148. Cho S, Yang HC, Rhee WJ. Simultaneous multiplexed detection of exosomal microRNAs and surface proteins for prostate cancer diagnosis. Biosens Bioelectron [Internet]. 2019;146:111749. Available from: https://www.sciencedirect.com/science/article/pii/S0956566319308280.
149. Alijaj N, Pavlovic B, Martel P, Rakauskas A, Cesson V, Saba K, et al. Identification of urine biomarkers to improve eligibility for prostate biopsy and detect high-grade prostate cancer. Cancers (Basel) [Internet]. 2022;14(5). Available from: https://www.mdpi.com/2072-6694/14/5/1135.
150. Bauckneht M, Ciccarese C, Laudicella R, Mosillo C, D'Amico F, Anghelone A, et al. Theranostics revolution in prostate cancer: basics, clinical applications, open issues and future perspectives. Cancer Treat Rev [Internet]. 2024;124:102698. Available from: https://www.sciencedirect.com/science/article/pii/S0305737224000161.
151. Scott E, Munkley J. Glycans as biomarkers in prostate cancer. Int J Mol Sci [Internet]. 2019;20(6). Available from: https://www.mdpi.com/1422-0067/20/6/1389.
152. Singh M, Vinayak A, Pranav P, Divya J, Shriya A, Sachchida Nand R, et al. A comprehensive review and androgen deprivation therapy and its impact on Alzheimer's disease risk in older men with prostate cancer. Degener Neurol Neuromuscul Dis [Internet]. 2024;14(null):33–46. Available from: https://www.tandfonline.com/doi/abs/10.2147/DNND.S445130.
153. Nasimi H, Madsen JS, Zedan AH, Malmendal A, Osther PJS, Alatraktchi FA. Protein biomarker detection in prostate cancer: a comprehensive review of electrochemical biosensors. Sens Actuators Rep [Internet]. 2023;6:100168. Available from: https://www.sciencedirect.com/science/article/pii/S2666053923000310.
154. Vermassen T, De Bruyne S, Himpe J, Lumen N, Callewaert N, Rottey S, et al. N-linked glycosylation and near-infrared spectroscopy in the diagnosis of prostate cancer. Int J Mol Sci [Internet]. 2019;20(7). Available from: https://www.mdpi.com/1422-0067/20/7/1592.
155. Robinson HS, Lee SS, Barocas DA, Tosoian JJ. Evaluation of blood and urine based biomarkers for detection of clinically-significant prostate cancer. Prostate Cancer Prostatic Dis [Internet]. 2025;28(1):45–55. Available from: https://doi.org/10.1038/s41391-024-00840-0.
156. Bilal M, Javaid A, Amjad F, Youssif TA, Afzal S. An overview of prostate cancer (PCa) diagnosis: potential role of miRNAs. Transl Oncol [Internet]. 2022;26:101542. Available from: https://www.sciencedirect.com/science/article/pii/S1936523322002017.
157. Hatakeyama S, Yoneyama T, Tobisawa Y, Yamamoto H, Ohyama C. Narrative review of urinary glycan biomarkers in prostate cancer. Transl Androl Urol. 2021;10(4):1850–64.
158. Aidoo-Brown J, Moschou D, Estrela P. Multiplexed prostate cancer companion diagnostic devices. Sensors [Internet]. 2021;21(15). Available from: https://www.mdpi.com/1424-8220/21/15/5023.

Electrochemical Biosensor for Prostate Cancer

4

Rahul Kumar, Anup Kumar Sirbaiya, Shriyansh Srivastava, and Gita Bhat

Abbreviations

Ag/AgCl	Silver/silver chloride electrode
AI	Artificial intelligence
AuNP	Gold nanoparticle
DRE	Digital rectal examination
LOD	Limit of detection
miRNA	microRNA
ML	Machine learning
MWCNT	Multi-walled carbon nanotube
PCA3	Prostate cancer antigen 3
PoC	Point-of-care
PSA	Prostate-specific antigen
PSMA	Prostate-specific membrane antigen
rGO	Reduced graphene oxide
SCE	Saturated calomel electrode

R. Kumar
Faculty of Pharmacy, Vidya University, Meerut, Uttar Pradesh, India

A. K. Sirbaiya
Department of Pharmacy, K.P Singh Memorial Institute of Pharmacy, Sitapur, Uttar Pradesh, India

S. Srivastava
Department of Pharmacy, School of Medical and Allied Sciences, Galgotias University, Greater Noida, Uttar Pradesh, India

G. Bhat (✉)
Department of Internal Medicine, Northern Ontario School of Medicine (NOSM) University, Thunder Bay, Canada

S. Srivastava et al. (eds.), *Biosensor Technologies for Prostate Cancer*, https://doi.org/10.1007/978-981-95-8644-8_4

4.1 Introduction

Prostate cancer ranks as one of the most common tumors among male patients worldwide, who mainly fall within ageing groups [1]. The prostate gland serves as the starting point for this type of cancer because it produces the seminal fluid. The World Health Organisation records prostate cancer as the second most prevalent cancer that leads to male cancer death [2]. Most prostate cancer cases remain indolent yet slow-growing, yet aggressive types can spread through the body, causing serious death if not recognized early [3]. The disease progresses at a steady pace, providing patients with an essential opportunity for early medical treatment [4]. Because prostate cancer shows significant differences in its clinical manifestations, it becomes challenging to distinguish between harmless benign masses and lethal, threatening ones. Medical professionals require precise diagnostic methods at early disease stages to support better therapeutic choices while decreasing unnecessary treatment practices [5]. Early disease detection remains vital for enhancing survival statistics while improving patient care. The doctor examines the prostate with a digital rectal examination (DRE) yet combines the test with prostate-specific antigen (PSA) testing and transrectal ultrasound-guided biopsy procedures [6]. Medical institutions often employ PSA testing as their primary method, although this approach can impact both the precision and reliability of diagnosis. PSA testing detects elevated levels that can stem from benign prostatic hyperplasia alongside prostatitis, thus triggering superfluous invasive procedures [7]. Patient management outcomes and survival statistics improve significantly when the diagnosis occurs at an early stage. The diagnostic instruments for prostate cancer evaluation consist of digital rectal examination (DRE) and prostate-specific antigen (PSA) testing combined with transrectal ultrasound-guided biopsy [8]. Correctly, among these diagnostic methods, PSA serves as the most commonly used one yet shows low performance levels for specificity and sensitivity tests [9]. The detection of elevated PSA stands in conflict with non-cancerous conditions such as benign prostatic hyperplasia and prostatitis, which results in improper diagnosis and intrusive medical procedures [10].

The medical research community focuses on creating new biomarkers combined with diagnostic technologies because they require enhanced accuracy levels [11]. The objective is to create accurate diagnostic methods that perform tests without surgery and provide dependable measurements in real time alongside high precision rates. The detection and monitoring of prostate cancer, facilitated by biosensor technology, show promise. The analytical devices detect biological responses by transmitting quantifiable electrical signals, enabling the rapid, sensitive, and specific detection of cancer biomarkers [12]. Electrochemical biosensors are preferred over other biosensor types because they offer a low cost, alongside portability, fast response times, and compatibility with microfabrication and point-of-care technology [13]. Electrochemical biosensors possess the

Table 4.1 Comparison between PSA and emerging biomarkers

Biomarker	Biological source	Sample type	Clinical utility	Advantages	Limits	References
PSA	Glycoprotein from prostate epithelial cells	Blood	Screening and monitoring	Widely available; sample assay	Low specificity false positives; overdiagnosis	[17]
PCA3	Non-coding RNA	Urine (post-DRE)	Decision aid for repeat biopsy	High specificity; non-invasive	Limited sensitivity	[18]
PSMA	Transmembrane protein	Tissue imaging	Diagnostic and therapeutic targeting	High expression in advanced cancers	Requires imaging tools or targeted ligands	[19]
miRNAs (e.g., miR-21, miR-141, miR-221)	Regulatory RNA	Blood, urine, tissue	Prognostic and diagnostic marker	Stable in fluids; multiplexing possible	Validation and standardization are required	[20]

capability to detect various prostate cancer markers, such as PSA, together with PCA3, PSMA, and specific microRNAs [14]. Random biorecognition entities, including antibodies, aptamers, and enzymes, alongside nucleic acids, permit the customization of biosensors to find ultra-low concentration targets selectively (Table 4.1) [15]. Electrochemical biosensors have gained additional analytical capabilities through the integration of nanotechnology with microfluidics and biosensing. These discoveries enable researchers to create complex miniaturized devices designed for real-time analysis either in hospitals or personal residences [16]. Electrochemical biosensors will change precision oncology through their expected ability to detect prostate cancer at an early stage and estimate patient prognosis, as well as match treatments specifically to each patient.

4.2 Biomarkers for Prostate Cancer

The early detection, diagnosis, and management of prostate cancer depend much on biomarkers. Found in blood, urine, or tissue, these biological markers help determine the presence and progression of the disease. Though it has some drawbacks, prostate-specific antigen (PSA) is the most well-known prostate cancer biomarker and is usually used in screening. PCA3, TMPRSS2-ERG gene fusion, and circulating tumor cells (CTCs), among other new biomarkers, are improving the precision of prostate cancer diagnosis and directing individualized treatment plans. Ongoing studies continue to discover new biomarkers with higher specificity and sensitivity, offering hope for improved patient outcomes.

4.2.1 Prostate-Specific Antigen (PSA)

The prostate gland produces prostate-specific antigen (PSA) as a glycoprotein enzyme that originates from prostate epithelial cells [21]. The substance functions naturally to liquefy semen, and elevated blood serum concentrations have become known indicators of prostate cancer development [22]. Healthcare professionals introduced PSA testing into clinical practice during the late 1980s to become the primary method for diagnosing and monitoring prostate cancer [17]. PSA utilization across medical practices faces notable drawbacks since it demonstrates inadequate precision, along with detectability issues [23]. Breaking down PSA levels above the threshold can result from both benign prostatic hyperplasia (BPH), prostatitis, and recent ejaculation, in addition to carcinoma. PSA testing generates false results because it fails to distinguish between harmless prostate cancers and aggressive growths, thus causing unnecessary medical interventions [24]. The diagnosis of PSA receives three enhancement attempts through assessments of free-to-total PSA ratio, PSA density, and PSA velocity measurements [25]. These diagnostic refinement techniques produce marginal improvements but do not provide definitive accuracy for diagnoses, which sustains the research effort for new or supporting biomarkers [26].

4.2.2 Emerging Biomarkers (e.g., PCA3, PSMA, miRNAs)

Research into new biomarkers has gained momentum because PSA proved inadequate in detecting prostate cancer specifically, while characterizing its nature, as shown in Table 4.1 [27]. *PCA3 (Prostate Cancer Antigen 3):* The non-coding RNA PCA3 appears in prostate cancer tissues at elevated levels. Urine collection after a digital rectal examination reveals the presence of this biomarker, making it an ideal non-invasive diagnostic tool [18]. Research has demonstrated that PCA3 diagnostic tests provide superior specificity performance compared to PSA tests, especially when evaluating the necessity of repeat biopsies [27]. *PSMA (Prostate-Specific Membrane Antigen):* The transmembrane protein PSMA presents high expression levels in prostate cancer tissue and shows maximum overexpression in tumors of high classification that metastasize [18]. The detection method functions to identify prostate cancer for both medical diagnosis and therapeutic applications involving radioligand and antibody-based therapies [19]. *MicroRNAs (miRNAs)* are post-transcriptional regulators that function as short messenger RNAs, controlling gene expression. Multiple research studies have confirmed that prostate cancer shows altered expression of miR-21, miR-141, and miR-221 [28]. These biomarkers exist in blood plasma and urinary excreta alongside tissues, and scientists can utilize their molecular signatures to make prognoses and therapeutic and diagnostic assessments. Research scientists continue studies on sarcosine as well as TMPRSS2-ERG gene fusion and circulating tumor cells (CTCs) because of their potential value for prostate cancer diagnostic tests.

Table 4.2 Clinical challenges in biomarker implementations

Challenge	Description	Impact on clinical use	References
Validation and standardization	Lack of consistent performance across populations and settings	Limits generalizability and reliability	[31]
Sensitivity and specificity	Improving one often compromises the other	Impacts diagnostic accuracy	[26]
Biological variability	Differences in tumor genetics and patient physiology	Reduce test reproducibility	[32]
Regulatory and economic barrier	Need for approvals and cost-effective integration into workflows	Slows clinical adoption	[33]

4.2.3 Clinical Relevance and Challenges

Biomarkers play an essential role in prostate cancer diagnosis as well as risk assessment during patient selection of appropriate treatments and disease tracking [29]. Table 4.2 shows the number of obstacles that affect the clinical implementation of new biomarkers in regular medical practice [30].

Validation and Standardization: Clinical validation of biomarkers requires extensive testing to generate dependable and precise results that work the same way among multiple population types and various clinical environments [31]. *Sensitivity and Specificity Trade-offs:* The introduction of new biomarkers tends to enhance biomarker performance in one area while sacrificing the opposite trait [32]. *Biological Variability:* The heterogeneity found in tumors alongside differences between patient cases influences biomarker detection methods and makes interpretation more difficult [34]. *Regulatory and Economic Considerations:* The implementation of new biomarkers depends on regulatory clearance, together with the ability to maintain cost-effectiveness and integration with medical algorithms for diagnosis [35]. Prospective improvements in both multi-biomarker analysis and biosensing technology development hold great promise for increasing the efficiency of prostate cancer diagnostic methods in the coming years [36].

4.3 Electrochemical Biosensing Principles

Electrochemical biosensing employs biological recognition elements that achieve specific detection, while electrochemical transduction measures the response sensitivity [37]. The biosensors establish operations through the measurement of electrical signals that emerge due to interactions between target analytes and a biorecognition element fixed on electrode surfaces [38]. The interpretation principle bases its operation on turning biochemical changes such as antigen–antibody interactions, enzymatic responses, and nucleic acid hybridization into electrical signals [39]. The biosensor generates detectable signals, which appear as current measurements in amperometry mode, voltage readings under potentiometry conditions, and impedance patterns in electrochemical impedance spectroscopy systems [40]. The measurement magnitude escalates based on analyte concentration levels, allowing for proper detection at low concentration thresholds [41]. Biosensors based on electrochemical principles offer several benefits, including high sensitivity, rapid response, affordable cost, and potential minimization and portability characteristics [42]. The identified characteristics of these sensors prove them convenient for in-field diagnostic functions with real-time feedback, especially within regions with limited resources [43]. An electrochemical biosensor consists of vital components, including the working electrode with nanomaterial modifications for improved performance, as well as a reference electrode and a counter electrode, alongside a bio-recognition layer [44]. The working electrode functions as the fundamental element that draws biomarkers for electrochemical reaction processing [45]. The device's functionality improves significantly when it integrates both microfluidics technology and digital signal processing units, which offer automated analysis capabilities and multiplex detection [46]. Prostate cancer and other cancer types benefit significantly from electrochemical biosensing technologies, as these systems provide highly sensitive and specific detection of biochemical markers, including PSA, PCA3, and PSMA, for diagnostic purposes [47]. Research focused on improving materials, together with design modifications, should extend their clinical utility.

4.3.1 Fundamentals of Electrochemical Detection

The analytical method of electrochemical biosensing uses biological recognition elements together with electrochemical signal transduction mechanisms to generate results [48]. These systems use a specific biological element (antibody, enzyme, aptamer, or nucleic acid) that recognizes target analytes, after which an electrode system measures the generated electrical signal [49]. Electrochemical detection functions by observing electrical parameters, including current, potential, and impedance, which change due to biochemical reactions on sensor interfaces. The changes occurring at the sensor interface display either direct or indirect correspondence to the target biomarker concentration [50]. The popularity of electrochemical biosensors stems from their easy implementation, together with minute detection boundaries and quick recognition, along with capabilities to create scaled-down devices [51]. Biosensors apply well to point-of-care diagnostics since they have features that enable them to work in these settings, particularly for prostate cancer detection and other diseases that need precise early diagnosis [52].

4.3.2 Types of Electrochemical Techniques

Biosensing makes use of multiple electrochemical methods (Fig. 4.1) that suit different requirements based on the intended application [53]. *Amperometry:* The technique measures oxidative or reductive reaction-generated current through a predetermined potential setting [54]. This method detects enzyme-based sensor

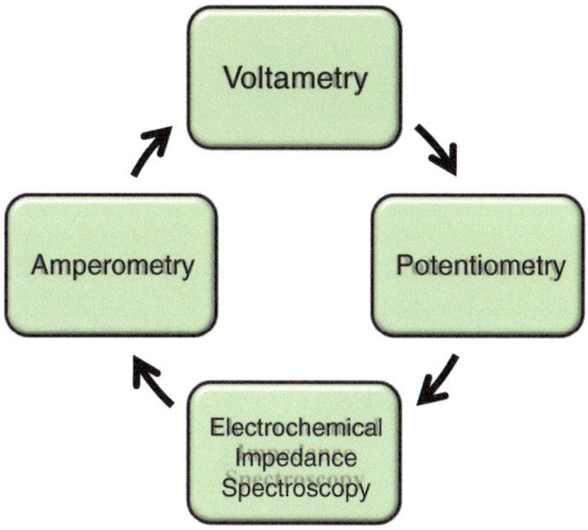

Fig. 4.1 Different electrochemical techniques

outputs through the enzymatic reaction that generates electroactive chemicals, such as H_2O_2. Voltammetry: The technique involves sweeping the potential across different values while recording the measured current response. The redox reaction research combined with sensor kinetic analysis is accomplished using voltametric techniques, including cyclic voltammetry (CV), differential pulse voltammetry (DPV), and square wave voltammetry (SWV) [55]. *Potentiometry:* The technique measures the potential difference between a working and a reference electrode under negligible current flow [56]. It is useful for ion-selective electrodes and pH sensors. *Electrochemical Impedance Spectroscopy (EIS):* The technique monitors the impedance of an electrochemical system over a range of frequencies [57]. EIS demonstrates high sensitivity toward surface alterations because it operates successfully without labels to detect rare cancer biomarkers.

The techniques provide adjustable functionality that matches sensors with their target reaction features for different biomedical testing needs [58].

4.3.3 Key Components of Electrochemical Biosensor

The integration of prostate cancer biomarkers (e.g., PSA, PCA3, PSMA, miRNAs) with electrochemical biosensing components, including working and reference electrodes, biorecognition elements, and signal processors, enables precise detection and diagnosis (Fig. 4.2). *Working Electrode (Transducer):* The biorecognition event occurs directly on the surface of this electrode. Phones commonly use conductive polymers in combination with carbon and gold, along with platinum materials, as working electrode materials [59]. The surface receives modifications through functional layers, along with nanomaterials, which enhance both sensitivity and bio-immobilization efficiency. *Biorecognition Element:* A molecule displays the capability to select and connect exclusively with the target analyte [60]. The recognition elements usually consist of antibodies used for immunosensor applications, combined with enzymes and aptamers, as well as nucleic acid probes. The detection needs accurate results to function properly; therefore, high specificity plays a vital

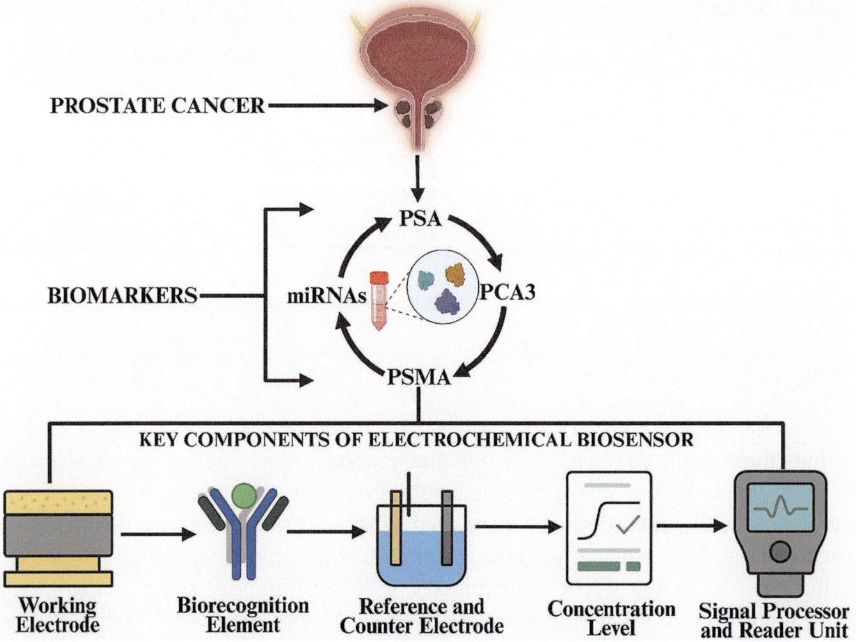

Fig. 4.2 Integrated pathway of electrochemical biosensing for prostate cancer diagnosis

role in achieving these results. *Reference Electrode:* The working electrode measures its potential value against this fixed reference electrode system. Ag/AgCl as well as saturated calomel electrodes (SCE) represent typical examples of reference electrodes [61]. *Counter (Auxiliary) Electrode:* The device finishes the electrical circuit for current functionality during measurement processes [62]. Platinum, along with carbon, serves as a typical inert component for this function. *Signal Processor and Reader Unit:* This unit converts the electrochemical response into readable data. This data acquisition and analysis system operates in portable and point-of-care environments with integrated digital or wireless components. Surface engineering and nanotechnology support biosensor development for prostate cancer diagnostics through their combined usage with these distinct components.

4.4 Design and Fabrication of an Electrochemical Biosensor

Electrochemical biosensors comprise the integration of a biorecognition element with an electrochemical transducer on a suitable substrate in the design and fabrication (Fig. 4.3) of the electrochemical biosensors [63]. The first step in the process is to identify the target analyte and an appropriate biological sensing component (e.g., an enzyme, an antibody, or nucleic acids) that associates with the analyte. The immobilization is done by adsorption, covalent bonding, or entrapment of this bioreceptor on the sensor surface to achieve stability and activity of this bioreceptor

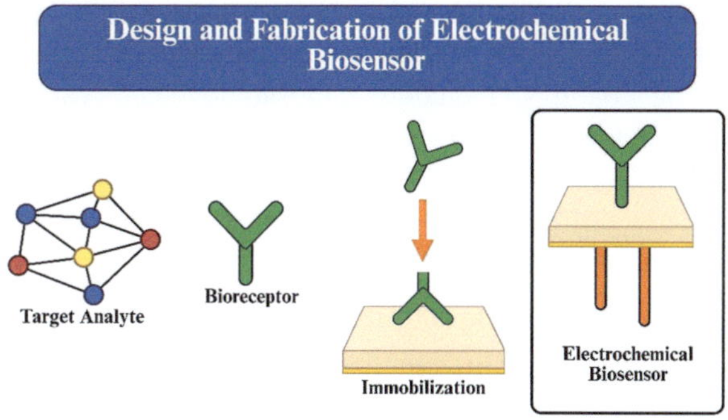

Fig. 4.3 Electrochemical biosensor development

[64]. Typically, the transducer or interface in the case comprises electrodes of gold, carbon, or platinum and derives electrical signals from the biochemical interaction [65]. Fabrication is performed with considerations of miniaturization, biocompatibility, sensitivity, and reproducibility; thus, these chips can be used for applications in clinical diagnostics as well as environmental monitoring [66].

4.4.1 Electrode Material and Modifications

Electrodes function as the main element of electrochemical biosensors because they both hold biorecognition elements for immobilization and transform biochemical responses into detectable electrical outputs [67]. The electrode material selection determines how well the sensor performs, affecting its sensitivity, stability, and signal-to-noise ratio measurements [68]. The four most widely utilized electrode materials used in electrochemical biosensors consist of gold alongside carbon (glassy carbon, carbon nanotubes, graphene), as well as platinum and indium tin oxide (ITO) [69]. The selected materials exhibit both excellent electrical conductivity properties and biocompatible performance. The analytical capabilities of electrodes are enhanced through the application of nanomaterials, including gold nanoparticles, carbon nanotubes, graphene oxide, and metal-organic frameworks, as these materials provide additional surface area, faster electron transfer, and multiple functional groups that support further chemical modifications [70]. By using screen printing and photolithography together with 3D printing methods, manufacturers can now produce affordable electrode structures that exhibit high repeatability [71].

4.4.2 Surface Functionalization Strategies

The device's surface needs specific modification because it determines how well biobased components stay bound to electrodes [72]. Introducing chemical groups or coatings enables the development of binding capacities for biorecognition elements through both covalent and non-covalent interactions [73]. Common strategies include the following [74]: Gold electrodes receive well-ordered reactive surfaces through self-assembled monolayers (SAMs), which interact with thiol (-SH) chemistry; Biomolecule binding and biocompatibility enhancement occur through polymeric coatings, including chitosan together with polyaniline and polypyrene; Nanomaterial composites provide functionalized materials with a large surface area contact and multiple binding sites to make better biomolecule attachments possible. Such alterations enable robust bonding functions and correct positioning of recognition molecules and activity retention [75].

4.4.3 Immobilization of Biorecognition Elements

The practice of attaching biological recognition elements, such as antibodies, enzymes, aptamers, and nucleic acids, onto electrodes represents immobilization [76]. A suitable immobilization technique allows biological activity preservation along with a strong and specific interaction between the target analyte. Common immobilization methods include the following [77]: Physical adsorption uses simple and inexpensive methods for immobilization yet produces unstable results; A strong and durable attachment occurs through covalent bonding by applying EDC/NHS crosslinkers for connecting carboxyl and amine groups; Affinity interactions, such as biotin-streptavidin binding, are useful for modular and reversible systems; The fabrication of electrodes involves encapsulation of biomolecules through either polymer or sol–gel matrix entrapment. The selection process happens through evaluation of the bioreceptor nature, as well as sensor stability requirements, along with application needs [78]. An optimized method for immobilization leads to superior sensor selectivity and sensitivity, and reproducibility outputs [79].

4.5 Recent Advances and Applications

The development of electrochemical biosensors through recent innovations improved their ability to detect prostate cancer, along with their sensitivity and real-time monitoring capabilities, and enhanced specificity [80]. The point-of-care device manufacturing, along with wearable technology development and implantable sensing platforms, achieved their advances via the fusion of nanomaterials and microfluidic systems with digital interfaces [81]. The research into these biomarkers, PSA and PCA3, developed methods for non-contact, quick, and specific biomarker testing, which helps monitor therapies and facilitates early diagnosis of prostate cancer [82]. Superior clinical verification with medical remote applications and home-based health monitoring leads to the progressive potential of electrochemical biosensors to shift prostate cancer management practices [83].

4.5.1 Point-of-Care Devices

Point-of-care (PoC) devices brought a significant change to prostate cancer diagnostics because they provide fast on-site examinations using small specimen amounts without requiring extensive centralized laboratory equipment [84]. These diagnostic tools provide easy operation in portable formats that demonstrate real-time tests, which fit perfectly into primary healthcare facilities and limited-resource situations [85]. PoC applications strongly favor electrochemical biosensors because they function with a small physical size and low power use, as well as quick analytical speeds [86]. Research in screen-printed electrodes coupled with microfluidics development and smartphone functionality advancements supported the development of inexpensive, disposable point-of-care systems [87]. Medical devices used in prostate cancer detection target PSA, along with microRNAs and exosomal proteins, through detection methods that include enzymes, label-free observations, and immunoaffinity systems [88]. Proposed commercial and prototype point-of-care devices achieve picomolar detection limits and accurate tumor identification skills between benign prostatic hyperplasia (BPH) and malignant tumors [89]. The diagnostic performance improves through signal amplification that results from using nanomaterials, including gold nanoparticles, carbon nanotubes, and graphene.

4.5.2 Wearable and Implantable Devices

Implantable and wearable devices have now become biosensors that allow continuous individualized monitoring of prostate cancer progression trajectory at a substan tial level. Biological markers are monitored by electrochemical sensors placed on the body by measuring changes in body fluids, such as sweat or saliva, or in interstitial fluid between tissues [90]. Biosensors have been incorporated into smartwatches, textile-based patches, and wearable devices that monitor medical indicators in real time for patients at outside medical facilities [91]. Implantable biosensors are the most efficient mode of surveillance over tumor-specific biomarkers since such devices are directly implanted into biological tissues and use live tissue for continuous observation of cancer conditions [92]. With the development of small-sized devices, biosensors have compatibility with the biological systems to work inside the body with wireless data exchange and self-sustenance by their own function of power generation [93]. Basically, three key components of flexible biosensors, including graphene oxide sensors, stretchable polymer composites, and biodegradable materials, were developed by past scientists to avoid surgical retrieval [94]. While these systems are still in their experimental phase, they show great promise as early cancer recurrence detection systems, cancer therapy progress monitoring tools, and precision medicine systems.

4.5.3 Case Studies and Clinical Validation

Electrochemical biosensors to clinically validate for prostate cancer are a crucial step to translation from bench to bedside [95]. These sensors have found numerous applications in the real world, where their effectiveness has been demonstrated in numerous case studies. For example, biosensors that have performed successfully in detecting ultrasensitive PSA in human serum with excellent concordance with standard ELISA-based assays, with faster turnaround times [96]. A dual-marker electrochemical platform was developed in another study for a more specific diagnostic capability to recognize PSA and PCA3 mRNA. Biosensors have also been evaluated for post-treatment surveillance, and when combined with PSA kinetics while patients are on hormone therapy or are undergoing radiation, a more detailed picture of PSA kinetics can be obtained than merely static readings of the PSA [97]. A few biosensors are connected with machine learning algorithms for the interpretation of complex signal patterns, which increases the diagnostic accuracy and minimizes the false positives [98]. These innovations are being explored, and academies, industry, and healthcare providers are collaborating to develop clinically robust, scalable biosensor platforms. The promising results raise the need for addressing the challenges of sensor reproducibility, stability, large-scale manufacturing, and regulatory compliance [99]. It is important to note that these goals are continuing efforts in standardization and multicenter validation studies.

4.6 Challenges and Future Directions

The wide range of restrictions has prevented electrochemical biosensors developed for prostate cancer diagnosis from reaching clinical acceptance [100]. High sensitivity along with high specificity measurements in biological samples remains the main scientific hurdle, while maintaining reproducibility and stability is a parallel challenge. Laboratory models need technical solutions to match large-scale manufacturing requirements, as well as regulatory compliance needs and healthcare system needs [101]. The advancement of this sector depends on heavy investment in nanotechnology while adding AI diagnostic abilities and flexible electronic functionalities to progress sensor capacity and enable individualized continuous healthcare observation [102]. The new inventions aim to replace current individual biomarker testing by developing robust, multiplexed platforms for improved disease profile outcomes. The current obstacles affecting electrochemical biosensors used in prostate cancer detection are analyzed in detail through Table 4.3, which also presents potential future solutions for these challenges. The table functions as a research instrument that facilitates scientists and stakeholders in creating superior biosensing systems for future utilization.

Table 4.3 Challenges and emerging solutions in electrochemical biosensing for prostate cancer

Challenge	Description	Emerging solutions	References
Sensitivity and detection limits	Challenges in finding biomarkers at extremely low (pico- to femtomolar) concentrations	Use of nanomaterials (e.g., AuNPs, graphene) and signal amplification techniques	[103]
Specificity and selectivity	Non-target compounds' cross-reactivity and interference	Functionalization with aptamers, antibodies, nanobodies, and multi-biomarker approaches	[104]
Reproducibility and stability	Inconsistent performance across samples and conditions	Standardized fabrication processes, robust surface chemistries	[105]
Sample complexity	Presence of interfering substances in real biological fluids	Advanced filtering, microfluidics, pre-concentration steps	[106]
Scalability and manufacturing	Difficulty transitioning from lab-scale to large-scale production	Printable electronics, roll-to-roll fabrication, low-cost sensor platforms	[107]
Regulatory and clinical validation	Long, costly approval processes and the need for large-scale validation	Collaborative clinical studies, early regulatory engagement, modular device certification	[105]
Data interpretation	Complex signals require experts' analysis	AI/ML algorithms for pattern recognition and decision support	[108]
User-friendliness and integration	Need for professional operation or lab settings	Smartphone-based readouts, point-of-care interfaces, wearable integrations	[109]
Invasiveness and patient compliance	Traditional tests are uncomfortable or inconvenient	Non-invasive sample collection (saliva, urine), wearable and implantable biosensors	[110]
Single biomarker limitation	Reliance on PSA alone may be insufficient for accurate diagnosis	Multiplexed biosensors targeting PSA, PCA3, microRNAs, exosomes, and metabolic markers	[111]

4.6.1 Sensitivity, Specificity, and Selectivity

The primary challenge lies in improving the sensitivity, specificity, and selectivity of electrochemical biosensing for prostate cancer [112]. Fluid-based matrices pose a challenge for sensing ultra-low concentrations of biomarkers, such as PSA or emerging targets, PCA3, or exosomal miRNAs, due to the presence of other biomarkers and interference. The performance of a sensor can be greatly affected by nonspecific binding, signal drift, and background noise [113]. However, although signal amplification, nanomaterials, and surface functionalization techniques have improved, reproducibility and stability are not in a satisfactory state. Distinguishing BPH from a malignant tumor also requires multiplexed platforms that simultaneously analyze multiple biomarkers with high precision of diagnosis [110].

Overcoming these limitations requires continuous biorecognition elements and signal enhancement methods to increase novel aptamers, nanobodies, and other biomolecule variants, as well as develop new and improved signal amplification methods that are needed to differentiate heaven from hell [114].

4.6.2 Commercialization Barriers and Regulatory Aspects

Although electrochemical sensors have promising laboratory results, their commercialization involves many difficulties. Besides the scalability of fabrication methods, immediate quality control at mass production and integration with standardized medical diagnostic workflows are the key barriers [115]. Therefore, sensors must pass consistent performance tests in large-scale patient populations and various sample types, making extensive clinical trials mandatory. Also, whether FDA or EMA approval is obtained, such drugs must meet very stringent safety, efficacy, and quality bar standards [33]. Other hurdles include navigating intellectual property rights, obtaining funds for development, and, at the same time, trying to keep the costs down [116]. The success of translating these technologies into clinical practice depends on the involvement of academic researchers, industry stakeholders, and regulatory agencies.

4.6.3 Future Trends in Prostate Cancer Biosensing

Several new innovative approaches help to define the progressive development of electrochemical biosensing technology for prostate cancer diagnosis [117]. AI and ML algorithms should work with this data to evaluate quality criteria because AI diagnosis predictions emerge from this integration system. Real-time biosensors that integrate within the body function as implanted and wearable devices to monitor prostate cancer development and therapeutic effects, thus ensuring unceasing patient surveillance [118]. Advanced personalized diagnoses emerge from combining biosensing devices that synchronize their operations to conduct integrated biomarker tests that quantify genomic, proteomic, and metabolomic information [119]. The combination of biodegradable materials with flexible electronics supported by wireless connections leads to the development of sustainable patient-centered design methods, according to adoption ideas [120]. Technology based on biosensing serves as a fundamental tool for distributed prostate cancer care, as its development meets the requirements of preventive health systems while enhancing its network capabilities.

4.7 Conclusion

The most often impacted group among elderly male patients is the main worldwide health issue of prostate cancer. Exact early detection of medical problems not only helps healthcare professionals choose appropriate treatment choices but also helps patients by reducing needless medical procedures brought on by overdiagnosis. Current diagnostic methods have particular and sensitive issues that require more research to produce more dependable diagnostic solutions for patient diagnosis. Preserving speed, sensitivity, and cost-effectiveness, the improved electrochemical sensors serve as developing diagnostic tools with the detection capacity for prostate cancer biomarkers. Biosensors' mix of biological recognition components, comprising enzymes, antibodies, nucleic acids, and aptamers, provides them with versatility for biomarker identification of PSA and PSMA and three important cancer markers: PSA, PCA3, and microRNAs. Rapid detection limits and reduced response times, along with steady operation, are produced via electrode design improvement and surface functionalizing techniques, as well as the usage of nanomaterials. Advancement of wearable devices that do multiplexed biosensing without labels makes feasible point-of-care testing advance toward clinical reality, with early screening, real-time monitoring, and personalized therapies. Despite continuous developments, researchers still have work to do to create clinical diagnostic standards from laboratory-based research prototypes. Integration of healthcare infrastructure with repeatability criteria calls for consideration, as they provide significant barriers to development in conjunction with the necessity for stability assessment and regulatory requirements. Integrating biosensors with digital health technology components, such as mobile interfaces and cloud-based analytics systems, will help precision cancer research in the future. Electrochemical biosensors have great potential to enhance techniques used to identify prostate cancer. Combining multidisciplinary research with clinical collaboration will remove current barriers, allowing these technologies to reach their greatest value for modern healthcare systems.

4.8 Summary

An extensive review of electrochemical biosensors in relation to the diagnosis of prostate cancer is provided in this chapter. It describes the structural and functional elements of biosensors, including signal processors, biorecognition elements, working, reference, and counter electrodes, as well as how they can be combined with nanotechnology to improve sensitivity and specificity. The diagnostic utility of prostate-specific biomarkers, such as PSA, PCA3, PSMA, and miRNAs, is examined. Along with discussing standardization, reproducibility, scalability, and regulatory barriers, the chapter also discusses new technological and methodological approaches to clinical translation, such as artificial intelligence, point-of-care platforms, and aptamer-based recognition. All things considered, this chapter highlights the potential of electrochemical biosensing as a rapid, straightforward, and cost-effective method for the early and precise diagnosis of prostate cancer.

Glossary

Aptamer Short single-stranded DNA or RNA molecules that bind to specific targets, used as biorecognition elements.

Biorecognition element Component of a biosensor that interacts specifically with the target analyte (e.g., antibody, aptamer).

Electrochemical biosensor Analytical device that converts a biological response into an electrical signal.

Limit of detection (LOD) The lowest concentration of an analyte that can be reliably detected.

Point-of-care (PoC) Medical diagnostic testing performed at or near the site of patient care.

Prostate-specific antigen (PSA) A protein produced by prostate cells, commonly used as a biomarker for prostate cancer.

Microfluidics Technology that processes small amounts of fluid using microscale channels, often integrated into biosensors.

Nanomaterials Materials with structural features at the nanoscale, used to enhance sensor sensitivity and surface area.

Transducer Converts the biorecognition event into a measurable signal in a biosensor.

References

1. Rawla P. Epidemiology of prostate cancer. World J Oncol. 2019;10(2):63.
2. Gandaglia G, Leni R, Bray F, Fleshner N, Freedland SJ, Kibel A, et al. Epidemiology and prevention of prostate cancer. Eur Urol Oncol. 2021;4(6):877–92.
3. Kim H, Park S, Jeong IG, Song SH, Jeong Y, Kim CS, et al. Noninvasive precision screening of prostate cancer by urinary multimarker sensor and artificial intelligence analysis. ACS Nano. 2020;15(3):4054–65.
4. Sartor O, De Bono JS. Metastatic prostate cancer. N Engl J Med. 2018;378(7):645–57.
5. Evans AJ. Treatment effects in prostate cancer. Mod Pathol. 2018;31:110–21. https://www.sciencedirect.com/science/article/pii/S0893395222011279
6. Gillessen S, Attard G, Beer TM, Beltran H, Bossi A, Bristow R, et al. Management of Patients with advanced prostate cancer: the report of the advanced prostate cancer consensus conference APCCC 2017. Eur Urol. 2018;73(2):178–211. https://www.sciencedirect.com/science/article/pii/S0302283817304979
7. Komura K, Sweeney CJ, Inamoto T, Ibuki N, Azuma H, Kantoff PW. Current treatment strategies for advanced prostate cancer. Int J Urol. 2018;25(3):220–31.
8. Sathianathen NJ, Konety BR, Crook J, Saad F, Lawrentschuk N. Landmarks in prostate cancer. Nat Rev Urol. 2018;15(10):627–42.
9. Gillessen S, Bossi A, Davis ID, de Bono J, Fizazi K, James ND, et al. Management of patients with advanced prostate cancer—metastatic and/or castration-resistant prostate cancer: report of the Advanced Prostate Cancer Consensus Conference (APCCC) 2022. Eur J Cancer. 2023;185:178–215.
10. Smith MR, Saad F, Chowdhury S, Oudard S, Hadaschik BA, Graff JN, et al. Apalutamide and overall survival in prostate cancer. Eur Urol. 2021;79(1):150–8.
11. Porter CM, Shrestha E, Peiffer LB, Sfanos KS. The microbiome in prostate inflammation and prostate cancer. Prostate Cancer Prostatic Dis. 2018;21(3):345–54.

12. Subramani IG, Ayub RM, Gopinath SCB, Perumal V, Fathil MFM, Arshad MKM. Lectin bioreceptor approach in capacitive biosensor for prostate-specific membrane antigen detection in diagnosing prostate cancer. J Taiwan Inst Chem Eng. 2021;120:9–16.
13. Zhao J, Ma H, Liu Y, Xu B, Song L, Han X, et al. SERS-based biosensor for detection of f-PSA%: implications for the diagnosis of prostate cancer. Talanta. 2023;261:124654.
14. Chen W, Li J, Wei X, Fan Y, Qian H, Li S, et al. Surface plasmon resonance biosensor using hydrogel-AuNP supramolecular spheres for determination of prostate cancer-derived exosomes. Microchim Acta. 2020;187:1–10.
15. Akbari jonous Z, Shayeh JS, Yazdian F, Yadegari A, Hashemi M, Omidi M. An electrochemical biosensor for prostate cancer biomarker detection using graphene oxide–gold nanostructures. Eng Life Sci. 2019;19(3):206–16.
16. Deswal R, Narwal V, Kumar P, Verma V, Dang AS, Pundir CS. An improved amperometric sarcosine biosensor based on graphene nanoribbon/chitosan nanocomposite for detection of prostate cancer. Sensors Int. 2022;3:100174.
17. Ferraro S, Bussetti M, Bassani N, Rossi RS, Incarbone GP, Bianchi F, et al. Definition of outcome-based prostate-specific antigen (PSA) thresholds for advanced prostate cancer risk prediction. Cancers (Basel). 2021;13(14):3381.
18. Rodríguez SVM, García-Perdomo HA. Diagnostic accuracy of prostate cancer antigen 3 (PCA3) prior to first prostate biopsy: A systematic review and meta-analysis. Can Urol Assoc J = J l'Association des Urol du Canada. 2020 May;14(5):E214–9.
19. Corpetti M, Müller C, Beltran H, de Bono J, Theurillat JP. Prostate-specific membrane antigen–targeted therapies for prostate cancer: towards improving therapeutic outcomes. Eur Urol. 2024;85(3):193–204. https://www.sciencedirect.com/science/article/pii/S0302283823032785.
20. Bilal M, Javaid A, Amjad F, Youssif TA, Afzal S. An overview of prostate cancer (PCa) diagnosis: potential role of miRNAs. Transl Oncol 2022;26:101542. https://www.sciencedirect.com/science/article/pii/S1936523322002017.
21. Nordström T, Akre O, Aly M, Grönberg H, Eklund M. Prostate-specific antigen (PSA) density in the diagnostic algorithm of prostate cancer. Prostate Cancer Prostatic Dis. 2018;21(1):57–63.
22. Moradi A, Srinivasan S, Clements J, Batra J. Beyond the biomarker role: prostate-specific antigen (PSA) in the prostate cancer microenvironment. Cancer Metastasis Rev. 2019;38:333–46.
23. Pathirana T, Sequeira R, Del Mar C, Dickinson JA, Armstrong BK, Bell KJL, et al. Trends in prostate specific antigen (PSA) testing and prostate cancer incidence and mortality in Australia: A critical analysis. Cancer Epidemiol. 2022;77:102093.
24. Gandaglia G, Albers P, Abrahamsson PA, Briganti A, Catto JWF, Chapple CR, et al. Structured population-based prostate-specific antigen screening for prostate cancer: the European Association of Urology position in 2019. Eur Urol 2019;76(2):142–150. https://www.sciencedirect.com/science/article/pii/S0302283819303471.
25. Farshchi F, Hasanzadeh M. Nanomaterial based aptasensing of prostate specific antigen (PSA): recent progress and challenges in efficient diagnosis of prostate cancer using biomedicine. Biomed Pharmacother. 2020;132:110878. https://www.sciencedirect.com/science/article/pii/S0753332220310702
26. Grammatikopoulou MG, Gkiouras K, Papageorgiou ST, Myrogiannis I, Mykoniatis I, Papamitsou T, et al. Dietary factors and supplements influencing prostate-specific antigen (PSA) concentrations in men with prostate cancer and increased cancer risk: An Evidence Analysis Review Based on Randomized Controlled Trials. Nutrients. 2020;12(10). https://www.mdpi.com/2072-6643/12/10/2985
27. Arrighetti N, Beretta GL. miRNAs as therapeutic tools and biomarkers for prostate cancer. Pharmaceutics. 2021;13(3). https://www.mdpi.com/1999-4923/13/3/380
28. Paschalis A, Sheehan B, Riisnaes R, Rodrigues DN, Gurel B, Bertan C, et al. Prostate-specific membrane antigen heterogeneity and DNA repair defects in prostate cancer. Eur Urol. 2019;76(4):469–78. https://www.sciencedirect.com/science/article/pii/S0302283819305202

29. Gandhi J, Afridi A, Vatsia S, Joshi G, Joshi G, Kaplan SA, et al. The molecular biology of prostate cancer: current understanding and clinical implications. Prostate Cancer Prostatic Dis. 2018;21(1):22–36. https://doi.org/10.1038/s41391-017-0023-8.
30. Matoso A, Epstein JI. Defining clinically significant prostate cancer on the basis of pathological findings. Histopathology. 2019;74(1):135–45.
31. Tonry C, Finn S, Armstrong J, Pennington SR. Clinical proteomics for prostate cancer: understanding prostate cancer pathology and protein biomarkers for improved disease management. Clin Proteomics. 2020;17(1):41. https://doi.org/10.1186/s12014-020-09305-7.
32. Haffner MC, Zwart W, Roudier MP, True LD, Nelson WG, Epstein JI, et al. Genomic and phenotypic heterogeneity in prostate cancer. Nat Rev Urol. 2021;18(2):79–92. https://doi.org/10.1038/s41585-020-00400-w.
33. Liu S, Xu Y, Jiang X, Tan H, Ying B. Translation of aptamers toward clinical diagnosis and commercialization. Biosens Bioelectron. 2022;208:114168.
34. Wallis CJD, Glaser A, Hu JC, Huland H, Lawrentschuk N, Moon D, et al. Survival and complications following surgery and radiation for localized prostate cancer: an international collaborative review. Eur Urol. 2018;73(1):11–20. https://www.sciencedirect.com/science/article/pii/S0302283817304955
35. von Eyben FE, Picchio M, von Eyben R, Rhee H, Bauman G. 68Ga-labeled prostate-specific membrane antigen ligand positron emission tomography/computed tomography for prostate cancer: A systematic review and meta-analysis. Eur Urol Focus. 2018;4(5):686–93. https://www.sciencedirect.com/science/article/pii/S2405456916301602
36. Cheng ML, Pectasides E, Hanna GJ, Parsons HA, Choudhury AD, Oxnard GR. Circulating tumor DNA in advanced solid tumors: clinical relevance and future directions. CA Cancer J Clin. 2021;71(2):176–90.
37. Afsarimanesh N, Mukhopadhyay SC, Kruger M. Electrochemical biosensor: point-of-care for early detection of bone loss, vol. 30. Springer; 2019.
38. Negahdary M, Angnes L. Application of electrochemical biosensors for the detection of microRNAs (miRNAs) related to cancer. Coord Chem Rev. 2022;464:214565.
39. Hu Y, Lv S, Wan J, Zheng C, Shao D, Wang H, et al. Recent advances in nanomaterials for prostate cancer detection and diagnosis. J Mater Chem B. 2022;10(26):4907–34.
40. Bertok T, Lorencova L, Chocholova E, Jane E, Vikartovska A, Kasak P, et al. Electrochemical impedance spectroscopy based biosensors: mechanistic principles, analytical examples and challenges towards commercialization for assays of protein cancer biomarkers. ChemElectroChem. 2019;6(4):989–1003.
41. Li CH, Chan MH, Chang YC, Hsiao M. Gold nanoparticles as a biosensor for cancer biomarker determination. Molecules. 2023;28(1). https://www.mdpi.com/1420-3049/28/1/364
42. Mohan B, Mehak, Virender, Kumar A, Modi K, Singh G, et al. Detecting cancer biomarkers using electrochemical composite nanomaterials tools. Vietnam J Chem. 2024;
43. Son MH, Park SW, Sagong HY, Jung YK. Recent advances in electrochemical and optical biosensors for cancer biomarker detection. BioChip J. 2023;17(1):44–67. https://doi.org/10.1007/s13206-022-00089-6.
44. Zhao B, Miao P, Hu Z, Zhang X, Geng X, Chen Y, et al. Signal-on electrochemical aptasensors with different target-induced conformations for prostate specific antigen detection. Anal Chim Acta. 2021;1152:338282. https://www.sciencedirect.com/science/article/pii/S0003267021001082
45. Mladenović M, Jarić S, Mundžić M, Pavlović A, Bobrinetskiy I, Knežević NŽ. Biosensors for cancer biomarkers based on mesoporous silica nanoparticles. Biosensors. 2024;14(7). https://www.mdpi.com/2079-6374/14/7/326
46. Palakollu VN, Veera Manohara Reddy Y, Shekh MI, Vattikuti SVP, Shim J, Karpoormath R. Electrochemical immunosensing of tumor markers. Clin Chim Acta. 2024;557:117882. https://www.sciencedirect.com/science/article/pii/S0009898124001232
47. Fu L, Zheng Y, Li X, Liu X, Lin CT, Karimi-Maleh H. Strategies and applications of graphene and its derivatives-based electrochemical sensors in cancer diagnosis. Molecules. 2023;28(18). https://www.mdpi.com/1420-3049/28/18/6719

48. Ho KV, Tatum DS, Watkinson L, Carmack T, Jia F, Mascioni A, et al. Single chelator–minibody theranostic agents for 89Zr PET imaging and 177Lu radiopharmaceutical therapy of PSMA-expressing prostate cancer. J Nucl Med. 2024;65(9):1435–42.
49. Afshary H, Amiri M, Marken F, McKeown NB, Amiri M. ECL sensor for selective determination of citrate ions as a prostate cancer biomarker using polymer of intrinsic microporosity-1 nanoparticles/nitrogen-doped carbon quantum dots. Anal Bioanal Chem. 2023;415(14):2727–36. https://doi.org/10.1007/s00216-023-04672-0.
50. Cameron M, Frame F, Maitland NJ, Hancock Y. Raman spectroscopy reveals oxidative stress-induced metabolic vulnerabilities in early-stage AR-negative prostate-cancer versus normal-prostate cell lines. Sci Rep. 2024;14(1):25388. https://doi.org/10.1038/s41598-024-70338-1.
51. Benjamin SR, Júnior EJMR. Recent advances in designing porous carbon nanomaterial based for electrochemical biosensing prostate cancer. In: Grace AN, Sonar P, Bhardwaj P, Chakravorty A, editors. Handbook of porous carbon materials. Singapore: Springer Nature Singapore; 2023. p. 1007–34. https://doi.org/10.1007/978-981-19-7188-4_36.
52. Liu X, Chen L, Li Y, He C, Zhang X, Zhou H, et al. Synthesis of novel DOTA−/AAZTA-based bifunctional chelators: solution thermodynamics, peptidomimetic conjugation, and radiopharmaceutical evaluation. Biomed Pharmacother. 2023;165:115114. https://www.sciencedirect.com/science/article/pii/S0753332223009058.
53. Noreen S, Ishaq I, Saleem MH, Ali B, Muhammad Ali S, Iqbal J. Electrochemical biosensing in oncology: a review advancements and prospects for cancer diagnosis. Cancer Biol Ther. 2025;26(1):2475581.
54. Hroncekova S, Lorencova L, Bertok T, Hires M, Jane E, Bučko M, et al. Amperometric miniaturised portable enzymatic Nanobiosensor for the ultrasensitive analysis of a prostate cancer biomarker. J Funct Biomater. 2023;14(3). https://www.mdpi.com/2079-4983/14/3/161
55. Nabok A, Abu-Ali H, Takita S, Smith DP. Electrochemical detection of prostate cancer biomarker PCA3 using specific RNA-based Aptamer labelled with Ferrocene. Chem Int. 2021;9(4). https://www.mdpi.com/2227-9040/9/4/59
56. Solovieva S, Karnaukh M, Panchuk V, Andreev E, Kartsova L, Bessonova E, et al. Potentiometric multisensor system as a possible simple tool for non-invasive prostate cancer diagnostics through urine analysis. Sensors Actuators B Chem. 2019;289:42–7. https://www.sciencedirect.com/science/article/pii/S0925400519304290
57. Pundir CS, Ritu D, Kumar P. Quantitative analysis of sarcosine with special emphasis on biosensors: a review. Biomarkers. 2019;24(5):415–22. https://doi.org/10.1080/1354750X.2019.1615124.
58. Chen H, Zhang J, Huang R, Wang D, Deng D, Zhang Q, et al. The applications of electrochemical immunosensors in the detection of disease biomarkers: A review. Molecules. 2023;28(8):3605.
59. Britto JSJ, Guan X, Tran TKA, Lei Z, Bahadur R, Patel V, et al. Emerging multifunctional carbon-nanomaterial-based biosensors for cancer diagnosis. Small Sci. 2024;4(3):2300221.
60. Badillo-Ramírez I, Carreón YJP, Rodríguez-Almazán C, Medina-Durán CM, Islas SR, Saniger JM. Graphene-based biosensors for molecular chronic inflammatory disease biomarker detection. Biosensors. 2022;12(4). https://www.mdpi.com/2079-6374/12/4/244
61. Bishnoi M, Deepika, Mody N, Jain A. Biomedical applications of nano-biosensor. In: Gopi S, Balakrishnan P, Mubarak NM, editors. Nanotechnology for biomedical applications [internet]. Singapore: Springer Singapore; 2022. p. 219–46. https://doi.org/10.1007/978-981-16-7483-9_10.
62. Tezcan T, Hsu CH. Nanotechnology in healthcare: nanoparticles for diagnostic and therapy. In: Biotechnology in healthcare. Elsevier; 2022. p. 55–69.
63. Rezaei Z, Alemzadeh I, Vossoughi M. Design and fabrication of an electrochemical-based nanofibrous immunosensor for detection of prostate cancer biomarker. PSMA Polym Adv Technol. 2022;33(6):1967–77.
64. Singh B, Ma S, Hara TO, Singh S. Nanomaterials-based biosensors for the detection of prostate cancer biomarkers: recent trends and future perspective. Adv Mater Technol. 2023;8(13):2201860.

65. Dehghani P, Karthikeyan V, Tajabadi A, Assi DS, Catchpole A, Wadsworth J, et al. Rapid near-patient Impedimetric sensing platform for prostate cancer diagnosis. ACS Omega. 2024 Mar 26;9(12):14580–91. https://doi.org/10.1021/acsomega.4c00843.
66. Alake J, Mahlalela MC, Mohite S, Partap S, Gafar MA, Adu DK, et al. Computational, microscale thermophoresis and electrochemical study of a hepta-peptide for a simple, sensitive electrochemical biosensor for PSA. Microchem J. 2024;206:111386. https://www.sciencedirect.com/science/article/pii/S0026265X2401498X
67. Sheydaei O, Khajehsharifi H, Rajabi HR. Rapid and selective diagnose of sarcosine in urine samples as prostate cancer biomarker by mesoporous imprinted polymeric nanobeads modified electrode. Sensors Actuators B Chem. 2020;309:127559. https://www.sciencedirect.com/science/article/pii/S0925400519317587
68. Mehrabi A, Rahimnejad M, Mohammadi M, Pourali M. Electrochemical detection of Flutamide as an anticancer drug with gold nanoparticles modified glassy carbon electrode in the presence of prostate cancer cells. J Appl Electrochem. 2021;51(4):597–606. https://doi.org/10.1007/s10800-020-01519-9.
69. Ibau C, Md Arshad MK, Gopinath SCB, Nuzaihan MNM, M. Fathil MF, Estrela P. Gold interdigitated triple-microelectrodes for label-free prognosticative aptasensing of prostate cancer biomarker in serum. Biosens Bioelectron. 2019;136:118–27. https://www.sciencedirect.com/science/article/pii/S0956566319303380
70. Yan L, Zhang C, Xi F. Disposable amperometric label-free Immunosensor on chitosan–graphene-modified patterned ITO electrodes for prostate specific antigen. Molecules. 2022;27(18). https://www.mdpi.com/1420-3049/27/18/5895
71. Thambiraj S, Vijayalakshmi R, Ravi Shankaran D. An effective strategy for development of docetaxel encapsulated gold nanoformulations for treatment of prostate cancer. Sci Rep. 2021;11(1):2808.
72. de Araujo JTC, Duarte JL, Di Filippo LD, Araujo VHS, Carvalho GC, Chorilli M. Nanosystem functionalization strategies for prostate cancer treatment: a review. J Drug Target. 2021;29(8):808–21.
73. Choksi AU, Khan AI, Lokeshwar SD, Segal D, Weiss RM, Martin DT. Functionalized nanoparticles targeting biomarkers for prostate cancer imaging and therapy. Am J Clin Exp Urol. 2022;10(3):142.
74. Yari H, Nkepang G, Awasthi V. Surface modification of liposomes by a lipopolymer targeting prostate specific membrane antigen for theranostic delivery in prostate cancer. Materials (Basel). 2019;12(5):756.
75. Barani M, Sabir F, Rahdar A, Arshad R, Kyzas GZ. Nanotreatment and nanodiagnosis of prostate cancer: recent updates. Nano. 2020;10(9):1696.
76. Gorgani L, Mohammadi M, Najafpour Darzi G, Raoof JB. Metal-organic framework (MOF)-based biosensors for miRNA detection. Talanta. 2024;273:125854. https://www.sciencedirect.com/science/article/pii/S0039914024002339
77. Noori R, Ahmad R, Sardar M. Nanobiosensor in health sector: the milestones achieved and future prospects. In: Mohsin M, Naz R, Ahmad A, editors. Nanobiosensors for agricultural, medical and environmental applications. Singapore: Springer Singapore; 2020. p. 63–90. https://doi.org/10.1007/978-981-15-8346-9_4.
78. Tabassum S, Kumar R. Advances in fiber-optic technology for point-of-care diagnosis and in vivo biosensing. Adv Mater Technol. 2020;5(5):1900792.
79. Padash M, Faridafshin M, Nouroozi A. Electrochemical biosensors. In: Sensors for next-generation electronic systems and technologies. CRC Press; 2023. p. 71–123.
80. Varaprasad GL, Gupta VK, Prasad K, Kim E, Tej MB, Mohanty P, et al. Recent advances and future perspectives in the therapeutics of prostate cancer. Exp Hematol Oncol. 2023;12(1):80. https://doi.org/10.1186/s40164-023-00444-9.
81. Zhao J, Zhang C, Wang W, Li C, Mu X, Hu K. Current progress of nanomedicine for prostate cancer diagnosis and treatment. Biomed Pharmacother. 2022;155:113714. https://www.sciencedirect.com/science/article/pii/S0753332222011039

82. Couñago F, López-Campos F, Díaz-Gavela AA, Almagro E, Fenández-Pascual E, Henríquez I, et al. Clinical applications of molecular biomarkers in prostate cancer. Cancers (Basel). 2020;12(6). https://www.mdpi.com/2072-6694/12/6/1550
83. Testa U, Castelli G, Pelosi E. Cellular and molecular mechanisms underlying prostate cancer development: therapeutic implications. Medicines. 2019;6(3). https://www.mdpi.com/2305-6320/6/3/82
84. Chan KM, Gleadle JM, O'Callaghan M, Vasilev K, MacGregor M. Prostate cancer detection: a systematic review of urinary biosensors. Prostate Cancer Prostatic Dis. 2022;25(1):39–46. https://doi.org/10.1038/s41391-021-00480-8.
85. Broomfield J, Kalofonou M, Bevan CL, Georgiou P. Recent electrochemical advancements for liquid-biopsy nucleic acid detection for point-of-care prostate cancer diagnostics and prognostics. Biosensors. 2024;14(9). https://www.mdpi.com/2079-6374/14/9/443
86. Le LTP, Nguyen AHQ, Phan LMT, Ngo HTT, Wang X, Cunningham B, et al. Current smartphone-assisted point-of-care cancer detection: towards supporting personalized cancer monitoring. TrAC Trends Anal Chem. 2024;174:117681. https://www.sciencedirect.com/science/article/pii/S0165993624001638
87. Hwang IM, Cantu CM, Chawla R, Kamei DT. Biosensor-based point-of-care devices: detection of infectious diseases and cancer. In: Borse V, Chandra P, Srivastava R, editors. BioSensing, Theranostics, and medical devices: from laboratory to point-of-care testing [internet]. Singapore: Springer Singapore; 2022. p. 105–32. https://doi.org/10.1007/978-981-16-2782-8_5.
88. Mandal N, Pakira V, Samanta N, Das N, Chakraborty S, Pramanick B, et al. PSA detection using label free graphene FET with coplanar electrodes based microfluidic point of care diagnostic device. Talanta. 2021;222:121581. https://www.sciencedirect.com/science/article/pii/S0039914020308729
89. Asci Erkocyigit B, Ozufuklar O, Yardim A, Guler Celik E, Timur S. Biomarker detection in early diagnosis of cancer: recent achievements in point-of-care devices based on paper microfluidics. Biosensors. 2023;13(3). https://www.mdpi.com/2079-6374/13/3/387
90. Li P, Lee GH, Kim SY, Kwon SY, Kim HR, Park S. From diagnosis to treatment: recent advances in patient-friendly biosensors and implantable devices. ACS Nano. 2021;15(2):1960–2004. https://doi.org/10.1021/acsnano.0c06688.
91. Hazra RS, Hasan Khan MR, Kale N, Tanha T, Khandare J, Ganai S, et al. Bioinspired materials for wearable devices and point-of-care testing of cancer. ACS Biomater Sci Eng. 2023 May 8;9(5):2103–28. https://doi.org/10.1021/acsbiomaterials.1c01208.
92. Sarac B, Yücer S, Sahin H, Unal M, Ciftci F. Wearable and implantable bioelectronic: biosensing contact lens and applications. Chem Eng J. 2024;491:152016. https://www.sciencedirect.com/science/article/pii/S1385894724035034
93. Kar A, Ahamad N, Dewani M, Awasthi L, Patil R, Banerjee R. Wearable and implantable devices for drug delivery: applications and challenges. Biomaterials. 2022;283:121435. https://www.sciencedirect.com/science/article/pii/S0142961222000746
94. Bakri MH, Özarslan AC, Erarslan A, Basaran Elalmis Y, Ciftci F. Biomedical applications of wearable biosensors. Next Mater. 2024;3:100084. https://www.sciencedirect.com/science/article/pii/S2949822823000849
95. Wang J, Huang X, Xie J, Han Y, Huang Y, Zhang H. Exosomal analysis: advances in biosensor technology. Clin Chim Acta. 2021;518:142–50. https://www.sciencedirect.com/science/article/pii/S000989812100111X
96. Wijayanti SD, Tsvik L, Haltrich D. Recent advances in electrochemical enzyme-based biosensors for food and beverage analysis. Foods. 2023;12(18). https://www.mdpi.com/2304-8158/12/18/3355
97. Joshi V, Upadhyay A, Amanullah A, Mishra R, Mishra A. Predicting E3 ubiquitin ligases as possible promising biomarkers for brain tumors. In: Shukla KK, Sharma P, Misra S, editors. Molecular diagnostics in cancer patients [internet]. Singapore: Springer Singapore; 2019. p. 43–72. https://doi.org/10.1007/978-981-13-5877-7_4.

98. Malode SJ, Ali Alshehri M, Shetti NP. Nanomaterial-based electrochemical sensors for the detection of pharmaceutical drugs. Chem Int. 2024;12(11). https://www.mdpi.com/2227-9040/12/11/234
99. Yamin M, Raza HG, Fatima I. Nanomaterial-based electrochemical sensors for the detection of pharmaceutical drugs. In: Masood N, Shakil Malik S, editors. Essentials of cancer genomic, computational approaches and precision medicine [internet]. Singapore: Springer Singapore; 2020. p. 3–33. https://doi.org/10.1007/978-981-15-1067-0_1.
100. Campuzano S, Pedrero M, Pingarrón JM. Non-invasive breast cancer diagnosis through electrochemical biosensing at different molecular levels. Sensors. 2017;17(9). https://www.mdpi.com/1424-8220/17/9/1993
101. Ragothaman M, Yoo SY. Engineered phage-based cancer vaccines: current advances and future directions. Vaccines. 2023;11(5). https://www.mdpi.com/2076-393X/11/5/919
102. Bai Y, Xu T, Zhang X. Graphene-based biosensors for detection of biomarkers. Micromachines. 2020;11(1). https://www.mdpi.com/2072-666X/11/1/60
103. Khan T, Altamimi MA, Hussain A, Ramzan M, Ashique S, Alhuzani MR, et al. Understanding of PSA biology, factors affecting PSA detection, challenges, various biomarkers, methods, and future perspective of prostate cancer detection and diagnosis. Adv Cancer Biol - Metastasis. 2022;5:100059. https://www.sciencedirect.com/science/article/pii/S2667394022000338
104. Pal M, Khan R. Graphene oxide layer decorated gold nanoparticles based immunosensor for the detection of prostate cancer risk factor. Anal Biochem. 2017;536:51–8. https://www.sciencedirect.com/science/article/pii/S0003269717303330
105. Jang HD, Kim SK, Chang H, Choi JW. 3D label-free prostate specific antigen (PSA) immunosensor based on graphene-gold composites. Biosens Bioelectron. 2015;63:546–51.
106. Heydari-Bafrooei E, Shamszadeh NS. Electrochemical bioassay development for ultrasensitive aptasensing of prostate specific antigen. Biosens Bioelectron. 2017;91:284–92.
107. Wei B, Mao K, Liu N, Zhang M, Yang Z. Graphene nanocomposites modified electrochemical aptamer sensor for rapid and highly sensitive detection of prostate specific antigen. Biosens Bioelectron. 2018;121:41–6. https://www.sciencedirect.com/science/article/pii/S0956566318306730
108. Alnaimi A, Al-Hamry A, Makableh Y, Adiraju A, Kanoun O. Gold nanoparticles-MWCNT based Aptasensor for early diagnosis of prostate cancer. Biosensors. 2022;12(12). https://www.mdpi.com/2079-6374/12/12/1130
109. Sengupta J, Hussain CM. Early detection of cancer utilizing biosensors based on "green graphene": an innovative and sustainable methodology for advancing cancer diagnosis. TrAC Trends Anal Chem. 2023;167:117254. https://www.sciencedirect.com/science/article/pii/S0165993623003412
110. Hemdan M, Ali MA, Doghish AS, Mageed SSA, Elazab IM, Khalil MM, et al. Innovations in biosensor technologies for healthcare diagnostics and therapeutic drug monitoring: applications, recent progress, and future research challenges. Sensors (Basel). 2024;24(16)
111. Hunt A, Slaughter G. Electrochemical detection of prostate cancer—associated miRNA-141 using a low-cost disposable biosensor. Biosensors. 2025;15(6). https://www.mdpi.com/2079-6374/15/6/364
112. Garg S, Sachdeva A, Peeters M, McClements J. Point-of-care prostate specific antigen testing: examining translational Progress toward clinical implementation. ACS Sensors. 2023;8(10):3643–58. https://doi.org/10.1021/acssensors.3c01402.
113. Mayoral-Peña K, González Peña OI, Orrantia Clark AM, Flores-Vallejo R del C, Oza G, Sharma A, et al. Biorecognition engineering Technologies for Cancer Diagnosis: A systematic literature review of non-conventional and plausible sensor development methods. Cancers (Basel) 2022;14(8). https://www.mdpi.com/2072-6694/14/8/1867
114. Sanko V, Kuralay F. Label-free electrochemical biosensor platforms for cancer diagnosis: recent achievements and challenges. Biosensors. 2023;13(3). https://www.mdpi.com/2079-6374/13/3/333

115. Moulahoum H, Ghorbanizamani F. The LOD paradox: when lower isn't always better in biosensor research and development. Biosens Bioelectron. 2024;264:116670. https://www.sciencedirect.com/science/article/pii/S0956566324006766
116. Ahmed Taha B, Kadhim AC, Addie AJ, Haider AJ, Azzahrani AS, Raizada P, et al. Advancing cancer diagnostics through multifaceted optical biosensors supported by nanomaterials and artificial intelligence: A panoramic outlook. Microchem J. 2024;205:111307. https://www.sciencedirect.com/science/article/pii/S0026265X2401419X
117. Thakur S, Kumari M, Kumar N, Kumar S, Gandhi S, Bhaduri GA, et al. Fundamentals, fabrication, engineering, and prototyping aspects of bioelectronics and biosensors for biomedical analysis. In: Mahato K, Chandra P, editors. Biosensors for personalized healthcare [internet]. Singapore: Springer Nature Singapore; 2024. p. 69–114. https://doi.org/10.1007/978-981-97-5473-1_4.
118. Yadav L, Yadav A, Chatterjee S, Tyeb S, Gupta RK, Sen P, et al. Red-emitting polyaniline-based nanoparticle probe for pH-sensitive fluorescence imaging. Biomater Adv. 2022;140:213088. https://www.sciencedirect.com/science/article/pii/S277295082200365X
119. Singh J, Nayak P, Singh G, Khandai M, Sarangi RR, Kar MK. Carbon nanostructures as therapeutic cargoes: recent developments and challenges. C. 2023;9(1). https://www.mdpi.com/2311-5629/9/1/3
120. Chaurawal N, Raza K. Nano-interventions for the drug delivery of docetaxel to cancer cells. Heal Sci Rev. 2023;7:100101. https://www.sciencedirect.com/science/article/pii/S2772632023000272

Optical Biosensor: Techniques and Applications Against Prostate Cancer

5

Sakshi Patel, Stuti Verma, Mohammed El-Tanani, and Sathvik Belagodu Sridhar

Abbreviations

PSA	prostate-specific antigen
SPR	surface plasmon resonance
CTC	circulating tumor cell
SERS	surface-enhanced Raman scattering
LOC	lab-on-a-chip
AI	artificial intelligence
miRNA	microRNA
DRE	digital rectal examination
FRET	Förster resonance energy transfer
CCD	charge-coupled device (used in optical detectors)
PHI	Prostate Health Index

S. Patel
Department of Pharmaceutical Technology, Meerut Institute of Engineering & Technology, Meerut, Uttar Pradesh, India

S. Verma
Department of Pharmacy, Aryakul College of Pharmacy and Research, Sitapur, Uttar Pradesh, India

M. El-Tanani · S. B. Sridhar (✉)
RAK College of Pharmacy, RAK Medical & Health Sciences University, Ras al Khaimah, United Arab Emirates
e-mail: eltanani@rakmhsu.ac.ae; sathvik@rakmhsu.ac.ae

S. Srivastava et al. (eds.), *Biosensor Technologies for Prostate Cancer*,
https://doi.org/10.1007/978-981-95-8644-8_5

5.1 Introduction

Prostate cancer ranks as one of the leading cancers that develops in men across the globe, predominantly among older male patients [1]. Prostate cancer develops from the prostate gland, which is the smallest yet essential reproductive system part of males, and it can evolve from harmless to life-threatening metastatic disease [2]. Prostate cancer occupies a position among the top cancer-related death causes that affect men throughout developed nations worldwide, based on global cancer data [3]. Advanced therapeutic approaches have improved, yet the disease stage at diagnosis remains the primary determinant of treatment effectiveness for patients [4]. The early detection of prostate cancer presents a problem since the condition frequently shows no warning signs during this stage [5]. DRE, digital rectal examination, together with prostate-specific antigen (PSA) testing and tissue biopsy, holds traditional prominence in prostate cancer diagnosis, yet falls short due to weak sensitivity, poor specificity, and invasive nature and risk of overdiagnosis [6]. Early detection of cancer remains essential, as early diagnosis can improve patient survival and minimize the need for intensive medical interventions while preserving the quality of the patient's lifestyle [7]. Due to widespread PSA screening, numerous erroneous results lead to both false positives and unnecessary biopsies [8]. The current diagnostic challenges underscore the urgent need to develop high-accuracy, non-invasive diagnostic methods [9]. The use of circulating tumor cells (CTCs), along with exosomal microRNAs and cancer-specific antigens, has been shown to effectively aid in developing more accurate diagnoses over the past several years [10]. Progress in biosensor development is one of the determinants of achieving appropriate detection of these biomarkers. Biosensors are analytical instruments that combine a biological recognition element with a physicochemical sensing mechanism to detect target molecules with enhanced sensitivity and selectivity [11]. The major characteristics that make optical biosensors shine are their rapid responses, unmarked detection, and the ability to scale down and support point-of-care operations [12].

Several medical devices monitor changes in blood, urine, and saliva samples using a combination of fluorescence analysis, surface plasmon resonance (SPR), and Raman scattering [13]. The integration of prostate-specific antigen assays with extracellular vesicles from cancer identified at an early stage, when prostate cancer is not yet manifested, enables optical biosensors to demonstrate high potential for detecting prostate cancer [14]. Current diagnostic research employs optical biosensors to enable real-time illness monitoring and to hasten treatment procedures, while also developing patient-centered care-based treatment plans [15]. The chapter is based on an analysis of how technical advances in optical biosensors and the knowledge they yield can enable early-stage clinical diagnosis of prostate cancer [16].

5.2 Fundamentals of Optical Biosensors

The optical biosensing field has developed novel analytical instruments that exploit light interactions with biological substances to detect specific substances with the highest possible sensitivity and deliver prompt, accurate results [17]. This section

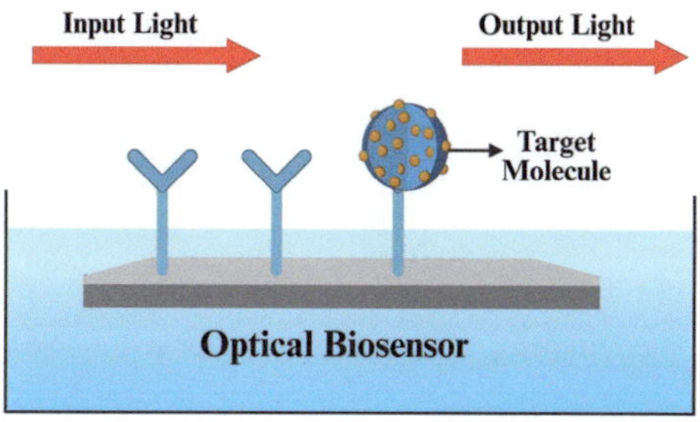

Fig. 5.1 Working principle of an optical biosensor

Table 5.1 Comparison of optical biosensing principles

Principle	Description	Key advantage	Limitation	Example of application	References
Label-free	No labels or dyes used	Real-time analysis	May require complex setup	SPR	[22, 23]
Label-based	Uses fluorescent/dye tags	High sensitivity	May alter biomolecule behavior	ELISA	[24]

begins by explaining fundamental optical biosensing principles (Fig. 5.1) that demonstrate how biological recognition enables the generation of measurable optical signals [18].

Surface plasmon resonance (SPR) joins fluorescence, Raman scattering, and interferometric methods as part of the diverse set of optical transduction techniques that offer specific advantages for particular applications [19]. The section outlines the fundamental elements and structural engineering principles of optical biosensors, explaining how these diagnostic tools are designed for early detection and monitoring of prostate cancer [20]. Table 5.1 outlines key aspects of optical biosensing principles, demonstrating the advantages and their corresponding limitations [21].

5.2.1 Principles of Optical Biosensing

Biosensing by means of light utilizes biological-analytical detection methods that employ molecular-light interactions for sensitive and specific detection of biochemical elements [25]. An optical biosensor enables the measurement of biological recognition events through optical signals arising from biological interactions, such as analyte-receptor binding [26]. Light signals generated during analysis display either intensity modification, wavelength alteration, index-of-refraction transformation, or polarization effects, depending on the selected optical detection method [27]. The success of optical biosensing depends on a biorecognition element affixed to the sensor surface that specifically binds target molecules [28]. A measured change in optical sensor properties occurs when an analyte interacts with it, correlating with particular changes in sample concentration [29]. The key advantage of optical biosensors stems from their ability to perform untagged detection, provide real-time

Table 5.2 Types of optical transduction techniques

Technique	Signal type	Sensitivity	Label required	Common use case	References
Fluorescence	Light intensity	High	Yes	DNA hybridization	[33]
SPR	Refractive index	High	No	Protein–ligand interaction	[30]
Interferometry	Phase shift	Moderate	No	Thin film detection	[34]
Colorimetry	Color change	Low–moderate	Sometimes	Glucose detection	[35]

analysis, and support multiple analysis modes simultaneously [23]. The high sensitivity, along with their non-invasive characteristics, makes fluorescent biosensors specifically suitable for cancer detection through clinical diagnosis because they enable accurate early biomarker identification.

5.2.2 Types of Optical Transduction Techniques

Different types of transduction mechanisms operate in optical biosensors, and each system is suited to applications with specific sensitivity requirements [30]. Key optical transduction techniques include [31]. Table 5.2 summarizes optical transduction methods and their application scope for biosensing [32].

Surface Plasmon Resonance (SPR): This technique exploits the resonance oscillation of conduction electrons at a metal-dielectric interface, using gold films [36]. The sensitivity of SPR detection changes when refractive index conditions fluctuate at sensor boundaries, enabling time-dependent biomolecular detection. *Fluorescence-Based Detection*: Biochemical sensors that use fluorescent components detect biochemical changes by emitting light upon excitation [37]. The instrument measures fluorescence emissions, providing easy-to-understand data on the targets of detection. Quantum dots and Förster Resonance Energy Transfer systems are generally used in research groups to improve detection sensitivity and specificity. *Raman and Surface-Enhanced Raman Scattering (SERS)*: The molecular fingerprints generated by Raman spectroscopy are the result of light scattering in accordance with the Raman and Surface-Enhanced Raman Scattering (SERS) technique [38]. Weak Raman signals can be expanded by several orders of magnitude when researchers use plasmonic nanostructures in SERS detection methods, enabling high-sensitivity detection of cancer biomarkers. *Interferometry and Photonic Crystal Biosensors*: Detecting small optical path variations as well as refractive index modifications is possible through sensors that leverage light interference effects together with their photonic crystal structures [39]. These devices are recognized for their high specificity and suitability for high-volume laboratory assays. The choice between these techniques depends on various factors, including the diagnostic application, the target molecule, and the required sensitivity and integration format [40].

5.2.3 Components and Architecture of Optical Biosensors

A standard optical biosensor system requires three fundamental operational parts: the biorecognition element and the optical transducer, followed by the signal processing unit [41]. The biorecognition element acts as a detection system through specific interactions between the sensor and the target analyte, using biomacromolecules such as antibodies, aptamers, and enzymes, as well as synthetic receptors [42]. Target-initiated sensing follows after the target binds selectively to an element immobilized on the sensor surface [43]. The biorecognition interaction becomes detectable optical signals through the operation of the optical transducer [44]. The transducer component selects its operating mode based on changes in light absorption, fluorescence, refractive index, and Raman scattering signals, depending on the optical biosensor type [45]. The selected transduction technique fundamentally affects how the sensor measures sensitivity, together with its specificity performance and detection threshold [46]. The signal processing unit obtains meaningful quantitative or qualitative data by receiving, amplifying, and analyzing optical signals [47]. Detectors made of photodiodes or CCD cameras, together with interpreter software, form the foundation of this analytical unit [48]. The complete system integrates these components to function as a small yet practical device that may appear as large-scale laboratory equipment or as compact portable systems for point-of-care diagnostics [49]. Optical biosensors require proper design and integration of their components to ensure performance, reliability, and clinical suitability for biomarker detection of prostate cancer and other diseases [50].

5.3 Optical Biosensing Techniques

Optical biosensing encompasses multiple methods that exploit light–matter interactions to monitor biological targets with high precision [51]. The techniques are beneficial for biomedical diagnostics because they operate without invasive procedures, exhibit high sensitivity, and have the potential to become more compact and enable real-time monitoring [51]. This section presents an exhaustive discussion of essential optical biosensing methods for early detection and monitoring of prostate cancer [52]. The main optical biosensor types have been comparatively analyzed in Table 5.3 [22].

5.3.1 Surface Plasmon Resonance (SPR)

The label-free biosensor SPR detects changes in refractive index by measuring the reflective properties of metal-dielectric interfaces, especially with gold [57]. The metal film detects specific conditions in polarized light that cause free electrons to oscillate as surface plasmons, thereby producing a deep dip in the reflected light intensity [58]. Sensor surface binding events shift the resonance condition, making it more sensitive to underlying molecular activities [59]. The widespread use

Table 5.3 Comparative analysis of optical biosensors

Biosensor type	Detection mechanism	Sensitivity	Label use	Application area	References
SPR	Refractive index change	High	No	Cancer biomarkers	[53]
Fluorescence	Emission intensity	Very high	Yes	Pathogen detection	[54]
Raman/SERS	Molecular vibration	High	No	Small molecule detection	[55]
Photonic crystal	Wavelength shift	Moderate	No	Environmental sensing	[56]

of SPR enables direct time-based observations of biomolecular interactions, including antigens with antibodies, DNA with proteins, and receptors with their ligands [60]. The detection capabilities of SPR in prostate cancer diagnostics include PSA, exosomes, and cancer-specific glycoproteins, using highly sensitive processes that do not require labeling [61]. The sensor's ability to measure binding kinetics facilitates biomarker confirmation and drug screening, making it suitable for these activities [62].

5.3.2 Fluorescence-Based Biosensors

Fluorescence-based biosensors are the leading optical platform due to their superior sensitivity, flexibility, and multiplexed detection [63]. The biosensors employ fluorophores that generate light upon exposure to a specific excitation wavelength [64]. Detection of target analyte concentration or presence relies on measuring fluorescent intensity and lifetime, or on measuring energy transfer [65]. Fluorescence biosensors are used in prostate cancer diagnostics to monitor PSA, microRNAs, and other tumor markers at very low concentrations [66]. The detection limits achieved highly depend on advanced detection methods that incorporate quantum dots, FRET systems, and nanomaterial-enhanced fluorescence, which have reached picomolar and femtomolar concentrations [67]. Aside from high-throughput screening, the platforms also use microfluidic systems for point-of-care diagnostics [68].

5.3.3 Raman and Surface-Enhanced Raman Scattering (SERS)

Molecular fingerprints obtained from inelastic scattering of monochromatic light enable Raman spectroscopy to serve as a vibrational spectroscopy technique [69]. Surface-enhanced Raman scattering (SERS) is a signal enhancement method that yields stronger Raman signals by placing analytes on nanostructured metal surfaces (silver or gold) [70]. The detection sensitivity of SERS-based biosensors is high, and they can detect cancer-related molecular changes at single-cell or single-molecule resolution [71]. Researchers use SERS techniques to detect trace levels of PSA, DNA mutations, and cancer-associated metabolites in serum and urine samples for prostate cancer analysis [72]. Through its exclusive identification capabilities and unlabeled operation, SERS offers exceptional utility for cancer diagnostics without invasive procedures [73].

5.3.4 Interferometric and Photonic Crystal Biosensors

Interferometric and photonic crystal biosensors function based on the concepts of light interference and diffraction [74]. These sensors detect tiny variations in the optical path length or resonance state induced by molecular binding at the sensor surface [33]. Biomolecular interactions cause phase shifts in light detected by interferometric biosensors such as Mach–Zehnder and Fabry–Perot interferometers [75]. Conversely, photonic crystal biosensors detect refractive index changes with high sensitivity via periodic nanostructures that alter light propagation [76]. Both are naturally label-free and provide precise measurements of analytes. Developed for the identification of cancer biomarkers, including PSA and exosomal proteins, they are well-suited to lab-on-chip systems [77]. Their capacity for multiplexing and incorporation into miniaturized devices makes them ideal for portable, real-time diagnostic applications. Optical biosensors consolidate diverse techniques and mechanisms into powerful diagnostic tools for prostate cancer. Figure 5.2 provides a unified graphical overview of these elements, including core biomarkers, sensing platforms, and real-world advantages such as speed, non-invasiveness, and portability.

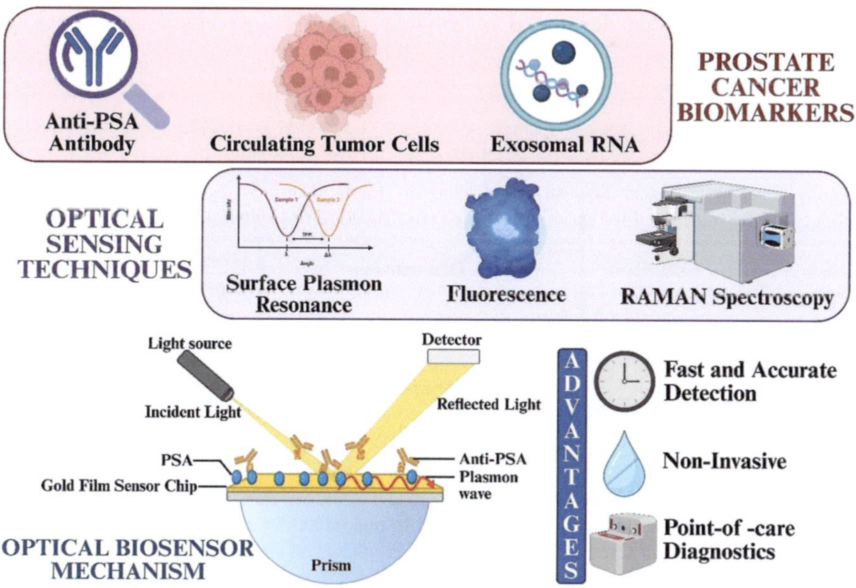

Fig. 5.2 Integrated overview of optical biosensors for prostate cancer detection

5.4 Biomarkers of Prostate Cancer

Prostate cancer needs biomarkers to detect the disease early, identify the condition, and track treatment outcomes for patients [78]. Scientists have identified multiple biomarkers through ongoing research to differentiate aggressive disease from indolent forms, help determine treatment approaches, and assess how treatments affect patients [79]. The consideration is based on key biomarkers that already exist and those that may be promising for the application of prostate cancer, explaining their current functionality and future contributions [80]. Figure 5.3 presents an overview of the categorization of these biomarkers by clinical use (diagnostic, prognostic, or predictive) and lists those biomarkers already in clinical use or in preclinical studies [81]. This graphical illustration highlights the heterogeneity and overlaps in biomarker functions, which can inform a personalized medicine approach to the management of prostate cancer.

5.4.1 Prostate-Specific Antigen (PSA)

Prostate-specific antigen (PSA) serves as both a benchmark for prostate cancer screening and patient management [82]. The prostate gland produces PSA, a glycoprotein, mainly from prostate epithelial cells, which is present in equal amounts in normal prostate tissue and malignant prostate cells [83]. Serum PSA elevations can signal prostate cancer, but they may similarly appear due to prostatitis or benign prostatic hyperplasia (BPH) [84]. The general adoption of PSA testing is limited because it has a poor ability to identify specific conditions [85] accurately. Multiple derivatives have been developed to enhance diagnostic accuracy by using PSA

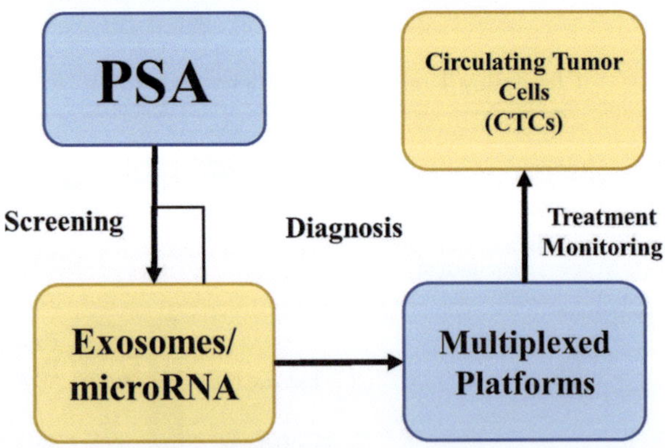

Fig. 5.3 The four key prostate cancer biomarkers that comprise PSA and circulating tumor cells (CTCs) and exosomes/microRNAs are presented in quadrants. Every category features its main clinical purposes: initial screening, diagnosis, and prognosis, along with oversight of treatments. The biomarkers and clinical choices interact through graphical arrows. The sections within the design use color codes to help readers better understand them (traditional biomarkers are blue, while emerging technologies are yellow)

density, PSA velocity, and the free-to-total PSA ratio [86]. These alterations seek to minimize pointless biopsies while offering better prostate cancer risk assessment for patients. The primary role of PSA lies in prostate cancer assessment at diagnosis and monitoring during active patient follow-up [87].

5.4.2 Circulating Tumor Cells (CTCs)

Tumor cells that originate at the primary site become circulating tumor cells and enter the bloodstream. CTCs enable physicians to monitor tumor behavior in real time via blood tests, an alternative to conventional tissue biopsies [88]. CTCs enable essential prognostic assessment because their detection is associated with worsening disease status, metastatic progression, and treatment resistance [89]. Research teams can analyze CTCs after technological advances have delivered systems for both capture and characterization [90]. The enumeration of CTCs proves beneficial for prostate cancer treatment by assessing patients' responses to androgen deprivation therapy and chemotherapy treatment [91]. The ongoing advancement of research makes CTC profiling a potential tool for identifying targeted therapies based on current tumor evolutionary patterns [92].

5.4.3 Exosomes and MicroRNAs

Exosomes are small vesicles released by cells that carry molecular cargo composed of proteins, lipids, and nucleic acids, including microRNAs (miRNAs) [93]. The vesicles serve as key mediators of cell-to-cell communication and promote tumor progression. Prostate cancer researchers have identified exosomes, together with the miRNAs they carry, as valuable diagnostic and prognostic biomarkers for the disease [94]. As short non-coding RNA molecules, microRNAs function to control how genes express themselves. It has been confirmed that certain miRNA molecular structures exhibit either high or low activity in prostate cancer tissues, and this activity is associated with the disease's developmental aspects, such as metastasis levels [95]. The research community investigates miR-141 and miR-375 as potential measurement tools for advanced prostate cancer severity because these microRNAs tend to increase during sophisticated disease stages [96]. Extracellular vesicle miRNA analysis allows doctors to identify cancer molecular alterations through non-invasive testing, thus supporting established diagnostic tools [97].

5.4.4 Multiplexed Biomarker Detection

Research teams developed combined biomarker detection systems to address issues with the independent use of biomarkers [98]. Modern scientific instruments enable the analysis of multiple biomarkers from a single patient's biological sample, thereby enhancing diagnostic accuracy and deepening understanding of disease

Table 5.4 Multiplexed detection platforms

Platform	No. of analysis	Detection method	Advantages	References
Luminex	50+	Fluorescence beads	High throughput	[101]
Microarray	100+	Fluorescence scanning	Parallel analysis	[102]
Lab-on-a-chip	Variable	Multiple integrated methods	Miniaturized, fast	[103]

[99]. Table 5.4 provides an overview of the newest biosensing platforms that demonstrate multiplex capabilities for prostate cancer detection [100].

Healthcare professionals can use multiplex assays to detect proteins, nucleic acids, and metabolites, thereby generating extensive information for prostate cancer profiling [103]. Clinical use of genomic panels, proteomic arrays, and next-generation sequencing platforms is now more widely available [104]. Tests such as the Prostate Health Index (PHI) and the 4Kscore evaluate multiple PSA isozyme patterns and combine them with clinical parameters, aiding doctors in patient biopsy risk assessments [101].

5.5 Recent Advances and Applications

Diagnostics and biomedical engineering have witnessed significant advancements in the present era due to the interplay of microfluidics and biosensing technologies, as well as advances in digital health [105, 106]. Recent scientific breakthroughs helped researchers develop portable, effective systems that improved diagnostic location and time performance [107]. Treatment of illnesses is currently being provided in clinical settings and at home using decentralized, user-centered devices, accelerating medical decision-making and enabling customized treatment opportunities worldwide [108]. The part analyzes current technological developments, clinical validation, and market trends as driving forces behind this development [109].

5.5.1 Point-of-Care Testing Devices

Drawing on their innovative nature, point-of-care testing devices have transformed the way tests are conducted by offering fast, on-the-spot testing close to health facilities [110]. Portable testing devices feature user-friendly interfaces to support immediate decision-making, which is vital for emergency work, remote healthcare, and pandemic response [111]. Modern smartphone-based microfluidic devices, combined with biosensor functionality, have improved the performance of point-of-care testing (POCT) devices and made them more accessible [112]. POCT devices now encompass three key examples: glucose meters, lateral flow immunoassays for infectious diseases, including COVID-19 and HIV, and handheld blood gas analyzers [113]. The development of multiplexing technologies and health information system interoperability, along with AI-enhanced result analysis, allows

Table 5.5 Point-of-care testing devices for prostate cancer

Device	Target biomarker	Detection method	Time to get results	Clinical use	References
PSA test strip	PSA	Colorimetric	10–15 min	Home clinical testing	[112]
SPR portable kit	PSA, CTCs	SPR	<30 min	Diagnostic clinics	[114]

point-of-care testing to establish itself as a fundamental preventive healthcare evaluation method [114]. Table 5.5 presents point-of-care testing (POCT) devices used in clinical prostate cancer diagnostic procedures [115].

5.5.2 Lab-on-a-Chip and Integrated Platforms

Scientists developed lab-on-a-chip (LOC) technology for single-chip laboratory miniaturization, which revolutionized biomedical diagnostics and analytical chemistry [116]. The integrated systems feature microfluidic capabilities that support small fluid volumes and enable the simultaneous running of multiple exams with minimal reagents, delivering faster results [102]. Science allows researchers to build self-contained systems that combine all preparation and reaction sequences with separation functions coupled with detection capabilities [117]. The system operates across various fields of genome research, including DNA sequencing, and also supports proteomic analyses, environmental testing, and food safety assessments [118]. The cost of acquiring LOC devices decreases, and their availability increases as scientists' inventive use of paper and 3D-printable materials increases [119]. Wireless data transmission and machine learning algorithms are advancing the field of smart diagnostics.

5.5.3 Clinical Studies and Case Examples

Medical settings and clinical laboratories demonstrate the assessed use of new diagnostic technologies, which is why they are becoming increasingly significant in everyday practice [120]. Outside the central lab has proved effective in providing useful solutions for a wide range of clinical applications, as evidenced by numerous research reports [121]. The first response teams have been effective in identifying pathogens in the mobile environment by using PCR machines that maintain the quality of laboratory findings through adherence to protocols [122]. Studies show that wearable biosensors for people with diabetes help enhance diabetes monitoring and related medical interventions [123]. Rapid antigen tests were useful for managing the spread of COVID-19 and for population-wide testing during the pandemic [124]. The reported examples confirm that developments in healthcare deliver better patient outcomes, with cost savings and improved administrative performance.

5.5.4 Commercialization and Market Trends

Diagnostic Technology has witnessed significant market growth as consumers increasingly require rapid testing alongside home testing diagnostic systems and telemedicine [125]. The POCT and LOC technologies attract investment through commercialization, as reflected in mergers and acquisitions in the field [126]. The market leaders seek frontier designs and regulatory standards to expand their manufacturing capacities and meet global demand [127]. According to contemporary market research, the global POCT market will exceed USD 50 billion in 2030, driven by chronic disease management in older populations and the emergence of digital health programs [128]. Regulatory nuances, cost-efficiency demands, and data surveillance issues are all vital in providing a clear direction for the industry's strategic path. Nanotechnology, information technology, and biotechnology are used to provide the sector with opportunities to achieve unprecedented growth in progress and influence [129].

5.6 Challenges and Future Directions

Rapid developments in diagnostic technologies pose multiple challenges to achieving full-scale implementation, including technical issues, regulatory complications, and strategic challenges [130]. The analysis of these barriers is necessary to improve innovation and reliability efforts and to speed up product development phases that lead to actual deployment [131]. Emerging technologies will deliver significant changes to future diagnostic possibilities, as the current horizon demonstrates great promise [132]. This section analyzes current diagnostic constraints and highlights upcoming breakthroughs that will address them [133].

5.6.1 Sensitivity and Specificity Issues

One of the most difficult tasks scientists have been working on for years is achieving the highest sensitivity and specificity during diagnostic development [134]. This sensitivity measures whether the tests correctly identify true positives or whether operators correctly identify true negatives [135]. For rapid diagnostic devices, such as laboratory chips and point-of-care systems, design compromises between sensitivity and specificity are made because they operate within sample-volume and target-concentration constraints [136]. The wrong results lead to two separate problems: not only do they cause unnecessary medical procedures and undue worry, but they also result in the loss of important treatment opportunities [137]. Issues such as an inability to isolate specific cancer-cell markers in the blood as proteins, biological variability, cross-reactivity, and environmental conditions compromise the test's accuracy [138]. These are all explored as methods by the research community to increase diagnostic accuracy: multiplexed assays, biosensors, machine learning, signal processing algorithms, and nanomaterial-enhanced biosensors [139].

5.6.2 Regulatory and Standardization Barriers

Multiple obstacles affect the process of moving prototypes into clinics due to complex regulatory processes and insufficient international standards [140]. The U.S. FDA, EMA, WHO, and many other regulatory bodies have strict guidelines to ensure device safety, efficacy, and quality, and they strongly endorse these guidelines. Many different attempts have been made, but with no benefit so far [141]. Most of these protocols are necessary, but they can add a very considerable length of time to development, particularly on novel or unconventional platforms [142]. Finally, companies looking to enter global markets face challenges due to disparities in regional approval processes and classification criteria [143]. Furthermore, there are no universally accepted benchmarks of performance evaluation to enable comparability and adoption. To accelerate innovation while maintaining public safety, companies must work with regulators from the outset, standardize their operations, and streamline their regulations [144].

5.6.3 Next-Generation Technologies

The development of advanced diagnostic tools progresses through innovative technological innovations that seek to resolve existing evaluation obstacles as they build enhanced instrument functionalities [145]. The most significant ones are as follows: *CRISPR-Based Diagnostics*: The application of gene-editing principles to detect biological markers of pathogens with high sensitivity and rapidity, which does not necessarily need complex laboratory facilities [146]. *Wearable Biosensor*: Medical sensors on clothing products detect biological signals by handling information collected by analyzing sweat, intercellular fluid, and saliva and then generating data that can be tested and verified. *Artificial Intelligence and Data Analytics*: Artificial intelligence helps make test interpretations more accurate by using predictive diagnostic features that link test results to electronic health records through data analytical systems [147]. *Quantum Dots and Nanophotonics*: When quantum dots are combined with nanophotonic principles that work on small platforms, they can detect many biomarkers at very high resolution levels [148]. *Synthetic Biology*: Engineers in synthetic biology create computerized systems that look for certain biomarkers and then make data that can be tested and confirmed [149]. These modern technologies, linked to mHealth and IoT operations, promise to make systems more accessible and improve disease detection, enabling personalized, large-scale medical treatments [150]. Table 5.6 describes some of the advanced technologies that may form the future biosensors [151].

Table 5.6 Emerging optical biosensing technologies

Technology	Principle	Expected advantage	Readiness level	References
Plasmonic nanostructures	Enhanced SPR	Higher sensitivity	Early development	[16]
Photonic crystal fibers	Light guiding	Compact format	Experimental	[32]
AI-based signal processing	Pattern recognition	Data accuracy	Growing adoption	[42]

5.7 Conclusion

The production of optical biosensors is one such step forward toward more precise, faster, and non-invasive devices for prostate cancer diagnosis. This chapter shows that continuous incidences of prostate cancer remain a global healthcare problem whose early detection would support improved treatment outcomes and survival rates. Surface plasmon resonance (SPR) optical biosensors, fluorescence-based systems, Raman spectroscopy, and photonic crystal sensors are examples of optical biosensors that hold great promise for detecting prostate-specific biomarkers, such as PSA, circulating tumor cells (CTCs), and exosomal RNAs. The core advantage of optical biosensors is that they can identify substances with high precision and provide results immediately, without labeling. Such functionalities are more effective than the conventional diagnostic instruments. The breakthrough of advanced technologies has enabled portable devices to offer user-friendly operations to both point-of-care analysis, decentralized testing, and continuous healthcare measurements outside the clinical setting. Despite progress, the popularization of optical biosensor technologies in the clinical setting remains a significant challenge. Solutions that address trade-offs among sensitivity and specificity, regulatory standardization, and cost are required to implement clinical routines successfully. Healthcare systems should be aware of the extensive interoperability requirements and regulate the flow of patient information, ensuring that patient data is easily accessible for use with such technologies. The use of medical technology in the future to detect prostate cancer will be advanced by next-generation collection procedures that integrate CRISPR-based detection with wearable biosensors, AI-based analytics, and nanophotonic enhancement technologies. Future healthcare solutions include individualized patient care, combining predictive health-monitoring systems with preventive therapies. Optical biosensors are a novel diagnostic method of detecting prostate cancer at an early stage and also in disease management. The integration of interdisciplinary disciplines and the development of a technology and policy framework will change the terms of cancer diagnosis, as these tools define personalized medicine as a new standard in modern medicine.

5.8 Summary

This chapter provides an extensive review of optical biosensors and their potential to improve prostate cancer monitoring and detection. The pathophysiology of prostate cancer and the necessity of early, non-invasive diagnostics are described first. This chapter covers, in detail, the principles, architecture, and varieties of optical biosensing techniques, including surface plasmon resonance (SPR), fluorescence, Raman/SERS, interferometry, and photonic crystals. These biosensors provide high sensitivity and real-time monitoring, especially for biomarkers such as exosomal RNAs, circulating tumor cells (CTCs), and PSA. The clinical relevance of multiplex detection platforms and point-of-care systems, including portable kits, lab-on-a-chip devices, and test strips, is examined. Additionally, recent developments in nanotechnology and the integration of artificial intelligence are reviewed. Sensitivity, standardization, and prospects such as wearable sensors, CRISPR, and AI-enhanced diagnostics are discussed in the chapter's conclusion.

Glossary

Biosensor An Analytical device that combines a biological element with a sensor.

Surface plasmon resonance (SPR) Optical detection method based on refractive index changes at a metal surface.

Fluorescence Emission of light by a substance that has absorbed light or electromagnetic radiation.

Raman spectroscopy A technique used to observe vibrational, rotational, and other low-frequency modes in a system.

Exosome Small extracellular vesicles carrying proteins, RNA, and other molecules.

CTC (circulating tumor cell) Cancer cells that have shed into the bloodstream from a primary tumor.

Microfluidics Technology that manipulates small volumes of fluids for biosensing or lab-on-chip applications.

Point-of-care (POC) Diagnostic testing performed at or near the site of patient care

References

1. Usman A. Nanoparticle-enhanced optical biosensing technologies for prostate-specific antigen biomarker detection. IEEE Rev Biomed Eng. 2020;15:122–37.
2. Paltusheva ZU, Ashikbayeva Z, Tosi D, Gritsenko LV. Highly sensitive zinc oxide fiber-optic biosensor for the detection of CD44 protein. Biosensors [Internet]. 2022;12(11). Available from: https://www.mdpi.com/2079-6374/12/11/1015.
3. Rasheed S, Kanwal T, Ahmad N, Fatima B, Najam-ul-Haq M, Hussain D. Advances and challenges in portable optical biosensors for onsite detection and point-of-care diagnostics. TrAC Trends Anal Chem [Internet]. 2024;173:117640. Available from: https://www.sciencedirect.com/science/article/pii/S0165993624001225.

4. Garzón V, Pinacho DG, Bustos RH, Garzón G, Bustamante S. Optical biosensors for therapeutic drug monitoring. Biosensors [Internet]. 2019;9(4). Available from: https://www.mdpi.com/2079-6374/9/4/132
5. Ahmad M, Hasan M, Tarannum N, Hasan M, Ahmed S. Recent advances in optical and photoelectrochemical nanobiosensor technology for cancer biomarker detection. Biosens Bioelectron X [Internet]. 2023;14:100375. Available from: https://www.sciencedirect.com/science/article/pii/S2590137023000729.
6. Hossain MB, Islam MM, Abdulrazak LF, Rana MM, Akib TBA, Hassan M. Graphene-coated optical fiber SPR biosensor for BRCA1 and BRCA2 breast cancer biomarker detection: a numerical design-based analysis. Photonic Sens [Internet]. 2020;10(1):67–79. Available from: https://doi.org/10.1007/s13320-019-0556-7.
7. Zhao S, Huang J, Yang L. Optical fiber peptide-sensor for ultrasensitive detection of prostate-specific antigen. Sensors Actuators B Chem. 2022;369:132317.
8. Shawky SM, Awad AM, Abugable AA, El-Khamisy SF. Gold nanoparticles–an optical biosensor for RNA quantification for cancer and neurologic disorders diagnosis. Int J Nanomedicine. 2018:8137–51.
9. Lino C, Barrias S, Chaves R, Adega F, Martins-Lopes P, Fernandes JR. Biosensors as diagnostic tools in clinical applications. Biochim Biophys Acta Rev Cancer [Internet]. 2022;1877(3):188726. Available from: https://www.sciencedirect.com/science/article/pii/S0304419X22000518.
10. Samadi Pakchin P, Fathi F, Samadi H, Adibkia K. Recent advances in receptor-based optical biosensors for the detection of multiplex biomarkers. Talanta [Internet]. 2025;281:126852. Available from: https://www.sciencedirect.com/science/article/pii/S0039914024012311.
11. Arshavsky-Graham S, Massad-Ivanir N, Segal E, Weiss S. Porous silicon-based photonic biosensors: current status and emerging Applications. Anal Chem [Internet]. 2019;91(1):441–67. Available from: https://doi.org/10.1021/acs.analchem.8b05028.
12. Alnaimi A, Al-Hamry A, Makableh Y, Adiraju A, Kanoun O. Gold nanoparticles-MWCNT based Aptasensor for early diagnosis of prostate cancer. Biosensors [Internet]. 2022;12(12). Available from: https://www.mdpi.com/2079-6374/12/12/1130.
13. Pourmadadi M, Moammeri A, Shamsabadipour A, Moghaddam YF, Rahdar A, Pandey S. Application of various optical and electrochemical nanobiosensors for detecting cancer antigen 125 (CA-125): a review. Biosensors [Internet]. 2023;13(1). Available from: https://www.mdpi.com/2079-6374/13/1/99
14. Amouzadeh Tabrizi M, Ferré-Borrull J, Marsal LF. An optical biosensor for the determination of cathepsin B as a cancer-associated enzyme using nanoporous anodic alumina modified with human serum albumin-thionine. Microchim Acta [Internet]. 2020;187(4):230. Available from: https://doi.org/10.1007/s00604-020-4188-9.
15. Sagar Shrikrishna N, Sharma R, Sahoo J, Kaushik A, Gandhi S. Navigating the landscape of optical biosensors. Chem Eng J [Internet]. 2024;490:151661. Available from: https://www.sciencedirect.com/science/article/pii/S1385894724031486.
16. Bari A, Aslam S, Khan HU, Shakil S, Yaseen M, Shahid S, et al. Next-generation optical biosensors: cutting-edge advances in optical detection methods. Plasmonics [Internet]. 2025; Available from: https://doi.org/10.1007/s11468-025-02870-3.
17. Xu L, Wen Y, Pandit S, Mokkapati VRSS, Mijakovic I, Li Y, et al. Graphene-based biosensors for the detection of prostate cancer protein biomarkers: a review. BMC Chem [Internet]. 2019;13(1):112. Available from: https://doi.org/10.1186/s13065-019-0611-x.
18. Kumari S, Saini SM. Optical biosensors for diagnostic applications. In: Nanomaterials-based sensing platforms. Apple Academic Press; 2022. p. 155–93.
19. Sharipov M, Azizov S, Kakhkhorov S, Yunuskhodjaev A, Lee YI. Emerging spectroscopic techniques for prostate cancer diagnosis. Appl Spectrosc Rev. 2019;54(10):829–55.
20. Purohit A, Jain S, Panda PK. Chapter 5 – Biosensors used for anticancer therapeutics. In: Hasnain MS, Nayak AK, Aminabhavi TM, editors. Applications of biosensors in healthcare [Internet]. Academic; 2025. p. 73–91. Available from: https://www.sciencedirect.com/science/article/pii/B9780443215926000239.

21. Rauta PR, Nayak D, Singh PK. Nanobiosensors and their biomedical applications. In: Nanotechnology in biology and medicine. CRC Press; 2019. p. 177–83.
22. Chen C, Wang J. Optical biosensors: an exhaustive and comprehensive review. Analyst. 2020;145(5):1605–28.
23. Pirzada M, Altintas Z. Recent progress in optical sensors for biomedical diagnostics. Micromachines [Internet]. 2020;11(4). Available from: https://www.mdpi.com/2072-666X/11/4/356
24. Sohrabi H, Bolandi N, Hemmati A, Eyvazi S, Ghasemzadeh S, Baradaran B, et al. State-of-the-art cancer biomarker detection by portable (Bio) sensing technology: a critical review. Microchem J [Internet]. 2022;177:107248. Available from: https://www.sciencedirect.com/science/article/pii/S0026265X22000765.
25. Guimarães CF, Cruz-Moreira D, Caballero D, Pirraco RP, Gasperini L, Kundu SC, et al. Shining a light on cancer—photonics in microfluidic tumor modeling and biosensing. Adv Healthc Mater. 2023;12(14):2201442.
26. Li M, Ding C, Zhang D, Chen W, Yan Z, Chen Z, et al. Distinguishable colorimetric biosensor for diagnosis of prostate cancer bone metastases. Adv Sci. 2023;10(32):2303159.
27. Maeda T, Kanamori R, Choi YJ, Taki M, Noda T, Sawada K, et al. Bio-interface on freestanding nanosheet of microelectromechanical system optical interferometric immunosensor for label-free Attomolar prostate cancer marker detection. Sensors [Internet]. 2022;22(4). Available from: https://www.mdpi.com/1424-8220/22/4/1356
28. Ivanov YD, Malsagova KA, Goldaeva KV, Kapustina SI, Pleshakova TO, Popov VP, et al. Nanoribbon biosensor-based detection of microRNA markers of prostate cancer. Sensors [Internet]. 2023;23(17). Available from: https://www.mdpi.com/1424-8220/23/17/7527
29. Chinchulkar SA, Patra P, Dehariya D, Appidi T, Rengan AK. 22 – Gold nanoparticle–based biosensing applications and fundamentals of sensor technology: principles and novel designs. In: Barhoum A, Altintas Z, editors. Fundamentals of sensor technology [Internet]. Woodhead Publishing; 2023. p. 669–723. (Woodhead Publishing Series in Electronic and Optical Materials). Available from: https://www.sciencedirect.com/science/article/pii/B9780323884310000144.
30. Vafadar A, AlaviManesh S, Maddahi ME, Alizadeh M, Movahedpour A, Savardashtaki A. Exosome biosensors for detection of prostate cancer. Clin Chim Acta [Internet]. 2025;571:120243. Available from: https://www.sciencedirect.com/science/article/pii/S0009898125001226.
31. Hasan MR, Ahommed MS, Daizy M, Bacchu MS, Ali MR, Al-Mamun MR, et al. Recent development in electrochemical biosensors for cancer biomarker detection. Biosens Bioelectron X [Internet]. 2021;8:100075. Available from: https://www.sciencedirect.com/science/article/pii/S259013702100011X.
32. Hajshahvaladi L, Kaatuzian H, Danaie M. Photonic crystal-assisted excitation of surface plasmons: a high-resolution refractive index sensor based on a gold spiral in a photonic crystal resonator. Opt Quant Electron. 2024;56(9):1417.
33. Mittal S, Saharia A, Ismail Y, Petruccione F, Bourdine AV, Morozov OG, et al. Spiral-shaped photonic crystal fiber-based surface plasmon resonance biosensor for cancer cell detection. Photonics [Internet]. 2023;10(3). Available from: https://www.mdpi.com/2304-6732/10/3/230
34. Liu LC, Wu C, Li W, Chen YA, Shao XP, Wilczek F, et al. Active optical intensity interferometry. Phys Rev Lett [Internet]. 2025;134(18):180201. Available from: https://link.aps.org/doi/10.1103/PhysRevLett.134.180201.
35. Wang Y, Wu C, Yu G, Yu S. Point-of-care detection of prostate cancer through surface protein profiling on extracellular vesicles using colorimetric 3D paper-based analytical devices. Biosens Bioelectron [Internet]. 2025;287:117695. Available from: https://www.sciencedirect.com/science/article/pii/S095656632500569X.
36. Eivazzadeh-Keihan R, Pashazadeh-Panahi P, Baradaran B, Maleki A, Hejazi M, Mokhtarzadeh A, et al. Recent advances on nanomaterial based electrochemical and optical aptasensors for detection of cancer biomarkers. TrAC Trends Anal Chem [Internet]. 2018;100:103–15. Available from: https://www.sciencedirect.com/science/article/pii/S0165993617304430.

37. Liao C, Wu Z, Lin C, Chen X, Zou Y, Zhao W, et al. Nurturing the marriages of urinary liquid biopsies and nano-diagnostics for precision urinalysis of prostate cancer. Smart Med. 2023;2(1):e20220020.
38. Qu H, Liu H, Jin Y, Cui Z, Han G. HUWE1 upregulation has tumor suppressive effect in human prostate cancer cell lines through c-Myc. Biomed Pharmacother [Internet]. 2018;106:309–15. Available from: https://www.sciencedirect.com/science/article/pii/S0753332218327653.
39. Amri C, Shukla AK, Lee JH. Recent advancements in nanoparticle-based optical biosensors for circulating cancer biomarkers. Materials (Basel) [Internet]. 2021;14(6). Available from: https://www.mdpi.com/1996-1944/14/6/1339.
40. Schatten H. Brief overview of prostate cancer statistics, grading, diagnosis and treatment strategies. In: Schatten H, editor. Cell & molecular biology of prostate cancer: updates, insights and new frontiers [Internet]. Cham: Springer International Publishing; 2018. p. 1–14. Available from: https://doi.org/10.1007/978-3-319-95693-0_1.
41. Banerjee A, Maity S, Mastrangelo CH. Nanostructures for biosensing, with a brief overview on cancer detection, IoT, and the role of machine learning in smart biosensors. Sensors [Internet]. 2021;21(4). Available from: https://www.mdpi.com/1424-8220/21/4/1253.
42. Kokabi M, Tahir MN, Singh D, Javanmard M. Advancing healthcare: synergizing biosensors and machine learning for early cancer diagnosis. Biosensors [Internet]. 2023;13(9). Available from: https://www.mdpi.com/2079-6374/13/9/884.
43. Appakkannu A, Govindaraj E, Balakrishnan K. Detection of abnormality in prostate tissues using two-dimensional photonic crystal tactile sensor. Plasmonics [Internet]. 2022;17(4):1451–62. Available from: https://doi.org/10.1007/s11468-022-01635-6.
44. Mostufa S, Rezaei B, Ciannella S, Yari P, Gómez-Pastora J, He R, et al. Advancements and perspectives in optical biosensors. ACS Omega [Internet]. 2024;9(23):24181–202. Available from: https://doi.org/10.1021/acsomega.4c01872.
45. Graça JS, Miyazaki CM, Shimizu FM, Volpati D, Mejía-Salazar JR, Oliveira JON, et al. On the importance of controlling film architecture in detecting prostate specific antigen. Appl Surf Sci [Internet]. 2018;434:1175–82. Available from: https://www.sciencedirect.com/science/article/pii/S0169433217330684.
46. Taha BA, Al-Tahar IA, Addie AJ, Mahdi AB, Haider AJ, Al Mashhadany Y, et al. Nanophotonic catheters: a lens into the body for biosensing and biomedical imaging. Appl Mater Today [Internet]. 2024;38:102229. Available from: https://www.sciencedirect.com/science/article/pii/S2352940724001744.
47. Khodaie A, Heidarzadeh H. Split ring resonator-based multimode Plasmonic optical biosensors for comprehensive antigen detection. Sens Imaging [Internet]. 2024;25(1):63. Available from: https://doi.org/10.1007/s11220-024-00514-0.
48. El-Sheikh SM, Sheta SM, Salem SR, Abd-Elzaher MM, Basaleh AS, Labib AA. Prostate-specific antigen monitoring using nano Zinc(II) metal–organic framework-based optical biosensor. Biosensors [Internet]. 2022;12(11). Available from: https://www.mdpi.com/2079-6374/12/11/931.
49. Kumar S, Singh H, Singh DK. Metasurfaces in optical biosensing: revolutionizing detection techniques and shaping the future. Photonics [Internet]. 2025;12(4). Available from: https://www.mdpi.com/2304-6732/12/4/360
50. Arshad F, Nabi F, Iqbal S, Khan RH. Applications of graphene-based electrochemical and optical biosensors in early detection of cancer biomarkers. Colloids Surfaces B Biointerfaces [Internet]. 2022;212:112356. Available from: https://www.sciencedirect.com/science/article/pii/S092777652200039X.
51. Funari R, Chu KY, Shen AQ. Multiplexed opto-microfluidic biosensing: advanced platform for prostate cancer detection. ACS Sensors [Internet]. 2024;9(5):2596–604. Available from: https://doi.org/10.1021/acssensors.4c00312.
52. Okhai TA, Idris AO, Feleni U, Snyman LW. Futuristic silicon photonic biosensor with nanomaterial enhancement for PSA detection. Photonics [Internet]. 2024;11(1). Available from: https://www.mdpi.com/2304-6732/11/1/97.

53. Mostufa S, Rezaei B, Azizi E, Wang YA, Li C, Gómez-Pastora J, et al. Characterizing the physicochemical properties of magnetic nanoparticles by a surface plasmon resonance approach. AIP Adv [Internet]. 2025;15(3):35022. Available from: https://doi.org/10.1063/9.0000856.
54. Nagdeve SN, Suganthan B, Ramasamy RP. Perspectives on the application of biosensors for the early detection of oral cancer. Sensors (Basel). 2025;25(5).
55. Song L, Xue F, Li T, Zhang Q, Xu X, He C, et al. Differential diagnosis of urinary cancers by surface-enhanced Raman spectroscopy and machine learning. Anal Chem [Internet]. 2025;97(1):27–32. Available from: https://doi.org/10.1021/acs.analchem.4c05287.
56. López JG, Muñoz M, Arias V, García V, Calvo PC, Ondo-Méndez AO, et al. Electrochemical and optical carbon dots and glassy carbon biosensors: a review on their development and applications in early cancer detection. Micromachines. 2025;16(2).
57. Mahani M, Alimohamadi F, Torkzadeh-Mahani M, Hassani Z, Khakbaz F, Divsar F, et al. LSPR biosensing for the early-stage prostate cancer detection using hydrogen bonds between PSA and antibody: molecular dynamic and experimental study. J Mol Liq [Internet]. 2021;324:114736. Available from: https://www.sciencedirect.com/science/article/pii/S0167732220369786.
58. Nanda BP, Rani P, Paul P, Aman, Ganti SS, Bhatia R. Recent trends and impact of localized surface plasmon resonance (LSPR) and surface-enhanced Raman spectroscopy (SERS) in modern analysis. J Pharm Anal [Internet]. 2024;14(11):100959. Available from: https://www.sciencedirect.com/science/article/pii/S209517792400056X.
59. Bellassai N, D'Agata R, Jungbluth V, Spoto G. Surface plasmon resonance for biomarker detection: advances in non-invasive cancer diagnosis. Front Chem. 2019;7:570.
60. Jazayeri MH, Aghaie T, Nedaeinia R, Manian M, Nickho H. Rapid noninvasive detection of bladder cancer using survivin antibody-conjugated gold nanoparticles (GNPs) based on localized surface plasmon resonance (LSPR). Cancer Immunol Immunother [Internet]. 2020;69(9):1833–40. Available from: https://doi.org/10.1007/s00262-020-02559-y.
61. Pinho S, Ferreira-Gonçalves T, Lopes J, Amaral MN, Viana AS, Coelho JMP, et al. A step forward for the treatment of localized prostate cancer using gold nanoparticles combined with laser irradiation. Int J Mol Sci [Internet]. 2024;25(8). Available from: https://www.mdpi.com/1422-0067/25/8/4488.
62. Tai J, Fan S, Ding S, Ren L. Gold nanoparticles based optical biosensors for cancer biomarker proteins: a review of the current practices. Front Bioeng Biotechnol. 2022;10:877193.
63. Ahmadi-Sangachin E, Mohammadnejad J, Hosseini M. Fluorescence self-assembled DNA hydrogel for the determination of prostate specific antigen by aggregation induced emission. Spectrochim Acta Part A Mol Biomol Spectrosc [Internet]. 2023;303:123234. Available from: https://www.sciencedirect.com/science/article/pii/S1386142523009198.
64. Yin Z, Zhu L, Lv Z, Li M, Tang D. Persistent luminescence nanorods-based autofluorescence-free biosensor for prostate-specific antigen detection. Talanta [Internet]. 2021;233:122563. Available from: https://www.sciencedirect.com/science/article/pii/S0039914021004847.
65. Williams RM, Lee C, Heller DA. A fluorescent carbon nanotube sensor detects the metastatic prostate cancer biomarker uPA. ACS Sensors [Internet]. 2018;3(9):1838–45. Available from: https://doi.org/10.1021/acssensors.8b00631.
66. He JH, Cheng YY, Zhang QQ, Liu H, Huang CZ. Carbon dots-based fluorescence resonance energy transfer for the prostate specific antigen (PSA) with high sensitivity. Talanta [Internet]. 2020;219:121276. Available from: https://www.sciencedirect.com/science/article/pii/S0039914020305671.
67. Zhao J, Wang J, Liu Y, Han XX, Xu B, Ozaki Y, et al. Detection of prostate cancer biomarkers via a SERS-based aptasensor. Biosens Bioelectron [Internet]. 2022;216:114660. Available from: https://www.sciencedirect.com/science/article/pii/S095656632200700X.
68. Jiang P, Bai Y, Yan L, Feng P, Huang K, Chen J, et al. Nanoarchitectonics-assisted simultaneous fluorescence detection of urinary dual miRNAs for noninvasive diagnosis of prostate cancer. Anal Chem [Internet]. 2023;95(19):7676–84. Available from: https://doi.org/10.1021/acs.analchem.3c00701.

69. Haroon M, Tahir M, Nawaz H, Majeed MI, Al-Saadi AA. Surface-enhanced Raman scattering (SERS) spectroscopy for prostate cancer diagnosis: a review. Photodiagnosis Photodyn Ther [Internet]. 2022;37:102690. Available from: https://www.sciencedirect.com/science/article/pii/S157210002100507X.
70. Rajput S, Pink D, Findlay S, Woolner E, Lewis JD, McDermott MT. Application of surface-enhanced Raman spectroscopy to guide therapy for advanced prostate cancer patients. ACS Sens [Internet]. 2022;7(3):827–38. Available from: https://doi.org/10.1021/acssensors.1c02551.
71. Ma Y, Chi J, Zheng Z, Attygalle A, Kim IY, Du H. Therapeutic prognosis of prostate cancer using surface-enhanced Raman scattering of patient urine and multivariate statistical analysis. J Biophotonics. 2021;14(1):e202000275.
72. Gaba F, Tipping WJ, Salji M, Faulds K, Graham D, Leung HY. Raman spectroscopy in prostate cancer: techniques, applications and advancements. Cancers (Basel) [Internet]. 2022;14(6). Available from: https://www.mdpi.com/2072-6694/14/6/1535.
73. Moisoiu V, Socaciu A, Stefancu A, Iancu SD, Boros I, Alecsa CD, et al. Breast cancer diagnosis by surface-enhanced Raman scattering (SERS) of urine. Appl Sci [Internet]. 2019;9(4). Available from: https://www.mdpi.com/2076-3417/9/4/806
74. Badawi KA, Hamed MM, Mohammed NA. An innovative biosensor harnessing the potential of photonic crystal technology to identify a multitude of cancer cells, distinguished by heightened quality factor and sensitivity. J Opt [Internet]. 2024;53(4):3246–58. Available from: https://doi.org/10.1007/s12596-023-01524-z.
75. Kaur B, Kumar S, Kaushik BK. Recent advancements in optical biosensors for cancer detection. Biosens Bioelectron [Internet]. 2022;197:113805. Available from: https://www.sciencedirect.com/science/article/pii/S0956566321008423.
76. Emon W, Chaki A, Mondal TP, Nayan MDF, Mahmud RR. Photonic crystal fiber-based SPR biosensor coated with Ag-TiO2 and Au-TiO2 for the detection of skin cancer: a comparison. Opt Quantum Electron [Internet]. 2024;56(8):1322. Available from: https://doi.org/10.1007/s11082-024-07250-5.
77. Moorthy DN, Dhinasekaran D, Rebecca PNB, Rajendran AR. Optical biosensors for detection of cancer biomarkers: current and future perspectives. J Biophotonics. 2024;17(12):e202400243.
78. Lamy PJ, Allory Y, Gauchez AS, Asselain B, Beuzeboc P, de Cremoux P, et al. Prognostic biomarkers used for localised prostate cancer management: a systematic review. Eur Urol Focus [Internet]. 2018;4(6):790–803. Available from: https://www.sciencedirect.com/science/article/pii/S2405456917300652.
79. Fredsøe J, Rasmussen AKI, Thomsen AR, Mouritzen P, Høyer S, Borre M, et al. Diagnostic and prognostic MicroRNA biomarkers for prostate cancer in cell-free urine. Eur Urol Focus [Internet]. 2018;4(6):825–33. Available from: https://www.sciencedirect.com/science/article/pii/S2405456917300664.
80. Li W, Xu W, Sun K, Wang F, Wong TW, Kong A. Identification of novel biomarkers in prostate cancer diagnosis and prognosis. J Biochem Mol Toxicol. 2022;36(9):e23137.
81. Boerrigter E, Groen LN, Van Erp NP, Verhaegh GW, Schalken JA. Clinical utility of emerging biomarkers in prostate cancer liquid biopsies. Expert Rev Mol Diagn. 2020;20(2):219–30.
82. Pérez-Ibave DC, Burciaga-Flores CH, Elizondo-Riojas MÁ. Prostate-specific antigen (PSA) as a possible biomarker in non-prostatic cancer: a review. Cancer Epidemiol [Internet]. 2018;54:48–55. Available from: https://www.sciencedirect.com/science/article/pii/S1877782118300936
83. Cho H, Oh CK, Cha J, Chung JI, Byun SS, Hong SK, et al. Association of serum prostate-specific antigen (PSA) level and circulating tumor cell-based PSA mRNA in prostate cancer. Prostate Int [Internet]. 2022;10(1):14–20. Available from: https://www.sciencedirect.com/science/article/pii/S2287888222000022
84. Yusim I, Krenawi M, Mazor E, Novack V, Mabjeesh NJ. The use of prostate specific antigen density to predict clinically significant prostate cancer. Sci Rep [Internet]. 2020;10(1):20015. Available from: https://doi.org/10.1038/s41598-020-76786-9.

85. Rönningås U, Fransson P, Holm M, Wennman-Larsen A. Prostate-specific antigen (PSA) and distress: – a cross-sectional nationwide survey in men with prostate cancer in Sweden. BMC Urol [Internet]. 2019;19(1):66. Available from: https://doi.org/10.1186/s12894-019-0493-1.
86. Mahal BA, Yang DD, Wang NQ, Alshalalfa M, Davicioni E, Choeurng V, et al. Clinical and genomic characterization of low–prostate-specific antigen, high-grade prostate cancer. Eur Urol [Internet]. 2018;74(2):146–54. Available from: https://www.sciencedirect.com/science/article/pii/S0302283818300988.
87. Sasaki T, Sugimura Y. The importance of time to prostate-specific antigen (PSA) nadir after primary androgen deprivation therapy in hormone-naïve prostate cancer patients. J Clin Med [Internet]. 2018;7(12). Available from: https://www.mdpi.com/2077-0383/7/12/565.
88. Enikeev D, Morozov A, Babaevskaya D, Bazarkin A, Malavaud B. A systematic review of circulating tumor cells clinical application in prostate cancer diagnosis. Cancers (Basel) [Internet]. 2022;14(15). Available from: https://www.mdpi.com/2072-6694/14/15/3802.
89. Cieślikowski WA, Antczak A, Nowicki M, Zabel M, Budna-Tukan J. Clinical relevance of circulating tumor cells in prostate cancer management. Biomedicines [Internet]. 2021;9(9). Available from: https://www.mdpi.com/2227-9059/9/9/1179.
90. Broncy L, Paterlini-Bréchot P. Clinical impact of circulating tumor cells in patients with localized prostate cancer. Cells [Internet]. 2019;8(7). Available from: https://www.mdpi.com/2073-4409/8/7/676.
91. Lu L, Hu W, Liu B, Yang T. Insights into circulating tumor cell clusters: a barometer for treatment effects and prognosis for prostate cancer patients. Cancers (Basel) [Internet]. 2022;14(16). Available from: https://www.mdpi.com/2072-6694/14/16/3985.
92. Yang M, Zhang X, Guo L, Liu X, Wu J, Zhu H. Research progress for the clinical application of circulating tumor cells in prostate cancer diagnosis and treatment. Biomed Res Int. 2021;2021(1):6230826.
93. Lorenc T, Klimczyk K, Michalczewska I, Słomka M, Kubiak-Tomaszewska G, Olejarz W. Exosomes in prostate cancer diagnosis, prognosis and therapy. Int J Mol Sci [Internet]. 2020;21(6). Available from: https://www.mdpi.com/1422-0067/21/6/2118
94. Barceló M, Castells M, Bassas L, Vigués F, Larriba S. Semen miRNAs contained in exosomes as non-invasive biomarkers for prostate cancer diagnosis. Sci Rep [Internet]. 2019;9(1):13772. Available from: https://doi.org/10.1038/s41598-019-50172-6.
95. Akoto T, Saini S. Role of exosomes in prostate cancer metastasis. Int J Mol Sci [Internet]. 2021;22(7). Available from: https://www.mdpi.com/1422-0067/22/7/3528.
96. Vlaeminck-Guillem V. Exosomes and prostate cancer management. Semin Cancer Biol [Internet]. 2022;86:101–11. Available from: https://www.sciencedirect.com/science/article/pii/S1044579X21002169.
97. Movahedpour A, Khatami SH, Karami N, Vakili O, Naeli P, Jamali Z, et al. Exosomal noncoding RNAs in prostate cancer. Clin Chim Acta [Internet]. 2022;537:127–32. Available from: https://www.sciencedirect.com/science/article/pii/S0009898122013523.
98. Timilsina SS, Jolly P, Durr N, Yafia M, Ingber DE. Enabling multiplexed electrochemical detection of biomarkers with high sensitivity in complex biological samples. Acc Chem Res [Internet]. 2021;54(18):3529–39. Available from: https://doi.org/10.1021/acs.accounts.1c00382.
99. Song J, Ma S, Sokoll LJ, Eguez RV, Höti N, Zhang H, et al. A panel of selected serum protein biomarkers for the detection of aggressive prostate cancer. Theranostics. 2021;11(13):6214–24.
100. Wu J, Ouyang L, Wadhawan N, Li J, Zhang M, Liao S, et al. A compact microfluidic system for cell migration studies. Biomed Microdevices. 2014;16:521–8.
101. Wong LCC, Jolly P, Estrela P. Development of a sensitive multiplexed open circuit potential system for the detection of prostate cancer biomarkers. Bionanoscience [Internet]. 2018;8(2):701–6. Available from: https://doi.org/10.1007/s12668-017-0408-0.
102. Umme S, Siciliano G, Primiceri E, Turco A, Tarantini I, Ferrara F, et al. Electrochemical sensors for liquid biopsy and their integration into lab-on-chip platforms: revolutioniz-

ing the approach to diseases. Chem Int. 2023;11(10). Available from: https://www.mdpi.com/2227-9040/11/10/517.
103. Kral M, Kurfurstova D, Zemla P, Elias M, Bouchal J. New biomarkers and multiplex tests for diagnosis of aggressive prostate cancer and therapy management. Front Oncol. 2025;15:1542511.
104. Liu S, Garcia-Marques F, Zhang CA, Lee JJ, Nolley R, Shen M, et al. Discovery of CASP8 as a potential biomarker for high-risk prostate cancer through a high-multiplex immunoassay. Sci Rep [Internet]. 2021;11(1):7612. Available from: https://doi.org/10.1038/s41598-021-87155-5.
105. Wang I, Song L, Wang BY, Rezazadeh Kalebasty A, Uchio E, Zi X. Prostate cancer immunotherapy: a review of recent advancements with novel treatment methods and efficacy. Am J Clin Exp Urol. 2022;10(4):210–33.
106. Feider CL, Krieger A, DeHoog RJ, Eberlin LS. Ambient ionization mass spectrometry: recent developments and applications. Anal Chem [Internet]. 2019;91(7):4266–90. Available from: https://doi.org/10.1021/acs.analchem.9b00807.
107. Cuocolo R, Cipullo MB, Stanzione A, Ugga L, Romeo V, Radice L, et al. Machine learning applications in prostate cancer magnetic resonance imaging. Eur Radiol Exp [Internet]. 2019;3(1):35. Available from: https://doi.org/10.1186/s41747-019-0109-2.
108. Akkilic N, Geschwindner S, Höök F. Single-molecule biosensors: recent advances and applications. Biosens Bioelectron [Internet]. 2020;151:111944. Available from: https://www.sciencedirect.com/science/article/pii/S095656631931022X.
109. Yang W, Liang H, Ma S, Wang D, Huang J. Gold nanoparticle based photothermal therapy: development and application for effective cancer treatment. Sustain Mater Technol [Internet]. 2019;22:e00109. Available from: https://www.sciencedirect.com/science/article/pii/S2214993719300399.
110. Hayes B, Murphy C, Crawley A, O'Kennedy R. Developments in point-of-care diagnostic technology for cancer detection. Diagnostics [Internet]. 2018;8(2). Available from: https://www.mdpi.com/2075-4418/8/2/39.
111. Malekjahani A, Sindhwani S, Syed AM, Chan WCW. Engineering steps for mobile point-of-care diagnostic devices. Acc Chem Res [Internet]. 2019;52(9):2406–14. Available from: https://doi.org/10.1021/acs.accounts.9b00200.
112. Meyer AR, Gorin MA. First point-of-care PSA test for prostate cancer detection. Nat Rev Urol [Internet]. 2019;16(6):331–2. Available from: https://doi.org/10.1038/s41585-019-0179-1.
113. Annese VF, Patil SB, Hu C, Giagkoulovits C, Al-Rawhani MA, Grant J, et al. A monolithic single-chip point-of-care platform for metabolomic prostate cancer detection. Microsystems Nanoeng. 2021;7(1):21.
114. Srinivasan B, Nanus DM, Erickson D, Mehta S. Highly portable quantitative screening test for prostate-specific antigen at point of care. Curr Res Biotechnol. 2021;3:288–99.
115. Marquez S, Morales-Narváez E. Nanoplasmonics in paper-based analytical devices. Front Bioeng Biotechnol. 2019;7:69.
116. Maciel Braga LA, Mota FB. Early cancer diagnosis using lab-on-a-chip devices: A bibliometric and network analysis. COLLNET J Sci Inf Manag. 2021;15(1):163–96.
117. Venkatesalu S, Dilliyappan S, Satish Kumar A, Palaniyandi T, Baskar G, Ravi M, et al. Prospectives and retrospectives of microfluidics devices and lab-on-A-chip emphasis on cancer. Clin Chim Acta [Internet]. 2024;552:117646. Available from: https://www.sciencedirect.com/science/article/pii/S0009898123004485.
118. Miccio L, Cimmino F, Kurelac I, Villone MM, Bianco V, Memmolo P, et al. Perspectives on liquid biopsy for label-free detection of "circulating tumor cells" through intelligent lab-on-chips. View. 2020;1(3):20200034.
119. Woo HK, Park J, Ku JY, Lee CH, Sunkara V, Ha HK, et al. Urine-based liquid biopsy: non-invasive and sensitive AR-V7 detection in urinary EVs from patients with prostate cancer. Lab Chip. 2019;19(1):87–97.
120. Siva S, Bressel M, Murphy DG, Shaw M, Chander S, Violet J, et al. Stereotactic Abative body radiotherapy (SABR) for Oligometastatic prostate cancer: a prospective clinical trial. Eur

Urol [Internet]. 2018;74(4):455–62. Available from: https://www.sciencedirect.com/science/article/pii/S0302283818304299.
121. Barsouk A, Padala SA, Vakiti A, Mohammed A, Saginala K, Thandra KC, et al. Epidemiology, staging and management of prostate cancer. Med Sci [Internet]. 2020;8(3). Available from: https://www.mdpi.com/2076-3271/8/3/28.
122. Boevé LMS, Hulshof MCCM, Vis AN, Zwinderman AH, Twisk JWR, Witjes WPJ, et al. Effect on survival of androgen deprivation therapy alone compared to androgen deprivation therapy combined with concurrent radiation therapy to the prostate in patients with primary bone metastatic prostate cancer in a prospective randomised clinical Tria. Eur Urol [Internet]. 2019;75(3):410–8. Available from: https://www.sciencedirect.com/science/article/pii/S0302283818306584.
123. Salami SS, Hovelson DH, Kaplan JB, Mathieu R, Udager AM, Curci NE, et al. Transcriptomic heterogeneity in multifocal prostate cancer. JCI Insight. 2018;3(21).
124. Jamaspishvili T, Berman DM, Ross AE, Scher HI, De Marzo AM, Squire JA, et al. Clinical implications of PTEN loss in prostate cancer. Nat Rev Urol [Internet]. 2018;15(4):222–34. Available from: https://doi.org/10.1038/nrurol.2018.9.
125. Srivastava A, Liu X, Maganty A, Kaufman SR, Shay A, Oerline M, et al. Commercial prices and their influence on urology practices: prostate cancer care among men with Medicare. Cancer. 2025;131(1):e35633.
126. Ostuni E, Taylor MRG. Commercial and business aspects of alpha radioligand therapeutics. Front Med. 2023;9:1070497.
127. Hughes T, Rai B, Madaan S, Chedgy E, Somani B. The availability, cost, limitations, learning curve and future of robotic systems in urology and prostate cancer surgery. J Clin Med [Internet]. 2023;12(6). Available from: https://www.mdpi.com/2077-0383/12/6/2268
128. Krstev S, Knutsson A. Occupational risk factors for prostate cancer: a meta-analysis. J Cancer Prev. 2019;24(2):91–111.
129. Omar MI, Roobol MJ, Ribal MJ, Abbott T, Agapow PM, Araujo S, et al. Introducing PIONEER: a project to harness big data in prostate cancer research. Nat Rev Urol. 2020;17(6):351–62.
130. Wang Y, Deng W, Li N, Neri S, Sharma A, Jiang W, et al. Combining immunotherapy and radiotherapy for cancer treatment: current challenges and future directions. Front Pharmacol. 2018;9:185.
131. Dagar G, Gupta A, Masoodi T, Nisar S, Merhi M, Hashem S, et al. Harnessing the potential of CAR-T cell therapy: progress, challenges, and future directions in hematological and solid tumor treatments. J Transl Med [Internet]. 2023;21(1):449. Available from: https://doi.org/10.1186/s12967-023-04292-3.
132. Bhullar KS, Lagarón NO, McGowan EM, Parmar I, Jha A, Hubbard BP, et al. Kinase-targeted cancer therapies: progress, challenges and future directions. Mol Cancer [Internet]. 2018;17(1):48. Available from: https://doi.org/10.1186/s12943-018-0804-2.
133. Kaur P, Singh A, Chana I. Computational techniques and tools for omics data analysis: state-of-the-art, challenges, and future directions. Arch Comput Methods Eng [Internet]. 2021;28(7):4595–631. Available from: https://doi.org/10.1007/s11831-021-09547-0.
134. Jones D, Friend C, Dreher A, Allgar V, Macleod U. The diagnostic test accuracy of rectal examination for prostate cancer diagnosis in symptomatic patients: a systematic review. BMC Fam Pract [Internet]. 2018;19(1):79. Available from: https://doi.org/10.1186/s12875-018-0765-y.
135. Perera M, Papa N, Roberts M, Williams M, Udovicich C, Vela I, et al. Gallium-68 prostate-specific membrane antigen positron emission tomography in advanced prostate cancer—updated diagnostic utility, sensitivity, specificity, and distribution of prostate-specific membrane antigen-avid lesions: a systematic review and meta. Eur Urol [Internet]. 2020;77(4):403–17. Available from: https://www.sciencedirect.com/science/article/pii/S0302283819300958.
136. Bass EJ, Pantovic A, Connor M, Gabe R, Padhani AR, Rockall A, et al. A systematic review and meta-analysis of the diagnostic accuracy of biparametric prostate MRI for prostate cancer in men at risk. Prostate Cancer Prostatic Dis. 2021;24(3):596–611.

137. Swift A, Heale R, Twycross A. What are sensitivity and specificity? Evid Based Nurs. 2020;23(1):2–4.
138. Evans JD, Jethwa KR, Ost P, Williams S, Kwon ED, Lowe VJ, et al. Prostate cancer–specific PET radiotracers: a review on the clinical utility in recurrent disease. Pract Radiat Oncol. 2018;8(1):28–39.
139. de Mendonça DPCM. Biosensors for the early diagnosis of acute myocardial infarction. Universidade de Aveiro (Portugal); 2016.
140. Ellis SD, Hwang S, Morrow E, Kimminau KS, Goonan K, Petty L, et al. Perceived barriers to the adoption of active surveillance in low-risk prostate cancer: a qualitative analysis of community and academic urologists. BMC Cancer [Internet]. 2021;21(1):649. Available from: https://doi.org/10.1186/s12885-021-08386-3.
141. Loeb S, Li R, Sanchez Nolasco T, Byrne N, Cheng HH, Becker D, et al. Barriers and facilitators of germline genetic evaluation for prostate cancer. Prostate. 2021;81(11):754–64.
142. Suri Y, Yasmeh JP, Basu A. Understanding the uptake and challenges of genetic testing guidelines for prostate cancer patients. Cancer Treat Res Commun [Internet]. 2022;32:100588. Available from: https://www.sciencedirect.com/science/article/pii/S2468294222000788.
143. Fox L, Wiseman T, Cahill D, Beyer K, Peat N, Rammant E, et al. Barriers and facilitators to physical activity in men with prostate cancer: a qualitative and quantitative systematic review. Psycho-Oncology. 2019;28(12):2270–85.
144. Saraç H, Morova T, Pires E, McCullagh J, Kaplan A, Cingöz A, et al. Systematic characterization of chromatin modifying enzymes identifies KDM3B as a critical regulator in castration resistant prostate cancer. Oncogene [Internet]. 2020;39(10):2187–201. Available from: https://doi.org/10.1038/s41388-019-1116-8.
145. Obinata D, Yamada Y, Sumiyoshi T, Tanegashima T, Watanabe R, Kobayashi H, et al. Recent advances in basic research on prostate cancer: where we are heading? Int J Urol. 2025;32(3):219–28.
146. Mohler ML, Sikdar A, Ponnusamy S, Hwang DJ, He Y, Miller DD, et al. An overview of next-generation androgen receptor-targeted therapeutics in development for the treatment of prostate cancer. Int J Mol Sci [Internet]. 2021;22(4). Available from: https://www.mdpi.com/1422-0067/22/4/2124.
147. Guelfi G, Cochetti G, Stefanetti V, Zampini D, Diverio S, Boni A, et al. Next generation sequencing of urine exfoliated cells: an approach of prostate cancer microRNAs research. Sci Rep [Internet]. 2018;8(1):7111. Available from: https://doi.org/10.1038/s41598-018-24236-y.
148. Valdés-Mora F, Clark SJ. Prostate cancer epigenetic biomarkers: next-generation technologies. Oncogene [Internet]. 2015;34(13):1609–18. Available from: https://doi.org/10.1038/onc.2014.111.
149. Gaglani S, Gonzalez-Kozlova E, Lundon DJ, Tewari AK, Dogra N, Kyprianou N. Exosomes as a next-generation diagnostic and therapeutic tool in prostate cancer. Int J Mol Sci [Internet]. 2021;22(18). Available from: https://www.mdpi.com/1422-0067/22/18/10131.
150. Nevedomskaya E, Baumgart SJ, Haendler B. Recent advances in prostate cancer treatment and drug discovery. Int J Mol Sci [Internet]. 2018;19(5). Available from: https://www.mdpi.com/1422-0067/19/5/1359.
151. Pirzada M, Altintas Z. Sensor technology: past, present, and future. In: Advanced sensor technology. Elsevier; 2023. p. 3–15.

Magnetic Biosensors: Innovations in the Detection of Prostate Cancer

6

Rahul Kumar, Priyanka Yadav, Deepika Sharma, and Rituparna Chetia

Abbreviations

AI	artificial intelligence
CTCs	circulating tumor cells
GMR	giant magnetoresistance
IoT	Internet of Things
LOD (LoD)	limit of detection
MNPs	magnetic nanoparticles
mpMRI	multiparametric magnetic resonance imaging
MPR	magnetic particle relaxation
PCa	prostate cancer
PCA3	prostate cancer antigen 3
POCT	point-of-care testing
PSA	prostate-specific antigen
TMR	tunnel magnetoresistance
TRUS	transrectal ultrasound

R. Kumar
Faculty of Pharmacy, Vidya University, Meerut, Uttar Pradesh, India

P. Yadav
Department of Pharmaceutical Chemistry, Faculty of Pharmacy, United University Jhalwa, Rawatpura, Prayagraj, Uttar Pradesh, India
e-mail: priyankayadav@unitedunivesity.edu.in

D. Sharma
Department of Pharmacy, School of Medical and Allied Sciences, Galgotias University, Greater Noida, Uttar Pradesh, India

R. Chetia (✉)
Department of Medical Oncology/Hematology, AIIMS, Guwahati, Assam, India

S. Srivastava et al. (eds.), *Biosensor Technologies for Prostate Cancer*,
https://doi.org/10.1007/978-981-95-8644-8_6

6.1 Introduction: The Need for Advanced Prostate Cancer Diagnostics

The disease of prostate cancer (PCa) stands as a substantial worldwide health problem because it emerges as one of the main types of cancer affecting men, while becoming a primary cause of male cancer mortality worldwide [1]. The diagnostic process faces multiple challenges that negatively affect patient care and quality, although therapy innovations yield better results for some patients [2]. Current diagnostic methods are limited because they cause diagnostic uncertainty that produces patient distress, together with the challenge of distinguishing important cancer from untreated harmless cases [3]. The complex environment reveals an immediate requirement for advanced diagnostic systems that can deliver precise and ideal invasive detection, together with characterization methods for prostate cancer [4]. A new technological solution is examined in this chapter because magnetic biosensors have displayed potential to solve vital diagnostic issues for prostate cancer detection [5].

6.1.1 Prostate Cancer Burden and Limitations of Current Diagnostics

A person experiencing suspected prostate cancer begins their clinical journey through tests consisting of both the prostate-specific antigen blood test and digital rectal examination [6]. The mass use of prostate-specific antigen (PSA) testing has helped doctors identify prostate cancer earlier, yet this major test also has major shortcomings that limit its effectiveness [7]. The prostate-specific protein called PSA originates from both normal and cancerous prostate cells, despite being non-specific for cancer cells [8]. The combination of benign prostate conditions, including benign prostatic hyperplasia (BPH) and prostatitis, increases false positive PSA results because these problems can cause PSA levels to rise [9]. Medical tests start follow-up examinations, which often require invasive biopsies to be performed on people with non-significant prostate cancer, leading to unwanted health expenses and procedure-related risks, together with patient anxiety [10]. In cases of aggressive cancers, the PSA levels might show decreased markers, so clinicians could miss the diagnosis [10]. Clinical assessment includes the DRE as a standard method, but it depends on the examiner's experience and shows limited ability to identify small early-stage tumors or those in anterior locations [10]. The utility of transrectal ultrasound (TRUS) in prostate cancer diagnosis lies in its use for medical procedures rather than direct diagnoses, since advanced imaging such as multiparametric magnetic resonance imaging (mpMRI) improves targeting but remains inaccessible and non-definitive [11]. Doctors consider prostate biopsy involving transrectal or transperineal needle extraction under TRUS or MRI guidance to be the definitive method for diagnosing PCa [12]. Prostate biopsy procedures trigger an array of medical risks that include bleeding, postoperative infection, and the experience of pain and discomfort for patients [13]. Standard biopsy protocols experience sampling errors, which result in both false negative diagnoses of clinically significant tumors and potentially labeling the patient with a diagnosis of low-grade cancers that will not endanger their life [14]. The separation of indolent from aggressive disease through biopsy analysis emerges as an unclear task [15].

6.1.2 Magnetic Biosensors: Principles and Potential

Magnetic biosensors have proven to be powerful diagnostic tools because regular cancer diagnostic methods have shown insufficient capability [16]. Biosensors unite magnetic materials with biorecognition elements, such as antibodies and nucleic acid probes, and magnetic nanoparticles (MNPs) to detect specific analytes [17]. When an analyte binds to the sensor system, it leads to changes in the magnetic properties of the detection method as well as disturbances in external magnetic fields [18]. Analysts employ susceptibility changes and GMR/TMR effects, relaxation time variations, and Hall voltage fluctuations to transmit signals through magnetic instruments [19]. Magnetic biosensors achieve high sensitivity measurement by utilizing biological solutions with minimal magnetism since this feature produces low noise alongside strong signal-to-noise ratios [20]. Biosensors based on magnetic detection enable scientists to identify specific biomarkers, such as prostate-specific antigen (PSA), along with other low-abundance disease indicators for early-stage prostate cancer (PCa) [21]. Biosensor systems require minimal sample preparation work because they function efficiently in complex testing fluids, such as blood and urine, thereby simplifying testing procedures [22]. The manipulation functions of MNPs under external magnetic fields enhance the analytical capabilities by producing target concentration and separation, leading to improved detection outcomes [23]. The GMR and TMR sensors, featuring magnetic sensing components, demonstrate compatibility with microfabrication processes, enabling their integration into portable lab-on-a-chip instruments. Point-of-care devices with real-time monitoring capabilities become possible through this compatible mechanism [24]. Magnetic biosensors provide an effective detection method for highly sensitive biomarker analysis through their ability to examine PCa biomarkers ranging from PSA isoforms to nucleic acids and circulating tumor cells and exosomes [25]. This section analyzes magnetic biosensor fundamentals along with present diagnostic systems, assessments of performance criteria, and their future integration within clinical operations [26]. Table 6.1 provides an overview of essential principles and components, detection methods, and applications of magnetic biosensors. This table explains the fundamental concepts and technology of magnetic biosensors, alongside an assessment of their clinical applications [27].

Table 6.1 Key concepts and applications of magnetic biosensors

Features	Description	References
Biosensor components	Magnetic materials, biorecognition elements (e.g., antibodies, nucleic acid probes), and magnetic nanoparticles (MNPs)	[28]
Detection mechanism	Changes in magnetic properties and disturbances in external magnetic fields upon analyte binding	[29]
Signal transduction	Susceptibility change, GMR/TMR effects, relaxation time variations, Hall voltage fluctuations	[30]
Sensitivity	High sensitivity with minimal magnetism from biological solutions	[31]
Application in cancer detection	Detection of biomarkers like PSA, low-abundance disease indicators for early-stage prostate cancer (PCa)	[32]
Sample preparation	Minimal sample preparation required; works efficiently in complex fluids (e.g., blood, urine)	[33]
Magnetic manipulation	MNPs under external magnetic fields enhance detection by producing target concentration and separation	[34]
Compatibility with microfabrications	GMR/TMR sensors can be integrated into portable lab-on-a-chip devices for real-time, point-of-care monitoring	[35]
Biosensor applications	Detection of biomarkers (e.g., PSA isoforms), nucleic acids, circulating tumor cells, and exosomes for highly sensitive biomarker analysis	[36]

6.2 Fundamentals of Magnetic Biosensors

Magnetic biosensors stand as next-generation diagnostic instruments because they use magnetic effects to assess biomolecular interactions [37]. The fundamental operational elements in magnetic biosensors consist of magnetic nanoparticles (MNPs) together with sophisticated magnetic detection systems [38]. The sensors present exceptional sensitivity alongside specificity that works optimally for analyzing complex biological samples like blood, serum, and urine without background biomagnetic interference [39]. The initial part shows the fundamental elements of magnetic biosensors, from their magnetic nanoparticles up to their essential detection approaches that produce superior biosensing capabilities [40]. The principal workflow of magnetic biosensors for prostate cancer, as outlined in Fig. 6.1, supports easier conceptual understanding [41].

6.2.1 Magnetic Nanoparticles (MNPs) in Biosensing

Magnetic nanoparticles (MNPs) work as nanomaterials based on iron oxide that present superparamagnetic properties because they become powerfully magnetized under external magnetic fields yet maintain no magnetic traces after these

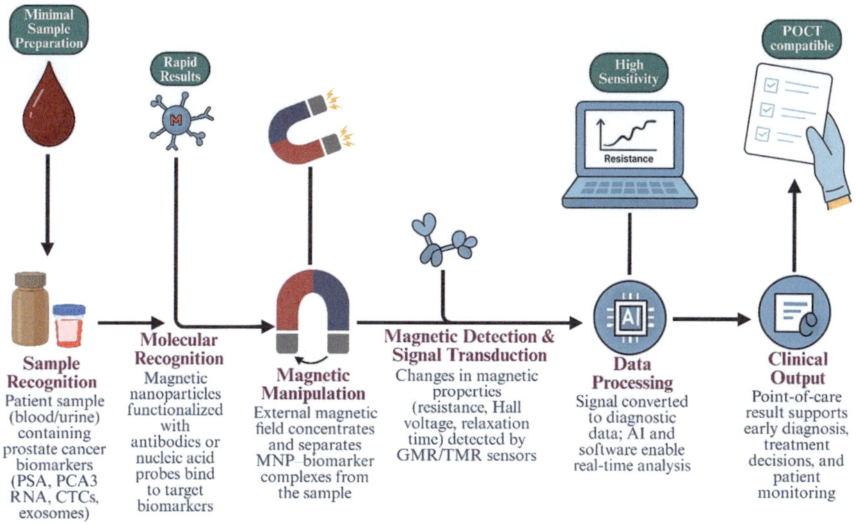

Fig. 6.1 Molecular-to-clinical workflow of magnetic biosensor-based prostate cancer detection

fields are withdrawn [42]. Their ability to be magnetically susceptible makes them suitable for biomedical uses [43]. MNPs serve as biosensing agents when modified with biorecognition elements such as antibodies together with aptamers or oligonucleotides for biomarker targeting [44]. The binding of target analytes causes nanoparticles to undergo alteration of both magnetic and physical characteristics that magnetic sensors can detect [45]. The use of MNPs in biosensing carries out several critical functions. The attachment of MNPs to targets allows researchers to both recognize and generate detectable signals, which yield high contrast [46]. Magnetic separation, along with concentration, relies on external magnetic fields that enable MNPs to become manipulatable tools for sample purification and analyte enrichment [47]. The magnetic response becomes enhanced using two methods; clustering effects and magnetic tagging systems to produce elevated detection sensitivity [48]. MNPs allow biosensing operations in challenging matrices by omitting expensive sample preparation protocols, which enables immediate and on-site diagnostic testing.

6.2.2 Key Magnetic Detection Technologies (GMR, TMR, MPR, etc.)

Magnetic biosensors turn biological interactions into measurable signals through different magnetic transduction procedures [49]. The most prominent methods include the following: *Giant Magnetoresistance (GMR)*: GMR sensors use electrical resistance changes that occur when magnetic layers align because of the presence of an external magnetic field [50]. The modification of electron spin alignment caused by MNP-labeled targets that bind near the sensor alters resistance levels at the local magnetic field location. The GMR sensors provide excellent sensitivity along with CMOS technology compatibility, which allows them to function well with miniature diagnostic devices. *Tunnel Magnetoresistance (TMR):* The functioning principle of TMR involves electron tunneling between two magnetic layers divided by an insulator. The sensor junction resistance levels off based on how two magnetic fields align in relation to one another [51]. Tunnel magnetoresistance becomes an excellent choice when higher sensitivity alongside better signal resolution is needed, yet its fabrication process remains challenging. *Magnetic Particle Relaxation (MPR)*: MPR determines the amount of time MNPs require to stop moving past the removal of an applied magnetic field. The target molecule detection causes changes in the relaxation behavior, which results from hydrodynamic volume variations [52]. The detection system supports real-time label-free recognition within turbid media through this method, which operates well with homogeneous assay systems. *Other Technologies*: The detection method utilizes magneto-optical properties to perform dual-mode sensing operations. The Hall effect produces voltage changes in magnetic sensors, which monitor field variations near bound MNPs. The different detection technologies provide distinct capabilities regarding signal detection, system expandability, and supporting capabilities [44]. The choice of magnetic detection system depends on both the diagnostic needs and the biomarkers and the required test method.

6.3 Target Biomarkers in Prostate Cancer

The diagnosis and evaluation of prostate cancer (PCa) treatment effectiveness, as well as the estimation of clinical outcomes, heavily depend on biomarkers [53]. Precise medical practices require trustworthy biomarkers to support doctors during patient care and achieve better treatment outcomes. Biosensors based on magnetism offer an attractive technique for detecting biomarkers through minimally handled biological fluids, enabling precise identification. The section focuses on important biomarkers that aid both PCa detection and monitoring through analysis of their use within magnetic biosensing platforms [54].

6.3.1 Established and Emerging Biomarkers (PSA, PCA3, CTCs, Exosomes, etc.)

Prostate-Specific Antigen (PSA): PSA serves as the primary biomarker for prostate cancer screening, complemented by monitoring procedures. The protein functions as a serine protease that is expressed by prostate epithelial cells [55]. PSA levels become elevated in the diagnosis of PCa; however, this biomarker also rises in cases of prostatitis and benign prostatic hyperplasia (BPH), which affects its diagnostic accuracy. Studies demonstrate that magnetic biosensors offer effective detection of total PSA and specific isoforms, such as free PSA and [−2] proPSA, which achieve superior sensitivity and separation potential in the early diagnosis and relapse surveillance ranges. *Prostate Cancer Antigen 3 (PCA3)*: The non-coding RNA PCA3 shows extremely elevated expression levels in prostate cancer tissues. The PCA3 detection from urine samples collected after digital rectal examination enhances PCa diagnosis through better performance than PSA [3]. Non-invasive molecular diagnostics of PCA3 are possible through MNP-conjugated nucleic acid probes operating on magnetic biosensors, which can serve as point-of-care testing devices. *Circulating Tumor Cells (CTCs)*: Primary tumor cancer cells break away to enter the circulating bloodstreams and become known as CTCs. The detection of these cells signals both a risk of metastases and an indirect determination of therapy effectiveness and disease evolution outlook [56]. Antibody-functionalized MNPs enable the magnetic separation method to extract CTCs from blood samples. Magnetic sensing or molecular tests benefit from the initial magnetic separation process to enable CTC monitoring within clinical practice systems. *Exosomes and Extracellular Vesicles*: The cell origin determines what proteins, lipids, and nucleic acids will be found in exosomes, which are small vesicles secreted by cells. The diagnostic information contained in PCa-derived exosomes established through urine and blood analyses includes PSA, PCA3, and TMPRSS2-ERG gene fusion transcripts [57]. Biosensors with magnetic features can identify and analyze exosomes through particular surface markers (CD63 and EpCAM) in a system that detects multiple molecules while requiring minimal sample input. *Emerging Biomarkers*: Human cells contain microRNA (miRNA), which are short non-coding RNA molecules that show irregular expression patterns in prostate cancer [58]. The research community is exploring miR-141 and miR-21 signatures as potential diagnostic indicators that could also facilitate clinical risk assessment. Gene fusions (e.g., TMPRSS2-ERG): These fusions are detected in a significant subset of PCa cases, particularly through RNA analysis in urine or tissue [59]. Multi-analysis panels containing protein molecules offer better diagnostic performance than individual biomarkers. Magnetic biosensor systems with miniaturized design and multi-analyte detection capability show strong potential to improve the detection of prostate cancer and its risk stratification, as well as treatment monitoring capability [60]. The biomarkers provide foundational knowledge for creating upcoming non-invasive diagnostic equipment, which will be examined in the following sections.

6.4 Magnetic Biosensor Platforms for Prostate Cancer Applications

Magnetic biosensor platforms bring a complete transformation to the diagnostic and monitoring practices of prostate cancer (PCa) [61]. Prostate cancer diagnosis benefits from magnetic biosensors by utilizing magnetic nanoparticles that can identify biomarkers regardless of fluid complexity [62]. Practical applications of magnetic biosensing in prostate cancer assessment include testing proteins and nucleic acids and extracting circulating tumor cells and exosomes during investigations of complex biological fluids with the help of multiplexed sensing platforms [63].

6.4.1 Detecting Circulating Tumor Cells (CTCs) and Exosomes

Biosensors based on magnetism serve widespread detection of protein biomarkers, including prostate-specific antigen (PSA), along with its isoforms, together with nucleic acids such as PCA3 mRNA and gene fusions (e.g., TMPRSS2-ERG) [64]. MNPs receive protein detection capability through integration of antibody functionalities, which allow specific protein binding. When MNPs interact with the sensor, they modify the magnetic field properties, which enable the detection of signals by TMR, GMR, or a Hall effect sensor [65]. The systems deliver low-picogram sensitivity combined with swift results, which makes them optimal for early identification and monitoring patients after treatment [3]. The binding capability of oligonucleotide-functionalized MNPs matches specific RNA or DNA sequences associated with PCa [61]. MNP clustering, as well as magnetic relaxation signal shift detection systems, are used in current detection platforms during hybridization. The techniques eliminate the need for PCR amplification to deliver precise point-of-care molecular detection solutions [66].

6.4.2 Detecting Circulating Tumor Cells (CTCs) and Exosomes

Madge, microscale objects named circulating tumor cells (CTCs) possess strong medical significance despite their scarce occurrence [67]. Whole blood analysis of CTCs becomes possible through magnetic biosensor platforms by adding epithelial marker-tagged MNPs (e.g., EpCAM) for isolation and detection purposes [68]. The gradient of magnetic fields used for cell separation allows the enumeration of labeled cells directly on the chip or enables additional molecular assessments to guide treatment decisions [69]. Exosomes contain specific proteins and nucleic acids that are tumor-dependent. A magnetic biosensor can detect exosomes through MNPs, which are conjugated with exosome surface antibodies such as CD63, CD9, or EpCAM [70]. The analysis of PCa biomarkers becomes possible once the vesicles get captured through magnetic signal changes in a minimally invasive, rapid diagnostic method [71]. The methods raise diagnostic efficiency by recognizing tumor metastatic possibilities in the early stages while conducting continuous treatment monitoring.

6.4.3 Multiplexed Detection Approaches

It is heterogeneous, as binucleate cancer of the prostate, and therefore, the detection of many biomarkers by multiplexed screening delivers essential benefits in diagnosing and creating individualized treatment plans [72]. Present-day platforms that utilize multiple magnetic sensors to detect various biomarkers simultaneously are also examples of magnetic array platforms [73]. This array consists of functionalized sites where the capture agents specifically bind to the target MNP [74]. This detection method provides a quantitative analysis of both PSA and PCA3 in a single biological sample, utilizing miRNAs and exosomal markers. Advantages of multiplexing include the following [3]: It improves diagnostic accuracy through multimarker signatures; It is also able to shorten the test time while requiring fewer sample amounts; Panel tests that express disease aggressiveness potential or therapeutic outcomes may be included in magnetic sensors; Combining the biological elements within microfluidic systems with magnetic biosensing is made possible by these microfluidic systems and smartphone readers to develop pocket-sized diagnostic tools. Magnetic biosensor platforms offer a top diagnostic approach for prostate cancer with fast, responsive tests requiring little sample that can provide for today's need for precise as well as individualized medical practices [75]. Later sections will discuss both field examples and clinical confirmation attempts to prove that laboratory breakthroughs do, in fact, lead to implementation in the hospital.

6.5 Performance, Validation, and Comparison

Rigid evaluation of the analytical performance and clinical relevance of magnetic biosensors for prostate cancer (PCa) diagnostics is a key step in the translational path of magnetic biosensors for PCa diagnostics [76]. It requires understanding their sensitivity, specificity, and limit of detection (LoD) so as to compare them with other conventional diagnostic methods [77]. Furthermore, they are validated (head-to-head comparisons), and reliability is established to be able to get regulatory approval and clinical adoption [78].

6.5.1 Key Performance Metrics (Sensitivity, Specificity, LoD)

Sensitivity and specificity are two main diagnostic parameters of the biosensor utility. Sensitivity is a measure of the sensor's capacity for correct determination of true positive cases; that is, it is very important for the detection of low-abundance biomarkers, such as, for example, PSA isoforms, PCA transcripts, and circulating tumor cells (CTCs) at early stages of disease [79]. Part of specificity's contribution comes from eliminating non-cancer cases, a measure critical given PSA's well-known lack of specificity [80].

Using magnetic biosensors, giant magnetoresistance (GMR) or magnetic particle relaxation (MPR)-based techniques, such magnetic biosensors can achieve sensitivities in the picomolar to femtomolar range and are able to differentiate signals amid insignificant amounts of non-specific background interference, even in complicated biological matrices such as serum or blood [81]. Performance Metrics for Magnetic Biosensor Systems SPECS provides the clarification of key evaluation parameters (such as sensitivity, specificity, and LoD) (Table 6.2) [82]. This metric defines the lowest concentration of an analyte that can be reliably distinguished from the absence of signal (limit of detection or LoD [83]). That biosensors are capable of detecting PCa biomarkers with magnetic LoD values of 1 to a few pg/mL for PSA and sub-attomolar ranges for nucleic acids puts these biosensors in a good

Table 6.2 Performance metrics for magnetic biosensor systems

Metric	Definition	Ideal range	Importance	References
Sensitivity	Ability to detect low levels	>90%	Early detection	[35]
Specificity	Ability to exclude non-targets	>90%	Reduce false positives	[30]
LoD (limit of detection)	Minimum detectable amount	<1 ng/ml	Critical for the early stage	[32]

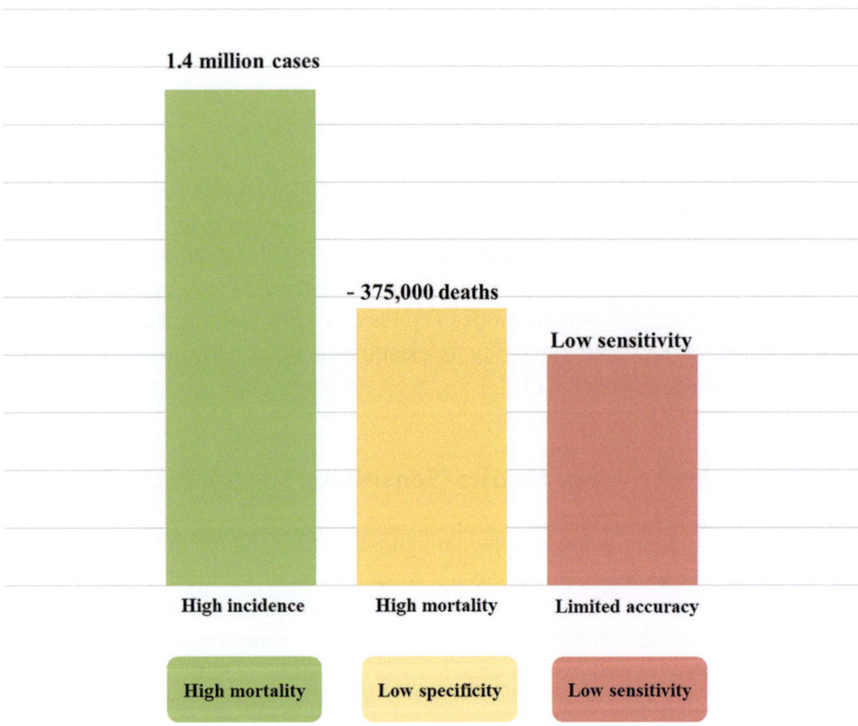

Fig. 6.2 Global prostate cancer burden and diagnostic limitations. The high incidence (~1.4 million cases) and mortality (~375,000 deaths) of prostate cancer and its inherent limitations in current diagnostics are also depicted in the figure, including low sensitivity, low specificity, and limited overall accuracy

position as early diagnosis and surveillance devices. However, prostate cancer is still one of the major global health problems, with about 1.4 million new cases and nearly 375,000 deaths per year. Current diagnostics are not specific and sensitive enough to prevent both overtreatment and missed diagnosis (Fig. 6.2); yet, the prevalence makes it a very common occurrence. Additional performance criteria include [84] dynamic range (linear response over a wide concentration range), reproducibility (low coefficient of variation), response time (often within 10–30 minutes), and sample volume requirements (typically <100 μL).

6.5.2 Validation and Comparison to Standard Methods

Validation is a crucial step in the development of any diagnostic or sensing technology, particularly for new biosensors and analytical systems [85]. These systems must be rigorously compared to ensure the reliability, specificity, and sensitivity of these systems are comparable to established gold standard methods, including ELISA (enzyme-linked immunosorbent assay), PCR (polymerase chain reaction), and mass spectrometry [86]. This analytical validation includes the evaluation of the limit of detection (LoD), linearity, dynamic range, repeatability, reproducibility, and selectivity in relation to interfering substances [87]. Conversely, clinical validation assesses performance in real-world scenarios using patient samples as a parameter to evaluate diagnostic sensitivity and specificity, positive and negative predictive values, and comparative outcome accuracy [88]. Emerging technologies excel in competing with established processes, such as requiring smaller sample volumes, shorter turnaround times, and simpler operating procedures. While these benefits exist, standardization, regulatory compliance, and batch-to-batch consistency are major challenges to be overcome before such clinical adoption.

6.6 Innovations and Advanced Systems

Today, sensor, data analytics, and materials science technology have progressed so rapidly that we have an entirely new generation of diagnostic and monitoring systems that are smarter, more responsive, and highly incorporated into multiple healthcare environments [89]. A summary presents the discussed innovations and clinical integration strategies, as shown in Table 6.3 [90].

6.6.1 Integration with Microfluidics and Point-of-Care (POCT) Systems

Validation is a critical phase in the development of any analytical system, but especially for a biosensor(s) or analytical system that is novel [1]. These systems must make sure to be reliable, specific, and sensitive to these gold standard methods like ELISA (enzyme-linked immunosorbent assay), PCR (polymerase chain reaction), and mass spectrometry [99]. The analytical validation evaluated includes limits of detection (LOD), linearity, dynamic range, repeatability, reproducibility, and selectivity against interfering substances [100]. In terms of clinical validation, they take performance in real-world situations, on how they perform on patient samples, in particular, of diagnostic sensitivity and specificity, as well as positive vs. negative predictive values and comparative outcome accuracy [100]. Emerging technologies

Table 6.3 Innovations and integration strategies in advanced biosensor systems

Category	Description and significance	References
Integration with POCT and microfluidics	Advanced biosensor platforms are being miniaturized and integrated into point-of-care testing (POCT) tools and lab-on-chip systems for rapid diagnostics	[91]
Validation parameters	Validation involves both analytical (LOD, linearity, dynamic range, reproducibility, selectivity) and clinical (sensitivity, specificity, predictive value) metrics	[92]
Comparison with gold standards	Novel biosensors must match or surpass standards like ELISA, PCR, and mass spectrometry but provide benefits in speed, sample volume, and process simplicity	[93]
Challenges for clinical translation	Key challenges include standardization, regulatory approval, and batch-to-batch consistency, which delay widespread clinical adoption	[94]
Emerging nanomaterials	Materials such as graphene, gold nanoparticles, and stimuli-responsive polymers enhance sensitivity and enable real-time adaptability	[95]
Flexible and wearable sensor designs	Innovations in flexible/stretchable electronics enable continuous health monitoring via wearable or implantable biosensors	[96]
Advanced data analytics	Use of machine learning, cloud computing, and IoT for real-time data interpretation, improving diagnostic accuracy and patient-specific insights	[97]
Future vision	Integration of multidisciplinary innovations enables predictive diagnostics, personalized medicine, and early disease intervention strategies	[98]

are usually more attractive when benchmarked against conventional methods because they demand less sample volume, shorter turnaround times, and less complicated life cycle processes [101]. While this has benefits, challenges range from standardization and regulatory compliance to batch-to-batch consistency, which are still very big obstacles to unreserved clinical adoption [102].

6.6.2 Novel Materials, Sensor Designs, and Data Analysis

Innovation in materials, sensor architectural design, and intelligent processing of signals are key components for performance improvement of modern diagnostic systems [103]. Nanomaterials such as graphene or gold nanoparticles can improve signal transduction and increase the surface area for biomolecular interactions, and smart polymers give such stimuli-responsive behavior with real-time adaptability [104]. New developments of medical devices based on electronic technology, which offer flexibility and stretchability, can continuously track health conditions with wearable implantable systems [105]. Equal power of transformation is delivered from emerging data analysis capabilities to the simultaneous advancement in hardware development [106]. Table 6.4 provides highlights of cutting-edge designs and materials, along with their impact on biosensor performance [107].

Table 6.4 Tabulating emerging materials and sensor designs

Innovation	Purpose	Impact on performance	References
Graphene-based sensors	Enhanced conductivity	Improved signal-to-noise	[108]
3D magnetic structures	Higher field interaction	Better sensitivity	[109]
AI-driven data analysis	Pattern recognition	Accurate classification	[110]

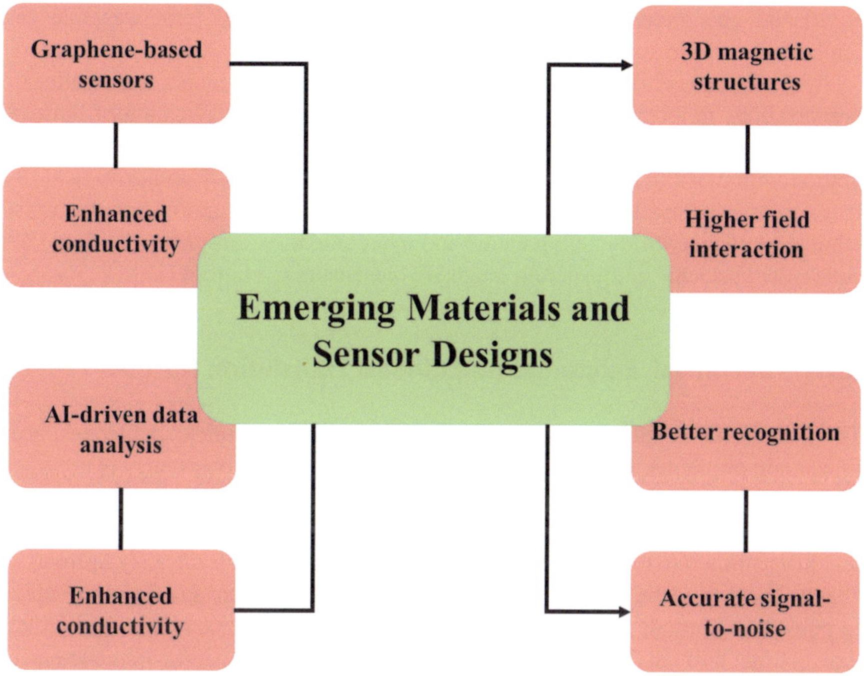

Fig. 6.3 Innovative materials and sensor architectures

This also makes biological signals real-time monitored and aggregated with machine learning applicable for the interpretation of complex biological signals using cloud computing and the Internet of Things (IoT) [111]. This enables an increase in the reliability and robustness of the diagnostic procedures when integrating multiple sensor data. To push boundaries towards patient-specific disease prediction and disease management before they take place, many medical breakthroughs unite together [112]. "Improvements in diagnostic performance and miniaturisation (Fig. 6.3) have been achieved by recent innovations such as integration of novel materials at scale, such as graphene, carbon nanotubes, and AI-assisted signal processing." Advances in these types are redefining magnetic biosensor platform sensitivity, speed, and adaptability for clinical use.

6.7 Challenges and Future Outlook

Even with the great potential of advanced biosensing and diagnostic platforms, there are a number of very significant challenges in the translation of these technologies from the controlled research laboratory prototype state to practical clinical application [113]: satisfying the needs for scalable, cost-effective manufacturing while maintaining high quality; ensuring the robustness and reliability of sensors under real-world patient conditions rather than a stable laboratory bench environment; and guaranteeing biocompatibility and safety in long-term wearable and implantable device applications [114].

Additionally, getting new technologies adopted by individuals and healthcare organizations in a complex corporate environment requires navigation of intricate regulatory approval processes, extensive clinical validation of efficacy, smooth integration with existing healthcare data systems, and data security and privacy [118]. It is essential to successfully translate this promising sensor innovation to routine clinical tools that will benefit patients and overcome these obstacles [2]. Table 6.5 shows the obstacles in translating magnetic biosensors to clinics [119].

6.7.1 Technical, Economic, and Clinical Translation Hurdles

The lack of diagnostic technology advancements due to technical challenges faces three main problems: sensor stability, biocompatibility, and consistency in accuracy under the complex biological environment [120]. Such considerations from an economic point of view include scalability of production, cost-effectiveness, and seamless integration into the current healthcare infrastructure [121]. Literally millions of "hands" have tried the product, failed, and then tried the product again and attempted to publish in journals that will not accept it [122]. Regulatory and clinical hurdles, like getting through FDA/EMA approval processes, establishing reimbursement pathways, and getting acceptance and use from clinicians, are really barriers that prevent widespread use [123]. These multifaceted challenges are surmountable only through great interdisciplinary collaboration amongst engineers, clinicians, regulators, and economists to bring laboratory innovation from the laboratory to the bedside in the form of a medical product [124].

Table 6.5 Challenges in translating magnetic biosensors to clinics

Challenge area	Specific issue	Suggested solutions	References
Technical	Signal drift	Calibration algorithms	[115]
Economic	High fabrication costs	Scalable production	[116]
Clinical	Lack of validation studies	Multicenter trials	[117]

6.7.2 Future Directions and Potential Impact on Patient Care

The biosensing and diagnostic platforms are evolving toward personalized medicine, whereby personalized data collection in real time is gathered from the patient [3]. The advances made in this area are largely due to wearable and implantable diagnostics that facilitate the monitoring of diseases over days, weeks, months, or even years [125]. Additionally, the combination of these AI-supported decision support systems in supporting early detection of disease as well as optimizing treatment plans will be extremely helpful [126]. With these mature technologies, healthcare will be revolutionized as they will drastically reduce diagnostic turnaround times, lead to considerable savings in overall costs, and enable better patient outcomes through timely interventions [127]. Moreover, they can enhance access to essential care, particularly for underserved populations, and pave the way for the era of smart, responsive, and patient-centric healthcare by integrating biosensing, data science, and system integration [128].

6.8 Conclusion

This chapter highlights the significant drawbacks in existing diagnostic strategies for prostate cancer (PCa) detection, particularly the lack of specificity in PSA screening, which necessitates improving specificity and reducing the invasiveness of PCa detection. The emergence of magnetic biosensors as a technology frontier holds significant promise to satisfy this clinical need with the advantages of good sensitivity and possibilities for miniaturization appropriate for advanced diagnostics. Turning to these sensors, we have explored the fundamental principles of these sensors, starting from their basic components, magnetic nanoparticles (MNPs), which serve as mediators of detection, as well as other important transduction techniques, such as GMR, TMR, and MPR. Magnetic biosensors are versatile in their targeting of a range of PCa biomarkers, including established markers such as PSA, new indicators including PCA3, circulating tumor cells (CTCs), and exosomes in the same review. This technology was utilized for discussing various platform configurations designed to detect proteins, nucleic acids, and cellular targets, including highly sophisticated multiplexed systems. The analysis of two essential performance metrics, sensitivity and specificity, and limit of detection, along with the critical processes for validation and benchmarking versus clinical standards, was done to emphasize the rigor of clinical translation. It also reviewed the most significant revolutionary advancements in the field, including the integration of magnetic biosensors with microfluidics to achieve point-of-care testing (POCT), the incorporation of complex materials and sensor designs, and the application of advanced analytics to enhance diagnostic accuracy. These advancements, however, do not overcome the biological and clinical challenges that hinder the translation of these technologies into routine patient care. Finally, the development and refinement of magnetic biosensors for the future look very promising for changing how PCa is diagnosed. We identify overcoming the present challenges as a means by which practically sensitive, specific, and potentially less invasive diagnostic tools could lead to earlier detection, make possible a more personalized approach to treatment, reduce overdiagnosis and attendant unnecessary procedures, and hopefully improve patient outcomes in prostate cancer management. The progression of nanotechnology, bioengineering, and clinical oncology through magnetic biosensing represents a potential future paradigm for more effective and patient-centric cancer care in clinical oncology.

6.9 Summary

This chapter provides an extensive examination of magnetic biosensors as potential new diagnostic instruments for prostate cancer (PCa). It starts by outlining the shortcomings of conventional PSA screening techniques and highlighting the demand for more precise, minimally invasive diagnostics. When it comes to identifying PCa biomarkers like PSA, PCA3, exosomes, and circulating tumor cells (CTCs), magnetic biosensors that use magnetic nanoparticles (MNPs) have excellent sensitivity and specificity. In order to enhance performance, the chapter covers integration with wearable technology, microfluidic systems, and AI-driven analytics in addition to outlining the mechanisms of magnetic detection techniques (GMR, TMR, and MPR). Also, issues such as a lack of clinical validation, high production costs, and signal drift are reviewed. Future directions for PCa management indicate a paradigm shift toward real-time, personalized monitoring solutions.

Glossary

Biosensor A device that uses biological molecules to detect chemical or biological targets.

Magnetic nanoparticles (MNPs) Nanoscale particles with magnetic properties used for detection and manipulation in biosensing.

GMR (giant magnetoresistance) A magnetoresistive effect used in sensors for detecting small magnetic field changes.

TMR (tunnel magnetoresistance) A sensing technique that uses electron tunneling for magnetic field detection.

MPR (magnetic particle relaxation) A method that detects relaxation time changes in MNPs to identify molecular binding.

Exosomes Nano-sized vesicles secreted by cells that carry molecular information like proteins and RNA.

CTCs (circulating tumor cells) Cancer cells that have detached from a primary tumor and circulate in the bloodstream.

POCT (point-of-care testing) Diagnostic testing performed at or near the site of patient care.

Lab-on-a-chip Miniaturized devices integrating multiple laboratory functions on a single chip.

AI (artificial intelligence) The simulation of human intelligence by machines for tasks like data interpretation and prediction.

References

1. Bernstein DE, Piedad J, Hemsworth L, West A, Johnston ID, Dimov N, et al. Prostate cancer and microfluids. Urol Oncol Semin Orig Investig. 2021;39(8):455–70. Available from: https://www.sciencedirect.com/science/article/pii/S1078143921001204.
2. Kim TJ, Lee YH, Koo KC. Current status and future perspectives of androgen receptor inhibition therapy for prostate cancer: a comprehensive review. Biomolecules. 2021;11(4). Available from: https://www.mdpi.com/2218-273X/11/4/492
3. Chen HMHYHHH, Zhang JJJJ, Huang R, Wang DDXDDD, Deng D, Zhang QQQQQQ, et al. Nanomaterial-based electrochemical sensors for the detection of pharmaceutical drugs. Schatten H, editor. Cancers (Basel). 2022;14(1):35. Available from: https://www.sciencedirect.com/science/article/pii/S0039914020305671
4. Lorenc T, Klimczyk K, Michalczewska I, Słomka M, Kubiak-Tomaszewska G, Olejarz W. Exosomes in prostate cancer diagnosis, prognosis and therapy. Int J Mol Sci. 2020;21(6). Available from: https://www.mdpi.com/1422-0067/21/6/2118
5. Gillessen S, Bossi A, Davis ID, de Bono J, Fizazi K, James ND, et al. Management of patients with advanced prostate cancer. Part I: intermediate–/high-risk and locally advanced disease, biochemical relapse, and side effects of hormonal treatment: report of the Advanced Prostate Cancer Consensus Conference 2022. Eur Urol. 2023;83(3):267–93.
6. Kelly SP, Anderson WF, Rosenberg PS, Cook MB. Past, current, and future incidence rates and burden of metastatic prostate cancer in the United States. Eur Urol Focus. 2018;4(1):121–7.
7. Williams IS, McVey A, Perera S, O'Brien JS, Kostos L, Chen K, et al. Modern paradigms for prostate cancer detection and management. Med J Aust. 2022 Oct;217(8):424–33.
8. Van Poppel H, Albreht T, Basu P, Hogenhout R, Collen S, Roobol M. Serum PSA-based early detection of prostate cancer in Europe and globally: past, present and future. Nat Rev Urol. 2022;19(9):562–72.
9. Pulumati A, Pulumati A, Dwarakanath BS, Verma A, Papineni RVL. Technological advancements in cancer diagnostics: improvements and limitations. Cancer Rep. 2023;6(2):e1764.
10. Bleyer A, Spreafico F, Barr R. Prostate cancer in young men: an emerging young adult and older adolescent challenge. Cancer. 2020;126(1):46–57.
11. Smith Palmer J, Takizawa C, Valentine W. Literature review of the burden of prostate cancer in Germany, France, the United Kingdom and Canada. BMC Urol. 2019;19:1–16.
12. Faria R, Soares MO, Spackman E, Ahmed HU, Brown LC, Kaplan R, et al. Optimising the diagnosis of prostate cancer in the era of multiparametric magnetic resonance imaging: a cost-effectiveness analysis based on the prostate MR imaging study (PROMIS). Eur Urol. 2018;73(1):23–30.
13. Ström P, Kartasalo K, Olsson H, Solorzano L, Delahunt B, Berney DM, et al. Artificial intelligence for diagnosis and grading of prostate cancer in biopsies: a population-based, diagnostic study. Lancet Oncol. 2020;21(2):222–32.
14. Fenton JJ, Weyrich MS, Durbin S, Liu Y, Bang H, Melnikow J. Prostate-specific antigen–based screening for prostate cancer: evidence report and systematic review for the US Preventive Services Task Force. JAMA. 2018;319(18):1914–31.
15. Panebianco V, Barchetti G, Simone G, Del Monte M, Ciardi A, Grompone MD, et al. Negative multiparametric magnetic resonance imaging for prostate cancer: what's next? Eur Urol. 2018;74(1):48–54.

16. Narlawar S, Coudhury S, Gandhi S. Chapter 10 - Magnetic properties-based biosensors for early detection of cancer. In: Khan R, Parihar A, Sanghi SK, editors. Biosensor based advanced cancer diagnostics. Academic Press; 2022. p. 165–78. Available from: https://www.sciencedirect.com/science/article/pii/B9780128234242000107
17. Hosu O, Tertis M, Cristea C. Implication of magnetic nanoparticles in cancer detection, Screening and Treatment. Magnetochemistry. 2019;5(4). Available from: https://www.mdpi.com/2312-7481/5/4/55
18. Calatayud DG, Neophytou S, Nicodemou E, Giuffrida SG, Ge H, Pascu SI. Nano-theranostics for the sensing, imaging and therapy of prostate cancers. Front Chem. 2022;10:830133.
19. Mostufa S, Rezaei B, Yari P, Xu K, Gómez-Pastora J, Sun J, et al. Giant magnetoresistance based biosensors for cancer screening and detection. ACS Appl Bio Mater. 2023;6(10):4042–59. https://doi.org/10.1021/acsabm.3c00592.
20. Kavetskyy T, Alipour M, Smutok O, Mushynska O, Kiv A, Fink D, et al. Magneto-immunoassay of cancer biomarkers: recent progress and challenges in biomedical analysis. Microchem J. 2021;167:106320. Available from: https://www.sciencedirect.com/science/article/pii/S0026265X21004045
21. Uhlirova D, Stankova M, Docekalova M, Hosnedlova B, Kepinska M, Ruttkay-Nedecky B, et al. A rapid method for the detection of sarcosine using SPIONs/au/CS/SOX/NPs for prostate cancer sensing. Int J Mol Sci. 2018;19(12). Available from: https://www.mdpi.com/1422-0067/19/12/3722
22. Dehghani P, Salehirozveh M, Tajabadi A, Yeung CC, Lam M, Leung HY, et al. Next-gen point-of-care tool for ultra-sensitive detection of urinary spermine for prostate cancer diagnosis. ACS Sens. 2025;10(4):2640–51. https://doi.org/10.1021/acssensors.4c03250.
23. Khan R, Arshad F, Hassan IU, Naikoo GA, Pedram MZ, Zedegan MS, et al. Advances in nanomaterial-based immunosensors for prostate cancer screening. Biomed Pharmacother. 2022;155:113649. Available from: https://www.sciencedirect.com/science/article/pii/S0753332222010381
24. Haleem A, Javaid M, Singh RP, Suman R, Rab S. Biosensors applications in medical field: a brief review. Sensors Int. 2021;2:100100.
25. Li CH, Chan MH, Chang YC, Hsiao M. Gold nanoparticles as a biosensor for cancer biomarker determination. Molecules. 2023;28(1). Available from: https://www.mdpi.com/1420-3049/28/1/364
26. Wang Q, Liu J, Zeng J, Yang Z, Ran F, Wu L, et al. Determination of miRNA derived from exosomes of prostate cancer via toehold-aided cyclic amplification combined with HRP enzyme catalysis and magnetic nanoparticles. Anal Biochem. 2021;630:114336.
27. Yang Q, Li N, Li Q, Chen S, Wang HL, Yang H. Amperometric sarcosine biosensor based on hollow magnetic Pt–Fe3O4@ C nanospheres. Anal Chim Acta. 2019;1078:161–7.
28. Issadore D, Min C, Liong M, Chung J, Weissleder R, Lee H. Miniature magnetic resonance system for point-of-care diagnostics. Lab Chip. 2011;11(13):2282–7. https://doi.org/10.1039/C1LC20177H.
29. Zhao F, He J, Li X, Bai Y, Ying Y, Ping J. Smart plant-wearable biosensor for in-situ pesticide analysis. Biosens Bioelectron. 2020;170:112636. Available from: https://www.sciencedirect.com/science/article/pii/S0956566320306266.
30. Connolly MR, Chiu KL, Giblin SP, Kataoka M, Fletcher JD, Chua C, et al. Gigahertz quantized charge pumping in graphene quantum dots. Nat Nanotechnol. 2013;8(6):417–20. https://doi.org/10.1038/nnano.2013.73.
31. Gu GY, Wang X, Zhou HL, Liu BL. Progresses of magnetic relaxation switch sensor in medical diagnosis and food safety analysis. Chinese J Anal Chem. 2018;46(8):1161–70. Available from: https://www.sciencedirect.com/science/article/pii/S1872204018611028.
32. Rho J, Jang W, Hwang I, Lee D, Lee CH, Chung TD. Multiplex immunoassays using virus-tethered gold microspheres by DC impedance-based flow cytometry. Biosens Bioelectron. 2018;102:121–8. Available from: https://www.sciencedirect.com/science/article/pii/S0956566317307558.

33. Lee H, Sun E, Ham D, Weissleder R. Chip–NMR biosensor for detection and molecular analysis of cells. Nat Med. 2008;14(8):869–74. https://doi.org/10.1038/nm.1711.
34. Mostufa S, Rezaei B, Azizi E, Wang YA, Li C, Gómez-Pastora J, et al. Characterizing the physicochemical properties of magnetic nanoparticles by a surface plasmon resonance approach. AIP Adv. 2025;15(3):35022. https://doi.org/10.1063/9.0000856.
35. Gaster RS, Hall DA, Nielsen CH, Osterfeld SJ, Yu H, Mach KE, et al. Matrix-insensitive protein assays push the limits of biosensors in medicine. Nat Med. 2009;15(11):1327–32. https://doi.org/10.1038/nm.2032.
36. Deng Y, Liu SY, Chua SL, Khoo BL. The effects of biofilms on tumor progression in a 3D cancer-biofilm microfluidic model. Biosens Bioelectron. 2021;180:113113. Available from: https://www.sciencedirect.com/science/article/pii/S0956566321001500.
37. Cheng K, Shun W, Jian-Wei Y, Si-Yu C, Hai-Long W, Chang-Hong X, et al. Applications of biosensors in bladder cancer. Crit Rev Anal Chem. 1–20. https://doi.org/10.1080/10408347.2024.2373923.
38. Rusling JF, Forster RJ. Biosensors designed for clinical applications. Biomedicine. 2021;9(7). Available from: https://www.mdpi.com/2227-9059/9/7/702
39. Li P, Long F, Chen W, Chen J, Chu PK, Wang H. Fundamentals and applications of surface-enhanced Raman spectroscopy–based biosensors. Curr Opin Biomed Eng. 2020;13:51–9. Available from: https://www.sciencedirect.com/science/article/pii/S2468451119300273.
40. Abdel-Karim R. Nanotechnology-enabled biosensors: a review of fundamentals, materials, applications, challenges, and future scope. Biomed Mater Devices. 2024;2(2):759–77. https://doi.org/10.1007/s44174-023-00147-z.
41. Klebes A, Ates HC, Verboket RD, Urban GA, von Stetten F, Dincer C, et al. Emerging multianalyte biosensors for the simultaneous detection of protein and nucleic acid biomarkers. Biosens Bioelectron. 2024;244:115800. Available from: https://www.sciencedirect.com/science/article/pii/S095656632300742X.
42. Farzin A, Etesami SA, Quint J, Memic A, Tamayol A. Magnetic nanoparticles in cancer therapy and diagnosis. Adv Healthc Mater. 2020;9(9):1901058.
43. Kim HS, Lee JS, Il KM. Poly-γ-glutamic Acid/Chitosan hydrogel nanoparticles entrapping glucose oxidase and magnetic nanoparticles for glucose biosensing. J Nanosci Nanotechnol. 2020;20(9):5333–7.
44. Su D, Wu K, Saha R, Peng C, Wang JP. Advances in magnetoresistive biosensors. Micromachines. 2020;11(1). Available from: https://www.mdpi.com/2072-666X/11/1/34
45. Parmanik A, Bose A. Magnetic nanoparticles used in biosensors. In: Materials and components of biosensors in healthcare. Elsevier; 2025. p. 165–74.
46. Wang M, Jin L, Hang-Mei Leung P, Wang-Ngai Chow F, Zhao X, Chen H, et al. Advancements in magnetic nanoparticle-based biosensors for point-of-care testing. Front Bioeng Biotechnol. 2024;12:1393789.
47. Zimina TM, Sitkov NO, Gareev KG, Fedorov V, Grouzdev D, Koziaeva V, et al. Biosensors and drug delivery in oncotheranostics using inorganic synthetic and biogenic magnetic nanoparticles. Biosensors. 2022;12(10). Available from: https://www.mdpi.com/2079-6374/12/10/789
48. Altintas Z. Applications of magnetic nanomaterials in biosensors and diagnostics. In: Biosens Nanotechnol Appl Health Care Diagnost; 2018. p. 277–96.
49. Usman F, Ghazali KH, Muda R, Johari NH, Dennis JO, Tamam N, et al. Magnetoresistance and magneto-plasmonic sensors for the detection of cancer biomarkers: a bibliometric analysis and recent advances. Sens Actuators Rep. 2023;6:100172. Available from: https://www.sciencedirect.com/science/article/pii/S2666053923000358
50. Dey P, Roy JN. Spintronics applications. In: Spintronics: fundamentals and applications. Singapore: Springer Singapore; 2021. p. 223–67. https://doi.org/10.1007/978-981-16-0069-2_10.
51. Ghemes C, Dragos-Pinzaru OG, Tibu M, Lostun M, Lupu N, Chiriac H. Tunnel magnetoresistance-based sensor for biomedical application: proof-of-concept. Coatings. 2023;13(2). Available from: https://www.mdpi.com/2079-6412/13/2/227

52. Ren C, Bayin Q, Feng S, Fu Y, Ma X, Guo J. Biomarkers detection with magnetoresistance-based sensors. Biosens Bioelectron. 2020;165:112340. Available from: https://www.sciencedirect.com/science/article/pii/S0956566320303353.
53. Coman RA, Schitcu VH, Budisan L, Raduly L, Braicu C, Petrut B, et al. Evaluation of miR-148a-3p and miR-106a-5p as biomarkers for prostate cancer: pilot study. Genes (Basel). 2024;15(5). Available from: https://www.mdpi.com/2073-4425/15/5/584
54. Wüstemann T, Haberkorn U, Babich J, Mier W. Targeting prostate cancer: prostate-specific membrane antigen based diagnosis and therapy. Med Res Rev. 2019;39(1):40–69.
55. Wang X, Zhang L, Cheng L, Wang Y, Li M, Yu J, et al. Extracellular vesicle-derived biomarkers in prostate cancer care: opportunities and challenges. Cancer Lett. 2024;601:217184. Available from: https://www.sciencedirect.com/science/article/pii/S0304383524005792.
56. Tang S, Cheng H, Zang X, Tian J, Ling Z, Wang L, et al. Small extracellular vesicles: crucial mediators for prostate cancer. J Nanobiotechnol. 2025;23(1):230. https://doi.org/10.1186/s12951-025-03326-w.
57. Liao C, Wu Z, Lin C, Chen X, Zou Y, Zhao W, et al. Nurturing the marriages of urinary liquid biopsies and nano-diagnostics for precision urinalysis of prostate cancer. Smart Med. 2023;2(1):e20220020.
58. Janjua KA, Shahzad R, Shehzad A. Development of novel cancer biomarkers for diagnosis and prognosis. In: Cancer biomarkers in diagnosis and therapeutics. Springer; 2022. p. 277–343.
59. Ionescu F, Zhang J, Wang L. Clinical applications of liquid biopsy in prostate cancer: from screening to predictive biomarker. Cancers (Basel). 2022;14(7). Available from: https://www.mdpi.com/2072-6694/14/7/1728
60. Doultsinos D, Mills IG. Derivation and application of molecular signatures to prostate cancer: opportunities and challenges. Cancers (Basel). 2021;13(3). Available from: https://www.mdpi.com/2072-6694/13/3/495
61. Liu HE, Vuppalapaty M, Hoerner CR, Bergstrom CP, Chiu M, Lemaire C, et al. Detecting androgen receptor (AR), AR variant 7 (AR-V7), prostate-specific membrane antigen (PSMA), and prostate-specific antigen (PSA) gene expression in CTCs and plasma exosome-derived cfRNA in patients with metastatic castration-resistant prostate cance. BMC Cancer. 2024;24(1):482. https://doi.org/10.1186/s12885-024-12139-3.
62. Aydın M, Aydın EB, Sezgintürk MK. Functionalized magnetic nanoparticles for electrochemical magneto biosensing of PSMA cancer biomarker. New J Chem. 2024;48(13):5769–81.
63. Feng Z, Zhi S, Guo L, Zhou Y, Lei C. An integrated magnetic microfluidic chip for rapid immunodetection of the prostate specific antigen using immunomagnetic beads. Microchim Acta. 2019;186:1–14.
64. Isebia KT, Dathathri E, Verschoor N, Nanou A, De Jong AC, Coumans FAW, et al. Characterizing circulating tumor cells and tumor-derived extracellular vesicles in metastatic castration-naive and castration-resistant prostate cancer patients. Cancers (Basel). 2022;14(18). Available from: https://www.mdpi.com/2072-6694/14/18/4404
65. Hussein MA, Munirathinam G. Gene expression and DNA methylation as prognostic markers in metastatic castration-resistant prostate cancer: analysis of circulating tumor cells and paired plasma-derived exosomes. Cancers (Basel). 2023;15(22). Available from: https://www.mdpi.com/2072-6694/15/22/5325
66. Aghamir SMK, Rahimnia A, Zadeh SST, Roudgari H. Chapter 5 - Circulating tumor cells and DNAs in prostate tumors. In: Aghamir SMK, editor. Liquid biopsy in urogenital cancers and its clinical utility. Academic Press; 2022. p. 67–99. Available from: https://www.sciencedirect.com/science/article/pii/B9780323998840000021.
67. Nimir M, Ma Y, Jeffreys SA, Opperman T, Young F, Khan T, et al. Detection of AR-V7 in liquid biopsies of castrate resistant prostate cancer patients: a comparison of AR-V7 analysis in circulating tumor cells, circulating tumor RNA and exosomes. Cells. 2019;8(7). Available from: https://www.mdpi.com/2073-4409/8/7/688
68. Zavridou M, Strati A, Bournakis E, Smilkou S, Tserpeli V, Lianidou E. Prognostic significance of gene expression and DNA methylation markers in circulating tumor cells and paired

plasma derived exosomes in metastatic castration resistant prostate cancer. Cancers (Basel). 2021;13(4). Available from: https://www.mdpi.com/2072-6694/13/4/780
69. Gerdtsson AS, Setayesh SM, Malihi PD, Ruiz C, Carlsson A, Nevarez R, et al. Large extracellular vesicle characterization and association with circulating tumor cells in metastatic castrate resistant prostate cancer. Cancers (Basel). 2021;13(5). Available from: https://www.mdpi.com/2072-6694/13/5/1056
70. Nanou A, Coumans FAW, van Dalum G, Zeune LL, Dolling D, Onstenk W, et al. Circulating tumor cells, tumor-derived extracellular vesicles and plasma cytokeratins in castration-resistant prostate cancer patients. Oncotarget. 2018;9(27):19283–93.
71. Saghezi BV, Mansouri K, Hallaj R. Microfluidic systems in cancer diagnosis: advancing exosome and CTC detection from laboratory research to clinical application. Nano Sel. 2025;6:e202400108.
72. Rajendran R, Beck RC, Waskasi MM, Kelly BD, Bauer DR. Digital analysis of the prostate tumor microenvironment with high-order chromogenic multiplexing. J Pathol Inform. 2024;15:100352. Available from: https://www.sciencedirect.com/science/article/pii/S2153353923001669.
73. Jones A, Dhanapala L, Kankanamage RNT, Kumar CV, Rusling JF. Multiplexed immunosensors and immunoarrays. Anal Chem. 2020;92(1):345–62. https://doi.org/10.1021/acs.analchem.9b05080.
74. Andreou C, Weissleder R, Kircher MF. Multiplexed imaging in oncology. Nat Biomed Eng. 2022;6(5):527–40. https://doi.org/10.1038/s41551-022-00891-5.
75. Blessin NC, Yang C, Mandelkow T, Raedler JB, Li W, Bady E, et al. Automated Ki-67 labeling index assessment in prostate cancer using artificial intelligence and multiplex fluorescence immunohistochemistry. J Pathol. 2023;260(1):5–16.
76. Thurtle D, Bratt O, Stattin P, Pharoah P, Gnanapragasam V. Comparative performance and external validation of the multivariable PREDICT Prostate tool for non-metastatic prostate cancer: a study in 69,206 men from Prostate Cancer data Base Sweden (PCBaSe). BMC Med. 2020;18(1):139. https://doi.org/10.1186/s12916-020-01606-w
77. Bulten W, Kartasalo K, Chen PHC, Ström P, Pinckaers H, Nagpal K, et al. Artificial intelligence for diagnosis and Gleason grading of prostate cancer: the PANDA challenge. Nat Med. 2022;28(1):154–63. https://doi.org/10.1038/s41591-021-01620-2.
78. Ma S, Xie H, Wang H, Han C, Yang J, Lin Z, et al. MRI-based radiomics signature for the preoperative prediction of extracapsular extension of prostate cancer. J Magn Reson Imaging. 2019;50(6):1914–25.
79. Kawada T, Shim SR, Quhal F, Rajwa P, Pradere B, Yanagisawa T, et al. Diagnostic accuracy of liquid biomarkers for clinically significant prostate cancer detection: a systematic review and diagnostic meta-analysis of multiple thresholds. Eur Urol Oncol. 2024;7(4):649–62. Available from: https://www.sciencedirect.com/science/article/pii/S2588931123002481.
80. Pantanowitz L, Quiroga-Garza GM, Bien L, Heled R, Laifenfeld D, Linhart C, et al. An artificial intelligence algorithm for prostate cancer diagnosis in whole slide images of core needle biopsies: a blinded clinical validation and deployment study. Lancet Digit Health. 2020;2(8):e407–16.
81. Antunes ME, Araújo TG, Till TM, Pantaleão E, Mancera PFA, de Oliveira MH. Machine learning models for predicting prostate cancer recurrence and identifying potential molecular biomarkers. Front Oncol. 2025;15:1535091.
82. Gaikwad PS, Banerjee R. Advances in point-of-care diagnostic devices in cancers. Analyst. 2018;143(6):1326–48.
83. Pothipor C, Wiriyakun N, Putnin T, Ngamaroonchote A, Jakmunee J, Ounnunkad K, et al. Highly sensitive biosensor based on graphene–poly (3-aminobenzoic acid) modified electrodes and porous-hollowed-silver-gold nanoparticle labelling for prostate cancer detection. Sensors Actuators B Chem. 2019;296:126657. Available from: https://www.sciencedirect.com/science/article/pii/S0925400519308573.
84. Hroncekova S, Bertok T, Hires M, Jane E, Lorencova L, Vikartovska A, et al. Ultrasensitive Ti3C2TX MXene/chitosan nanocomposite-based amperometric biosensor for detection of

potential prostate cancer marker in urine samples. PRO. 2020;8(5). Available from: https://www.mdpi.com/2227-9717/8/5/580
85. Belkahla S, Nahvi I, Biswas S, Nahvi I, Ben Amor N. Advances and development of prostate cancer, treatment, and strategies: a systemic review. Front Cell Dev Biol. 2022;10:991330.
86. Al-Zoubi RM, Yassin AA, Alwani M, Al-Qudimat A, Aboumarzouk OM, Zarour A, et al. A systematic review on the latest developments in testosterone therapy: innovations, advances, and paradigm shifts. Arab J Urol. 2021;19(3):370–5.
87. van Wijk Y, Halilaj I, van Limbergen E, Walsh S, Lutgens L, Lambin P, et al. Decision support systems in prostate cancer treatment: an overview. Biomed Res Int. 2019;2019(1):4961768.
88. Pucci C, Martinelli C, Ciofani G. Innovative approaches for cancer treatment: current perspectives and new challenges. Ecancermedicalscience. 2019;13:961.
89. Capuozzo M, Santorsola M, Ianniello M, Ferrara F, Zovi A, Petrillo N, et al. Innovative drug modalities for the treatment of advanced prostate cancer. Diseases. 2024;12(5). Available from: https://www.mdpi.com/2079-9721/12/5/87
90. Bhoir S, De Benedetti A. Beyond the horizon: rethinking prostate cancer treatment through innovation and alternative strategies. Cancers (Basel). 2025;17(1). Available from: https://www.mdpi.com/2072-6694/17/1/75
91. Sajid M, Kawde AN, Daud M. Designs, formats and applications of lateral flow assay: a literature review. J Saudi Chem Soc 2015;19(6):689–705. Available from: https://www.sciencedirect.com/science/article/pii/S131961031400129X.
92. Tishkov VI, Popov VO. Protein engineering of formate dehydrogenase. Biomol Eng. 2006;23(2):89–110. Available from: https://www.sciencedirect.com/science/article/pii/S1389034406000220.
93. Luppa PB, Müller C, Schlichtiger A, Schlebusch H. Point-of-care testing (POCT): current techniques and future perspectives. TrAC Trends Anal Chem. 2011;30(6):887–98. Available from: https://www.sciencedirect.com/science/article/pii/S0165993611000860.
94. Jung W, Han J, Choi JW, Ahn CH. Point-of-care testing (POCT) diagnostic systems using microfluidic lab-on-a-chip technologies. Microelectron Eng. 2015;132:46–57. Available from: https://www.sciencedirect.com/science/article/pii/S0167931714004316
95. Sun Q, Hong P, Wei D, Wu A, Tan K, Lu X. Chemoselectivity in Gold(I)-catalyzed propargyl ester reactions: insights from DFT calculations. Front Chem. 2019;7–2019. Available from: https://www.frontiersin.org/journals/chemistry/articles/10.3389/fchem.2019.00609
96. Ray TR, Choi J, Bandodkar AJ, Krishnan S, Gutruf P, Tian L, et al. Bio-integrated wearable systems: a comprehensive review. Chem Rev. 2019;119(8):5461–533. https://doi.org/10.1021/acs.chemrev.8b00573.
97. Topol EJ. High-performance medicine: the convergence of human and artificial intelligence. Nat Med. 2019;25(1):44–56. https://doi.org/10.1038/s41591-018-0300-7.
98. Ting DSW, Carin L, Dzau V, Wong TY. Digital technology and COVID-19. Nat Med. 2020;26(4):459–61. https://doi.org/10.1038/s41591-020-0824-5.
99. Yang SM, Lv S, Zhang W, Cui Y. Microfluidic Point-of-Care (POC) Devices in early diagnosis: a review of opportunities and challenges. Sensors. 2022;22(4). Available from: https://www.mdpi.com/1424-8220/22/4/1620
100. Wang D, Chan HN, Liu Z, Micheal S, Li L, Baniani DB, et al. Recent developments in microfluidic-based point-of-care testing (Poct) diagnoses. Nanotechnol Microfluid 2020;239–280.
101. Pillai S, Kwan JC, Yaziji F, Yu H, Tran SD. Mapping the potential of microfluidics in early diagnosis and personalized treatment of head and neck cancers. Cancers (Basel). 2023;15(15). Available from: https://www.mdpi.com/2072-6694/15/15/3894
102. Sibbitts J, Di Pietro L, Privitera A, Cardaci V, Maugeri S, Camarda M, et al. 3D bioprinting and microfluidic-based devices for cancer detection and drug treatment: focus on prostate cancer. Curr Med Chem. 2025.
103. Wen S, Wei Y, Zen C, Xiong W, Niu Y, Zhao Y. Long non-coding RNA NEAT1 promotes bone metastasis of prostate cancer through N6-methyladenosine. Mol Cancer. 2020;19(1):171. https://doi.org/10.1186/s12943-020-01293-4.

104. Gu P, Chen X, Xie R, Xie W, Huang L, Dong W, et al. A novel AR translational regulator lncRNA LBCS inhibits castration resistance of prostate cancer. Mol Cancer. 2019;18(1):109. https://doi.org/10.1186/s12943-019-1037-8.
105. de Barros HA, van Oosterom MN, Donswijk ML, Hendrikx JJMA, Vis AN, Maurer T, et al. Robot-assisted prostate-specific membrane antigen–radioguided salvage surgery in recurrent prostate cancer using a DROP-IN gamma probe: the first prospective feasibility study. Eur Urol. 2022;82(1):97–105. Available from: https://www.sciencedirect.com/science/article/pii/S0302283822016724.
106. Gandaglia G, Mazzone E, Stabile A, Pellegrino A, Cucchiara V, Barletta F, et al. Prostate-specific membrane antigen radioguided surgery to detect nodal metastases in primary prostate cancer patients undergoing robot-assisted radical prostatectomy and extended pelvic lymph node dissection: results of a planned interim analysis of a pro. Eur Urol. 2022;82(4):411–8. Available from: https://www.sciencedirect.com/science/article/pii/S0302283822024174
107. Wang H, Wang T, Yuan X, Wang Y, Yue X, Wang L, et al. Plasmonic nanostructure biosensors: a review. Sensors. 2023;23(19):8156.
108. Abdelwahab SI, Elhassan Taha MM, Sahli KA, Salem Alqhtani HA, Farasani A, Khamjan NA, et al. Graphene-based biosensors for PSA. Clin Chim Acta. 2025;576:120406. Available from: https://www.sciencedirect.com/science/article/pii/S0009898125002852
109. Huang Y, Zhou J, Feng H, Zheng J, Ma HM, Liu W, et al. A dual-channel fluorescent chemosensor for discriminative detection of glutathione based on functionalized carbon quantum dots. Biosens Bioelectron. 2016;86:748–55. Available from: https://www.sciencedirect.com/science/article/pii/S0956566316307102.
110. South BR, Mowery D, Suo Y, Leng J, Ferrández Ó, Meystre SM, et al. Evaluating the effects of machine pre-annotation and an interactive annotation interface on manual de-identification of clinical text. J Biomed Inform. 2014;50:162–172. Available from: https://www.sciencedirect.com/science/article/pii/S1532046414001191
111. Qiu W, Evans CA, Landels A, Pham TK, Wright PC. Phosphopeptide enrichment for phosphoproteomic analysis - a tutorial and review of novel materials. Anal Chim Acta. 2020;1129:158–80. Available from: https://www.sciencedirect.com/science/article/pii/S0003267020304803.
112. Luca BA, Brewer DS, Edwards DR, Edwards S, Whitaker HC, Merson S, et al. DESNT: a poor prognosis category of human prostate cancer. Eur Urol Focus. 2018;4(6):842–50. Available from: https://www.sciencedirect.com/science/article/pii/S2405456917300251.
113. Agrawal S, Vagha S, Agrawal Jr S. A comprehensive review of artificial intelligence in prostate cancer care: state-of-the-art diagnostic tools and future outlook. Cureus. 2024;16(8).
114. Li H, Lee CH, Chia D, Lin Z, Huang W, Tan CH. Machine learning in prostate MRI for prostate cancer: current status and future opportunities. Diagnostics. 2022;12(2). Available from: https://www.mdpi.com/2075-4418/12/2/289
115. Ilin A, Martyshov M, Forsh E, Forsh P, Rumyantseva M, Abakumov A, et al. UV effect on NO2 sensing properties of nanocrystalline In2O3. Sensors Actuators B Chem. 2016;231:491–6. Available from: https://www.sciencedirect.com/science/article/pii/S0925400516303458.
116. Daveri A, Paziani S, Marmion M, Harju H, Vidman A, Azzarelli M, et al. New perspectives in the non-invasive, in situ identification of painting materials: the advanced MWIR hyperspectral imaging. TrAC Trends Anal Chem. 2018;98:143–8. Available from: https://www.sciencedirect.com/science/article/pii/S0165993617302820.
117. Frénal K, Dubremetz JF, Lebrun M, Soldati-Favre D. Gliding motility powers invasion and egress in Apicomplexa. Nat Rev Microbiol. 2017;15(11):645–60. https://doi.org/10.1038/nrmicro.2017.86.
118. Bor G, Mat Azmi ID, Yaghmur A. Nanomedicines for cancer therapy: current status, challenges and future prospects. Ther Deliv. 2019;10(2):113–32.
119. Mohanan PV. Artificial intelligence and biological sciences. CRC Press; 2025.
120. Qu J, Kalyani FS, Liu L, Cheng T, Chen L. Tumor organoids: synergistic applications, current challenges, and future prospects in cancer therapy. Cancer Commun. 2021;41(12):1331–53.

121. Imber BS, Varghese M, Ehdaie B, Gorovets D. Financial toxicity associated with treatment of localized prostate cancer. Nat Rev Urol. 2020;17(1):28–40. https://doi.org/10.1038/s41585-019-0258-3.
122. He H, Liu L, Morin EE, Liu M, Schwendeman A. Survey of clinical translation of cancer Nanomedicines—lessons learned from successes and failures. Acc Chem Res. 2019;52(9):2445–61. https://doi.org/10.1021/acs.accounts.9b00228.
123. Đorđević S, Gonzalez MM, Conejos-Sánchez I, Carreira B, Pozzi S, Acúrcio RC, et al. Current hurdles to the translation of nanomedicines from bench to the clinic. Drug Deliv Transl Res. 2022;12(3):500–25. https://doi.org/10.1007/s13346-021-01024-2.
124. Gawne PJ, Ferreira M, Papaluca M, Grimm J, Decuzzi P. New opportunities and old challenges in the clinical translation of nanotheranostics. Nat Rev Mater. 2023;8(12):783–98. https://doi.org/10.1038/s41578-023-00581-x.
125. Fu J, Fu C, Wang RS, Geynisman DM, Ghatalia P, Lynch SM, et al. Current status and future direction to address disparities in diversity, equity, and inclusion in prostate cancer care. Curr Oncol Rep. 2023;25(7):699–708. https://doi.org/10.1007/s11912-023-01399-0.
126. Crawford ED, Heidenreich A, Lawrentschuk N, Tombal B, Pompeo ACL, Mendoza-Valdes A, et al. Androgen-targeted therapy in men with prostate cancer: evolving practice and future considerations. Prostate Cancer Prostatic Dis. 2019;22(1):24–38. https://doi.org/10.1038/s41391-018-0079-0.
127. Boettcher AN, Usman A, Morgans A, VanderWeele DJ, Sosman J, Wu JD. Past, current, and future of immunotherapies for prostate cancer. Front Oncol. 2019;9:884.
128. Tătaru OS, Vartolomei MD, Rassweiler JJ, Virgil O, Lucarelli G, Porpiglia F, et al. Artificial intelligence and machine learning in prostate cancer patient management—current trends and future perspectives. Diagnostics. 2021;11(2). Available from: https://www.mdpi.com/2075-4418/11/2/354

Nanotechnology-Based Biosensor Development for Prostate Cancer Detection

7

Nandani Jayaswal, Sakshi Patel, Saquib Tanweer, and Rakesh Sahu

Abbreviations

AuNPs	gold nanoparticles
CNTs	carbon nanotubes
CTC	circulating tumor cell
FET	field-effect transistor
L	limit of detection
miRNA	microRNA
MNPs	magnetic nanoparticles
MOFs	metal–organic frameworks
PCA3	prostate cancer antigen 3
POC	point-of-care
PSA	prostate-specific antigen
QDs	quantum dots
SAW	surface acoustic wave
SERS	surface-enhanced Raman spectroscopy
SPR	surface plasmon resonance

N. Jayaswal
Faculty of Pharmaceutical Sciences, Mahayogi Gorakhnath University Gorakhpur, Gorakhpur, Uttar Pradesh, India

S. Patel
Department of Pharmaceutical Technology, Meerut Institute of Engineering & Technology, Meerut, Uttar Pradesh, India

S. Tanweer
Department of Pharmaceutics, Faculty of Pharmacy, Jahangirabad Institute of Technology, Jahangirabad Forte, Barabanki, Uttar Pradesh, India

R. Sahu (✉)
School of Pharmacy, Sharda University, Knowledge Park III, Greater Noida, Uttar Pradesh, India

S. Srivastava et al. (eds.), *Biosensor Technologies for Prostate Cancer*, https://doi.org/10.1007/978-981-95-8644-8_7

7.1 Introduction

Men worldwide experience prostate cancer at high levels of diagnosis as a disease that kills numerous males in developed regions. The disease begins within the prostate, which constitutes a main part of the male reproductive system, while the main cancer manifestation occurs through adenocarcinoma subtype growth [1]. Early-phase prostate cancer development tends to remain symptomless until metastasis expands in patients, which leads to the delayed appearance of urinary problems, pelvic pain, or bone discomfort. The vulnerability to develop prostate cancer depends largely on age and family heritage, as well as ethnic identity, combined with lifestyle decisions, which require thorough and efficient screening protocols [2]. The combination of standard diagnostic tests, including PSA blood testing and digital rectal examination (DRE), faces limitations because they cannot accurately differentiate aggressive prostate cancer from less dangerous forms [3]. The uncertainty in prostate cancer diagnoses causes medical professionals to worry about unnecessary operations and medication, thus leading them to develop advanced examination methods with less invasiveness. The need to develop improved diagnostic tests is important because it will help detect prostate cancer early for better patient outcomes with prompt intervention [4]. Treatment options that offer a cure, such as radical prostatectomy and radiation therapy, as well as active surveillance, demonstrate optimal results if prostate cancer is detected within localized stages. Treatment success rates together with survival projections diminish when prostate cancer is identified in the later stages of development [4]. New diagnostic techniques emerging to address existing screening deficiencies use biosensors because these devices present exceptional potential for such applications [5]. Antigen–antibody reactions in biological processes are transformed into detectable signals through biosensors, which allow instant identification of disease markers. Biosensors serve as an effective diagnostic tool for prostate cancer through their examination of three significant biomarkers that include PSA, prostate cancer antigen 3 (PCA3), and circulating tumor cells (CTCs) [6]. Diagnostic biosensor capabilities have experienced substantial growth by incorporating nanotechnology into their design platforms [7]. Nanomaterials consisting of gold nanoparticles, carbon nanotubes, and graphene, alongside quantum dots, enhance the performance of sensors through improved organism compatibility, enlarged interfaces, and better electrical and optical properties. The acquired properties create biosensors that detect cancer in its initial stages, performing better, being more specific, and providing faster detection results. Biosensor arrays of miniature size can be produced using nanotechnology methods and should be integrated into point-of-care systems to deliver affordable diagnostic solutions in remote healthcare regions [8]. The research presents detailed information on the development of nanotechnology-based biosensors for prostate cancer detection and their contribution to addressing existing diagnostic practice limitations. Nanoscale biosensing technology leads to significant improvements in cancer diagnosis through the application of biomarkers implemented into sensor design fundamentals under medical-based analysis [9].

7.2 Fundamentals of Nanotechnology in Biosensing

Biosensing underwent fundamental changes through nanotechnology by developing nanomaterials and structures with special physical and chemical properties at the nanometer scale [10]. The nanosystems achieve higher sensitivity and speed up response intervals while demonstrating specificity suitable for identifying rare biomarkers that help detect prostate cancer [11]. Nanobiosensor technology relies on engineered nanomaterials because these nanomaterials combine high surface area to volume ratios with modifiable surface chemistry. Multiple nanobiosensor components are examined in this section, which includes nanomaterial properties alongside their built-in favorable characteristics, together with essential surface functionalization protocols. These elements jointly enable next-generation diagnostic platform development [12].

7.2.1 Nanomaterials for Biosensor Fabrication

Modern biosensor development relies fundamentally on nanomaterials, as they exhibit extraordinary physical, chemical, and biological properties [13]. The basis of highly sensitive and selective biosensing platforms is established through nanoparticle structures combined with nanowires and nanotubes, together with two-dimensional nanostructures [14]. The nanoscale structure leads to an enhanced surface-to-volume ratio, enabling higher capacity for biorecognition elements, including antibodies, nucleic acids, or aptamers. The improved sensor–analyte contact through this method helps strengthen the signal transmission process [15]. A wide range of nanomaterials serves biosensor fabrication, including gold nanoparticles (AuNPs), carbon nanotubes (CNTs), graphene, silica nanoparticles, and magnetic nanoparticles [16]. Table 7.1 summarizes commonly used nanomaterials in prostate cancer biosensor fabrication, highlighting their biosensing mechanisms and advantages. Scientists prefer AuNPs as nanomaterials because they possess superior electrical conductivity along with excellent biocompatibility for their use in creating optical and electrochemical sensors [17]. Carbon-based nanomaterials, such as graphene and CNTs, offer both robust mechanical properties and rapid electron movement, which enhances their electrochemical response performance. The separation process, together with the target molecule concentration for complex biological samples, becomes more efficient using magnetic nanoparticles. Different synthesis methods coupled with surface modifications enable scientists to precisely apply these nanomaterials into platforms that detect prostate cancer biomarkers in biosensors [18].

7.2.2 Unique Properties and Advantages of Nanoscale Systems

Nanoscale systems demonstrate superior performance features over typical materials because they are highly effective in biosensing applications [26]. Surface

Table 7.1 Types of nanomaterials used in prostate cancer biosensors

Nanomaterial	Key properties	Detection method enhanced	Target biomarker	Advantages in biosensing	References
Gold nanoparticles (AuNPs)	High conductivity, biocompatibility, surface plasmon resonance	Electrochemical, optical	PSA, PCA3	Signal amplification, surface functionalization, stability	[19, 20]
Carbon nanotubes (CNTs)	High surface area, electrical conductivity, mechanical strength	Electrochemical	PSA	Rapid electron transfer, enhanced sensitivity	[21]
Graphene	High electron mobility, 2D structure, flexibility	Electrochemical, FET-based	PSA, miRNAs	High carrier mobility, low detection limit	[22]
Magnetic nanoparticles (MNPs)	Super paramagnetism, surface modifiability	Magnetic, electrochemical	PSA, CTCs, exosomes	Easy separation, low background noise	[23]
Quantum dots (QDs)	Size-tunable fluorescence, photostability	Optical (fluorescence, FRET)	PCA3, miRNAs	Multiplex detection, high-resolution imaging	[24]
Metal–organic frameworks (MOFs)	High porosity, tunable structure	Electrochemical	PSA	Enhanced loading of biomolecules, signal enrichment	[25]

reactivity grows stronger because nanomaterials possess large quantities of atoms that span the surface region. The increased surface area produces better biomolecule bonding [27], which enhances the detection of scarce biochemical indicators [28]. Quantum confinement operates in materials with quantum dots, so scientists can modify electron and optical attributes through size-based adjustments. Biosensor platforms with selectable emission spectra could be developed through this concept because it satisfies the requirements of multiplexed detection systems. The exceptional electrochemical activities of nanomaterials result in lower operating potentials, along with accelerated electron transfer rates, which ultimately increase the signal-to-noise ratio of electrochemical biosensors [29]. The small dimensions of nanoscale systems enhance their flexibility, allowing wearable as well as implantable biosensors to be developed [30]. Photoacoustic biosensing and optical biosensing benefit from nanomaterials that demonstrate outstanding photothermal attributes along with plasmonic characteristics. These attributes collectively form a diverse methodology that yields highly effective biosensing instruments for detecting the early stages of prostate cancer [31].

7.2.3 Surface Functionalization and Biorecognition

Surface functionalization serves as an essential factor during nanobiosensor development because it determines how specific and stable the biorecognition process becomes [32]. Surface functionalization enables the attachment of bioreceptors that select prostate cancer biomarkers among PSA, PCA3, and exosomal proteins through surface modification of nanomaterials [32]. Surface modification occurs through silanization together with thiol–gold bonding and carbodiimide coupling (EDC/NHS chemistry), and polymer coating as separate chemical methods [33]. The applied modification strategies enable permanent biomolecule binding, which maintains their biological functionality. Thiol-modified antibodies bond covalently with gold nanoparticles, due to which the sensor achieves increased durability and consistent performance results [34]. Surface functionalization occurs through covalent binding, with the option to utilize non covalent interactions based on electrostatic forces, hydrogen bonding, and hydrophobic interactions [35]. The selected strategy is based on the characteristics of the target molecule, as well as the planned application goals. Through surface engineering processes, the bioreceptor maintains proper orientation and access to its targets, enabling it to detect and generate signals effectively.

7.3 Types of Nanobiosensors for Prostate Cancer

The development of biosensors has experienced a transformative change through nanotechnology, which produces more sensitive and specific detection in real time [36]. Various nanobiosensor platforms (as detailed in Table 7.2) operate in prostate cancer diagnostics, where individual nanoscale properties work to enhance biomarker detection [37]. This section demonstrates the principal nanobiosensors used for prostate cancer detection through an examination of operational guidelines alongside their benefits, along with restraining factors [38].

7.3.1 Electrochemical Biosensors

Electrochemical biosensors stand as the preferred choice for prostate cancer detection because their performance characteristics include high sensitivity and rapid response, low price, and simplified miniaturization features. Biosensors detect biomolecular electrode interactions through modifications in electrical parameters such as current or potential change and impedance variations [43]. Biosensors function more effectively when nanomaterials, such as gold nanoparticles, carbon nanotubes, graphene, and metal–organic frameworks (MOFs), enhance surface area availability and facilitate electron transfer processes and biomolecule attachment to the sensor surface [44]. The sensor modifications enable detection of prostate cancer biomarkers at significantly lower amounts, especially for prostate-specific antigen (PSA) and PCA3-related transcripts [45]. Industrial practice utilizes the following electrochemical methods, among others [46]: The amperometric sensor operates by measuring current modifications triggered by redox reactions; Electrical impedance changes caused by analyte binding trigger the operation of impedimetric sensors; Voltametric sensors obtain complete measurements of analyte redox profiles that help with quantification. Concepts in electrochemical nanobiosensing enable creators to produce compound instrumentation and portable measurement devices for on-site prostate cancer diagnostics.

7.3.2 Optical and Plasmonic Biosensors

Optical and plasmonic biosensors make use of changes in light characteristics such as absorbance, fluorescence, or scattering resulting from certain biomolecular interactions [47]. Nanotechnology integration, especially with plasmonic nanoparticles like gold and silver, increases the sensitivity of these optical biosensors to identify ultra-low concentrations of prostate cancer indicators. Important optical sensing techniques are as follows [48]: Detects refractive index changes near a sensor surface following biomarker attachment via surface plasmon resonance (SPR); Enables very sensitive molecular fingerprinting by using metallic nanostructures to magnify Raman signals; Optical readouts provide very particular biomarker detection using quantum dots, upconversion nanoparticles, or dye-doped nanocarriers in fluorescence-based sensors. For label-free, real-time analysis, plasmonic biosensors are especially useful since they reduce the requirement for thorough sample preparation [49]. Their great sensitivity makes them appropriate for finding uncommon prostate cancer-related targets, including exosomes, circulating tumor DNA (ctDNA), and certain miRNAs. Optical nanobiosensors are being pushed towards clinical translation by ongoing developments in miniaturization and multiplexing techniques [50].

Table 7.2 Nanobiosensor platforms for prostate cancer detection

Biosensor type	Operation principle	Nanomaterial used	Target biomarker	Detection limit	Strengths/Limitations	References
Electrochemical	Redox current or impedance change	AuNPs, CNTs, MOFs	PSA, PCA3	fM–pM	High sensitivity, portable; matrix interference possible	[20]
Optical (SPR, SERS)	Light absorption, scattering, or fluorescence	AuNPs, QDs	PSA, miRNAs, ctDNA	aM–fM	Label-free, real-time; expensive instrumentation	[39]
Magnetic	Magnetic relaxation or resistance change	MNPs	PSA, Exosomes	Low fM	Low noise, high specificity; needs external magnet	[40]
FET-based	Conductivity shifts with binding	Graphene, Si-nanowires	PSA, miRNAs	aM	Label-free, real-time; fabrication complexity	[41]
Piezoelectric/SAW	Mass change-induced frequency shift	Nanostructured quartz	PSA	pM	High sensitivity; sensitive to environmental noise	[42]

7.3.3 Magnetic Nanoparticle-Based Biosensors

Magnetic nanoparticle-based biosensors detect and isolate prostate cancer markers by leveraging the unique magnetic properties of nanoparticles. Often, these biosensors operate via magnetic relaxation switching, nuclear magnetic resonance (NMR), or magneto-resistive techniques. The main applications are as follows [51]: PSA, CTCs, or exosomes are selectively isolated from complex biological fluids using antibody-functionalized magnetic nanoparticles; Magneto-resistive sensors are used for monitoring variations in resistance brought on by magnetic labels linked to target analytes; Magnetic relaxation-based sensors are used for tracking variations in magnetic relaxation times related to biomarker binding. There are several advantages to magnetic nanobiosensors: Targeted magnetic capture offers outstanding specificity; minimal background noise, as biological samples often lack endogenous magnetic signatures; integration with microfluidic systems and non-invasive, in situ monitoring capability. Recent research has revealed extremely sensitive MNP-based methods for the simultaneous detection of many prostate cancer biomarkers, hence enhancing early diagnosis and disease categorization [52].

7.3.4 Novel Biosensor Modalities

New types of nanobiosensors are being researched for prostate cancer detection and are more effective than traditional electrochemical, optical, and magnetic biosensors. These innovative systems offer new approaches to enhance the usefulness, specificity, and sensitivity of detection. Among the remarkable new modalities are the following [53]: *Piezoelectric and acoustic biosensors*: These use nano-enhanced quartz crystal microbalances (QCM) and surface acoustic wave (SAW) sensors to detect small changes in mass when biomolecules attach, with very high sensitivity; *Thermal and calorimetric biosensors*: By employing nanomaterials that sense minute temperature changes caused by biological processes, biosensors offer indirect biomarker testing; *Field-effect transistor (FET)-based biosensors*: Driven by field-effect transistor (FET)-driven biosensors, they use nanowires or graphene sheets as channels whose electrical conductivity changes with target chemical binding. FET biosensors offer label-free, real-time detection with potential high-throughput screening; *Wearable and flexible biosensors*: These include nanoparticles in soft, flexible substrates to create skin-mounted or implanted devices for ongoing prostate cancer biomarker monitoring. Bringing together these new types of biosensors with artificial intelligence (AI) and data analysis is improving their features, allowing for better monitoring, predicting health issues, and understanding results in real time [23]. As material science, microfabrication, and bioengineering advance, these novel methods are expected to significantly influence the future landscape of prostate cancer diagnostics [23].

7.4 Biomarkers for Prostate Cancer Detection

Appropriately selected biomarkers would lead to highly sensitive and specific biosensors for prostate cancer [54]. A biomarker is a measurable indicator of the biological process occurring inside us, pathological changes, or response to the therapeutic intervention [55]. Ideally, a biomarker that allows early detection of prostate cancer, differentiates benign from malignant conditions, and allows monitoring of treatment efficacy would be most suitable for detecting prostate cancer [56]. By the detection of prostate cancer biomarkers at unprecedentedly low concentrations, one can leverage advances in nanotechnology to achieve diagnostic sensitivity and specificity of a previously unimaginable order of magnitude. The key biomarkers reviewed in this section include well-established prostate-specific antigen (PSA) tests, new genetic marker tests, PCA3, and multiplexed biomarker detection strategies that are being increasingly sought after [57].

7.4.1 Prostate-Specific Antigen (PSA)

Prostate-specific antigen (PSA) is the most commonly used biomarker for prostate cancer screening and monitoring. Serine protease PSA is a product of mainly the epithelial cells of the prostate gland [58]. Elevated PSA levels in blood represent an elevated risk for prostate cancer but are not necessarily cancer-associated (increased in noncancer conditions, including BPH, prostatitis, and other non-malignant conditions); overdiagnosis and overtreatment [59]. Improved sensitivity and lowered detection limits on the order of the femtomolar or attomolar range for PSA detection have been achieved with the use of nanotechnology-based biosensors. These include amplification of PSA detection signals through various mechanisms of surface plasmon resonance, electrochemical reaction, and fluorescence resonance with nanoscale materials such as gold nanoparticles, magnetic nanoparticles, carbon nanotubes, and quantum dots [60]. Also, attempts were made to differentiate the free PSA (fPSA) from the complexed PSA (cPSA) forms since the ratio of the latter can contribute to better diagnostic accuracy. New biosensors have become advanced enough to monitor a number of PSA isoforms at once, rendering an even more accurate evaluation of prostate cancer risk [61]. While its limitations hold, PSA is a cornerstone biomarker in which the innovations in nanotechnology continue to improve optimization for diagnostic and prognostic specificities.

7.4.2 PCA3 and Other Genetic Markers

Prostate cancer antigen 3 (PCA3) is a noncoding RNA that is highly overexpressed in prostate cancer tissues as opposed to normal prostate tissues [62]. Unlike PSA-based screening, the principle that drives PCA3 expression is highly specific to prostate cancer itself, implying that the PCA3 biomarker can largely reduce false positives associated with PSA-based screening [63]. When prostate secretions are enriched with digital rectal examination (DRE), PCA3 is most commonly detected in urine [64]. Nanotechnology-based biosensors for the detection of PCA3 RNA at very low concentrations will further enhance the non-invasive, highly specific prostate cancer diagnostics [65]. Using these nanostructured electrochemical and optical platforms, hybridization efficiency, amplification of the signal, and specificity in APA3 detection have been improved. However, besides PCA3, there are several other genetic and epigenetic markers that have been the object of publication, including gene fusion in TMPRSS2-ERG, which is seen in the majority of prostate cancers with accompanying disease progression [65]. Therefore, they are focusing on potential methylation patterns of genes, like GSTP1, APC, and RASSF1A, which can act as early indicators of malignant transformation. Dysregulated microRNAs (miRNAs) known to regulate gene expression, such as miR-21, miR-141, and miR-375, are found in prostate cancer. Integration of nanomaterials increases the sensitivity of biosensors to these genetic markers and allows for approaches to multi-modal diagnostics that enhance the sensitivity over classical protein biomarker detection.

7.4.3 Multiplexed Biomarker Detection Strategies

Prostate cancer is so heterogeneous that depending on a single biomarker does not always deliver adequate diagnostic resolution [66]. Thus, the ability to detect multiple biomarkers simultaneously (multiplexed biomarker detection)—simultaneously determining a variety of biomarkers—achieves more comprehensive and dependable diagnosis, prognosis, as well as monitoring of therapy [67]. Several platforms provided by nanotechnology are ideally suited to multiplexing, including the following [68]: They offer the ability to functionalize nanopillar/pillar and nanowire arrays with different capture probes for parallel detection; Distinct emission spectra result in the possibility that quantum dot-based systems can be used to simultaneously optically track multiple targets; By using magnetic nanoparticle arrays, it is possible to detect biomarkers label-free and in high throughput using magnetic sensing techniques; The combination of PSA isoforms, PCA3, TMPRSS2-ERG fusion transcripts, miRNAs, and protein biomarkers that are markers of inflammation and changes in the tumor microenvironment can be evaluated on multiplexed platforms. These systems allow a broader coverage of the biological picture, which improves the specificity and sensitivity in the detection of prostate cancer [69]. Additionally, machine learning and data analytics have been increasingly employed to interpret the complex dataset generated by the multiplexed biosensor to recognize patterns and model predictions to further enhance the diagnostic performance [70]. This is in line with the principles of precision medicine and the aim of multiplexed detection to identify subtypes of prostate cancer predisposing patients to metastasis and stratify them for more target-specific therapy [71].

7.5 Design and Fabrication Approaches

Innovative design and fabrication strategies based on new materials, architectures, and manufacturing strategies in order to make the new diagnostic platforms more sensitive, specific, faster, and more intuitive to use [72]. In these advancements, nanomaterials, microfluidic systems, and the reduction of sensor miniaturization techniques are central [73]. Together, these approaches create very compact, robust, and high-performance devices that can find application in the centralized laboratory as well as in point-of-care settings [74]. Figure 7.1 illustrates the design-to-deployment pipeline of nanobiosensors for prostate cancer diagnostics.

7.5.1 Nanomaterial Synthesis

As nanomaterials possess unique physicochemical properties such as a large (high) surface area with volume ratio and tenable surface chemistry, as well as quantum effects, they can be used to enhance the performance of diagnostic sensors [75]. *Industrial applications of nanomaterials*: The most commonly used materials include gold nanoparticles (AuNPs), carbon nanotubes (CNTs), graphene, quantum dots (QDs), and metal–organic frameworks (MOFs), with advantages and disadvantages in use for each specific application range [76]. *Synthesis techniques*: Chemical reduction, sol–gel methods, hydrothermal synthesis, and green synthesis approaches

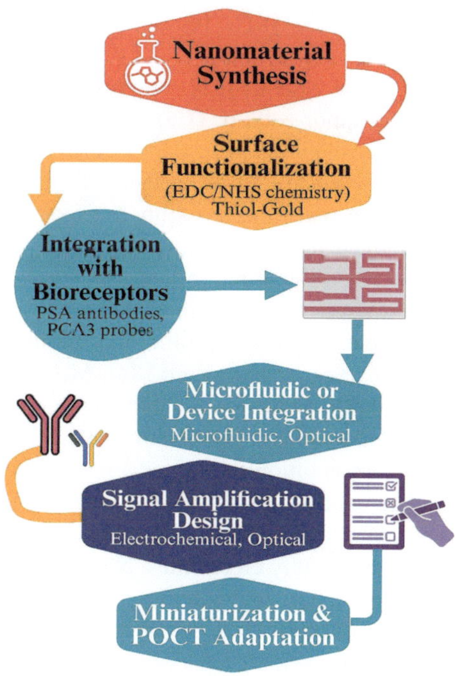

Fig. 7.1 Stepwise workflow for fabrication of nanobiosensors for prostate cancer

are all common synthesis techniques that have their chosen control over the size, shape, and surface functionalities of the nanomaterials [76]. *Surface functionalization*: Nanomaterials are tailored to bear the biorecognition elements, such as antibodies, aptamers, and enzymes, to increase the specificity and target the detection of biomolecules [77]. *Signal amplification*: Nanomaterials can act as signal amplifiers in electrochemical, optical, and colorimetric sensors, thereby increasing the signal and improving detection limits and reliability.

7.5.2 Integration with Microfluids

Converging nanotechnology-based biosensors with microfluidic systems is a revolutionary advancement for usage in prostate cancer diagnostics [78]. In microfluidics, a unique term coined as "lab on a chip" technology, the micromanipulation of minute volumes, from 1 to a few thousand liters, of biological fluids is made through the microscale channels. This integration provides significant improvement of biosensor function, including sample handling, reduced reagents, and multiplexed detection [79]. Microfluidic integration is one of the main advantages with regard to sensitivity and specificity. Microfluidic platforms give rise to confined microenvironments, which are beneficial for nanomaterial-based sensors such as gold nanoparticles, carbon nanotubes, or quantum dots [80]. In these controlled environments, reaction kinetics are optimized, and rapid binding of the analyte is enabled, as is necessary for the detection of low-abundance prostate-cancer biomarkers such as prostate-specific antigen (PSA) or prostate cancer antigen 3 (PCA3) [81]. In addition, automated sample preparation, including separation, concentration, and purification steps, can be accomplished in such microfluidic systems [82]. On-chip immunomagnetic separation could isolate circulating tumor cells (CTCs) or exosomes before they are detectable to enhance the diagnostic yield [83]. Capture efficiency can be further increased with integration into nanostructured surfaces within the microchannels and measurement of samples in real time. Possibly the most important advantage is the capacity for multiplexed analysis. Simultaneous quantification of multiple prostate cancer biomarkers on a single microfluidic chip is enabled by spatially segregating different sensing zones within a single microfluidic chip, thereby providing a more comprehensive diagnostic profile and minimizing false positives or negatives from single-marker measurement [84]. Moreover, microfluidic biosensor systems are well suited to point-of-care applications. This trend of small size, low power consumption, and short turnaround time fits perfectly with the market of distributed healthcare solutions designed for early diagnosis and long-term monitoring of prostate cancer outside of traditional lab settings [85]. There are yet many challenges that remain, such as fabrication reproducibility, biofouling, and integration with user-friendly electronics. Nevertheless, emerging fields of materials science, microfabrication technologies, and integrated device engineering are currently able to overcome these barriers for the creation of clinically viable integrated microfluidic-nanobiosensor hybrid platforms for detection.

7.5.3 Sensor Miniaturization and Portability

In revolutionizing prostate cancer diagnostics, nanotechnology-based biosensor miniaturization and portability are key for improving point-of-care (POC) testing, home monitoring, and decentralized healthcare [86]. Biosensors that use nanotechnology for miniaturization maintain performance and sensitivity, although the tools involved in achieving that scale are themselves nanotechnology [87]. The main reason for miniaturization relies on the high surface area to volume ratio of nanomaterials [88]. Nanostructures, including nanowires, graphene sheets, and nanoporous materials, can be utilized as sensors to assist highly sensitive detection on microscale platforms [89]. By facilitating efficient electron transport, signal amplification, rapid biomolecular recognition, and sensing of prostate cancer at its earliest stages, efficient electron transport, signal amplification, and biomolecular recognition are possible within the compact architectures [90]. However, miniaturized sensors can be incorporated with significantly extended utility in portable diagnostic devices [91]. These biosensors are integrated with readout systems based on handheld or wearable smartphones or provided with wireless data transmission capabilities that enable continuous monitoring and real-time data collection [92]. In particular, such portability is very useful for patients at risk of aggressive prostate cancer, as they can undergo more frequent examinations without having to return to the hospital several times. This trend can be exemplified by several recent innovations. Electrochemical biosensors using nanocomposites have been used for highly accurate PSA detection with handheld devices [93]. Likewise, optical biosensors are being miniaturized to be used in compact systems with simple user interfaces; optical biosensors are based on nanoparticle-enhanced fluorescence or plasmonic effects [94]. Also, for portability, battery-powered or battery-harvestable devices are developed that sustain continuous performance under resource-limited environments. Additionally, the integration of microfluidic sample handling in portable formats simplifies the testing process to a great extent, encountering external laboratory equipment [95]. Unfortunately, sensor miniaturization creates problems of maintaining sensor stability and reproducibility across manufacturing batches, as well as reducing signal noise [96]. Challenges in such applications can be addressed by using nanomaterials engineering, microelectronic, data processing algorithms and a user-centered design approach [97]. Overall, advancements in miniaturization and portability of the sensors are expected to enable significantly improved early detection, prognostic assessment, and personalized management of prostate cancer, which all fall within the general scope of precision medicine and accessible healthcare [98].

7.6 Clinical Applications and Case Studies

The successful translation of any novel diagnostic technology or biomarker from the research laboratory to routine clinical practice hinges on rigorous evaluation of its performance, validation in relevant patient populations, and assessment of its practical utility in real-world healthcare settings [99]. Now, it turns to the critical aspects of clinical application, the key metrics used for the evaluation of diagnostic accuracy, and the methods of clinical validation through trials, along with the possibility of point-of-care deployment [100]. Illustrative case studies, either hypothetical or based on research already extracted for the core topic of the chapter, can also illustrate these concepts [101].

7.6.1 Sensitivity and Specificity Metrics

A fundamental accuracy needs to be quantified [before a diagnostic test [or biomarker/method] can be considered for clinical use] [102]. Two cornerstone metrics of this evaluation are sensitivity and specificity. Specifically, these measures are the test's ability to classify correctly those who do and do not have the condition of interest [103]. Table 7.3 outlines reported sensitivity and specificity metrics using nanobiosensors in prostate cancer diagnosis. The true positive rate (TPR), also called sensitivity, measures the proportion of individuals with the target condition correctly identified by the test [104]. It answers the question: How often will the test be positive if a person has the disease? Mathematically, it is calculated as follows:

$$\text{Specificity} = \frac{\text{True Negatives}(TN)}{\text{True Negatives}(TN) + \text{False Positive}(FP)}$$

When the implications of the false positive result (e.g., risk to patient, anxiety, cost) are high, high specificity is critical. In other words, a positive test is highly specific for ruling out the disease (SpPIn) in [105].

Interplay and clinical context: Sensitivity and specificity are in a trade-off relationship in most cases: sensitivity may be improved at the expense of specificity or vice versa. ROC curves are a good visualization of this relationship. The balance should be such in the clinical context [111]. An example would be that a screening test with high sensitivity to identify as many possible cases as possible takes lower specificity, whereas the subsequent confirmatory test has high specificity for the

Table 7.3 Comparative metrics of sensitivity and specificity for nanobiosensors

Biosensor type	Target biomarker	Sensitivity (%)	Specificity (%)	Detection limit	References
Electrochemical (AuNPs)	PSA	96.5	92.1	1.3 pg/mL	[106]
Optical (SPR, QDs)	PCA3, miRNAs	94.0	90.5	10 aM	[107]
Magnetic (MNP-based)	Exosomes, PSA	93.7	95.2	0.5 pg/mL	[108]
FET-based (graphene)	PSA, miR-21	98.2	93.8	0.2 fM	[109]
SERS-based microfluidic	PSA, CTCs	91.5	89.6	0.01 ng/mL	[110]

reduction of false positives. *Beyond sensitivity and specificity*: However, these metrics are entirely fundamental but not exclusively predictive of clinical utility. The preceding two values, predictive values, namely positive predictive value (PPV) and negative predictive value (NPV), are also important because they interpret test results in the context of disease prevalence in the tested population [112].

$$PPV = \frac{TP}{TP = FP}$$

The probability that you have a negative test does not mean that you truly do not have the condition; this is called NPV [113].

$$NPV = \frac{TN}{TN + FN}$$

7.6.2 Clinical Validation and Trials

Clinical validation and trials are evaluated on the basis of accuracy, precision, limits of detection, and clinical validation (clinical validation follows from the analytical performance measures, which determine whether a test, biomarker, or method is able to provide meaningful and reliable information in the relevant patient population and in the clinical context) [114]. This process involves several phases [115]: *Proof of concept*: Early studies showing a power link between the test result and the clinical condition that is, the clinical condition proves as expected by the test result; *Clinical performance evaluation*: Retrospective or prospective studies to evaluate clinical performance, clinical sensitivity, clinical specificity, clinical PPV, and clinical NPV, using well-characterized patient cohorts and a gold standard; *Clinical utility assessment (if a randomized clinical trial is done)*: It recognizes that the test offers improvements in patient outcomes or decision-making by such means as randomized controlled trials (RCTs); *Ongoing monitoring (post-market surveillance)*: It continues to monitor in the real world to ensure habitual usefulness and continuing effectiveness in the real world. The essential trial design is rigorous, such as the following [116]: clear definition of the target population with appropriate inclusion and exclusion criteria; reliable reference standard for comparison; such an amount of sample size to carry out power statistics; reducing bias, for example, by blinding; endpoints, which are clinically relevant endpoints that represent meaningful patient outcomes [117]; ethical approval and informed consent in line with human research guidelines; the support for approval and clinical use with agencies such as the FDA or the EMA [118].

7.6.3 Point-of-Care Testing Potential

Point-of-care testing (POCT) is performed within the patient care setting, close to the site of care, rather than in a central laboratory [119]. As shown in Table 7.4, several portable nanobiosensor systems have demonstrated utility for decentralized

Table 7.4 Integration of nanotechnology with point-of-care testing devices

Device/System	Nanomaterial used	Target biomarker	Integration platform	Point-of-care suitability	References
Smartphone-integrated electrochemical sensor	AuNPs, CNTs	PSA	Mobile app + Bluetooth reader	High (portable, user-friendly)	[121]
Microfluidic chip with SERS detection	AgNPs, QDs	PSA, CTCs	Pump-free chip with optical reader	Medium (low-cost but fragile)	[122]
FET biosensor patch	Graphene nanoribbons	miR-21	Wearable skin patch	High (continuous monitoring possible)	[123]
Magnetic bead-based lateral flow device	Magnetic nanoparticles	PSA	Handheld magnetic reader	High (low background, rapid detection)	[124]
Dual-mode aptasensor with smartphone output	AuNPs + DNA aptamers	PSA, PCA3	Colorimetric + Fluorescence	High (dual-mode validation)	[125]

prostate cancer diagnostics. Because of the increasing demand for rapid, actionable diagnostic information in diverse clinical settings (e.g., ED, outpatient clinics, rural health centers, and even home care), a tremendous development in POCT technologies has taken place. The advantages of POCT are as follows [120]: *Rapid turnaround time*: POCT leads to reporting of immediate or almost immediate results, so that physicians can reach clinical decisions faster and streamline workflow; *Faster intervention*: The decrease of diagnostic delays allows for quicker intervention that could lead to improved outcomes, especially in acute care (for example, cardiac markers in suspected myocardial infarction); *Decentralized testing capability*: POCT decentralized testing capability provides access to diagnostics in remote or resource-limited settings in the presence of traditional lab infrastructure; *Enhanced patient engagement*: POCT can also enhance patient engagement in other areas such as diabetes or infectious disease management, where the patient can now be empowered to monitor and manage the condition themselves.

POCT offers a great deal of benefits, but for their successful clinical use, they should be taken into consideration. Here are some clinical integration considerations [126]: *Validation*: The analytical and clinical validations for POCT devices are rigorous to demonstrate accuracy, precision, sensitivity, and specificity similar to laboratory-based methods; *Quality assurance programs*: By converting these POCT tests into "spectrographic" instruments and applying the rules for quality assurance programs that apply to them, sample misidentification and confusion during transfers can be eliminated; *Integration and connectivity*: The integration of patient data-driven and EHRs is required for maintaining care continuity and making data decisions; *Quality and safety*: Quality and safety standards of use of POCT devices should be met; *Cost-effectiveness*: Economic aspects should be evaluated in both direct costs and the resultant indirect savings by better performance on clinical outcomes and operational efficiency. Trends and case studies on the rise in indications in infectious disease diagnostics for illnesses such as COVID-19, influenza, and HIV show how POCT may support outbreak control and encourage prompt treatment at initial points: *Chronic disease monitoring*: A portable HbA1c analyzer or a portable lipid profile device can be used for immediate chronic disease assessment and management; *Digital tools for POCT*: Digital tools are being implemented on the wearable and smartphone-integrated devices to provide real-time monitoring, automated interpretation, and remote sharing of data in other devices. Although such POCT is becoming more and more crucial in individualized and precision medicine, there is a significant possibility for POCT to even further reduce its impact [127]. Future POCT systems are predicted to be less mistake-prone, multifunctional, and seamless in-patient care stagnation as continuous innovation in biosensors, microfluidics, and data analytics stretches the horizon [128]. Maintaining a balance between accessibility, analytical rigor, and usefulness to the doctor will be somewhat difficult.

7.7 Challenges and Future Perspective

Although major progress has been made, a number of limitations still impede the clinical uptake and optimization of diagnostic technologies [129]. Such issues as variability in test performance across populations, interoperability with health care systems, regulatory hurdles, and the requirement for replicated validation frameworks are also included [130]. Furthermore, there is a continued struggle between innovativeness and cost-effectiveness. Some future developments may be to improve the accuracy of the diagnosis and improve the performance of the miniaturization and automation by utilizing artificial intelligence and the use of digital health tools to interpret real-time data in personalized care [131]. In the course of more decentralized and patient centric diagnostics, the stakes become ever higher that each patient will have equitable access and that clinical standards remain true to the rigorous clinical standards to which we hold in the laboratory setting [132].

7.7.1 Technical and Regulatory Hurdles

While great progress has been achieved in the development of nanotechnology-based biosensors, there is still a long way to go before they can be widely applied in clinical practice [133]. The reproducibility and stability of nanobiosensors are technical problems, although there is a way to implement an intrinsic self-test [134]. On the other hand, the inherent complexity of fabricating nanomaterials with consistent size, shape, and functional property requires the development of nanomaterial properties that are not sensitive to bias in terms of size, shape, and property [135]. Furthermore, biological recognition elements should be integrated into nanostructured surfaces and must provide long-term stability and bioactivity under different physiological and environmental conditions [136]. Being of novel materials and a novel mechanism, nanobiosensors are subjected to extremely strict regulation from a regulatory point of view [137]. Safety, biocompatibility, and efficacy are validated as comprehensively as regulatory agencies like the FDA and EMA would like them to be, and usually with costly and time-consuming clinical trials [138]. In addition, there are currently no common protocols to assess the performance of nanobiosensors, and this impedes regulatory approval and delays the delivery from the bench to bedside [139]. However, the solutions to address these issues will require a synchronized strategy by developers and regulatory bodies and clear regulatory frameworks and harmonized evaluation criteria that will guide their strategies for achieving convergence.

7.7.2 Commercialization Prospects

Nanobiosensor commercialization for prostate cancer detection has promising opportunities but also many obstacles [140]. With increasing demand for rapid, accurate, and non-invasive diagnostic tools to aid early detection as well as real-time monitoring, the market interest is growing [141]. There is a compelling value proposition to healthcare systems and investors that placing nanobiosensors in point-of-care (POC), wearable, and telemedicine ecosystems has the potential to allow for integration [142]. Nevertheless, scalability in relation to production with regard to consistency, affordability, and quality has been a challenge [143]. Physical and chemical properties of nanomaterials need to be stringently controlled, and translation of lab-scale prototypes to mass-producible forms that require redesign and reengineering can be required for large-scale manufacturing of nanomaterials [144]. High development costs, IP issues, and the presence of pre-existing diagnostic technology in the market may also discourage investment and slow commercialization. However, these barriers will have to be overcome by collaborations among academia, industry, and healthcare providers in order to speed the development of innovative diagnostic solutions [145].

7.7.3 Personalized Medicine and AI Integration

Assuming that the future of biosensing is based on nanotechnology, the convergence of personalized medicine with digital health is about to come into play [146]. Genetically and clinically, prostate cancer is heterogeneous, and the one-size-fits-all approach is becoming inefficient [147]. The contribution of nanobiosensors to precision oncology is made easier, possible through the ability to perform real-time and multiplexed detection of individual-specific biomarkers, which has the potential to support more precise treatment decisions based on a patient's individual molecular profile [148]. Additionally, integrating AI and ML into biosensor platforms is going to enormously increase diagnostic accuracy, data interpretation, and predictive analytics [149]. This makes AI algorithms especially useful for processing large datasets generated by sensor networks, in which an AI algorithm can identify subtle patterns and trends that could easily go unnoticed by a human. In particular, it is very useful for longitudinal monitoring, early relapse detection, and treatment response assessment [150]. AI-powered nanobiosensors could serve as the main platform for the development of smart diagnostic ecosystems that are based on connecting biosensing devices with corresponding cloud-based health databases and clinical DGSPs (decision support and providers). This will not just raise the diagnostic precision but will also lighten the load on the health structure to increase accessibility and benefit advanced cancer diagnoses in a patient-oriented way.

7.8 Conclusion

Due to conventional diagnostic challenges, biosensor technology combines nanotechnology solutions to detect prostate cancer at early stages and monitor it by using innovative biosensor designs. Biosensors demonstrate superior capacity to detect prostate cancer biomarkers PSA and PCA3 by implementing a nanotechnology-based framework of gold nanoparticles with quantum dots, carbon nanotubes, and magnetic nanostructures. The modern technological advancements demonstrate substantial potential for usage within both laboratory testing frameworks and microscopic healthcare units that strive to get rid of healthcare availability gaps between urban and rural locations. The performance of nanobiosensors depends on selecting appropriate material components combined with surface engineering and shrinking device dimensions and approval procedures for medical implementation, according to this chapter. Different sensing platforms that use electrochemistry, optics, and magnetism provide specific benefits that drive the advancement of individualized, accurate cancer diagnostic methods. Biosensors that can be integrated with microfluidics, as well as data analytics and AI-driven decision systems, are further extended to next-generation healthcare systems. The exceptional results of medical innovation are obstructed by enduring issues involving reliable testing procedures, medical approval protocols, and commercial application procedures. Current difficulties demand coordinated action between research teams, together with medical professionals, as well as regulatory authorities, for their resolution. The deployment needs a thorough assessment of ethical matters and long-term biocompatibility tests before it can be implemented safely and equally. Prostate cancer diagnosis benefits substantially from nanotechnology-based biosensors, as early detection facilitates more effective treatment through personalized treatment plans. Then existing smart diagnostic platforms will serve as the basis for the subsequent development of future oncology once they achieve the precision medicine goal and meet accessible global health targets.

7.9 Summary

The use of nanotechnology in the creation of biosensors for the early and precise detection of prostate cancer is examined in this chapter, with particular attention paid to prostate-specific antigen (PSA) and new biomarkers such as PCA3, miRNAs, and circulating tumor cells (CTCs). It highlights how nanomaterials, including graphene, quantum dots, carbon nanotubes, gold nanoparticles, and magnetic nanoparticles, can improve the sensitivity, specificity, and portability of sensors. Particular focus is placed on point-of-care (POC) devices that are integrated with electrochemical and optical sensing platforms. Additionally covered are developments in wearable, microfluidic, and FET-based biosensing technologies, emphasizing their potential for real-time cancer diagnosis in the future as well as their clinical utility.

Glossary

Biosensor A device that uses biological molecules to detect chemical or biological analytes.

Nanoparticle A microscopic particle with dimensions measured in nanometers, often used to enhance sensor performance.

Point-of-care (POC) Diagnostic testing at or near the site of patient care.

Electrochemical sensing A detection method based on changes in electrical properties due to analyte interaction.

Surface plasmon resonance (SPR) An optical technique for detecting molecular interactions in real time.

Field-effect transistor (FET) A sensor type that detects changes in electrical conductivity from biomolecule binding.

Aptamer A short DNA or RNA sequence that selectively binds to a specific target molecule.

References

1. Nasrollahpour H, Khalilzadeh B, Hasanzadeh M, Rahbarghazi R, Estrela P, Naseri A, et al. Nanotechnology-based electrochemical biosensors for monitoring breast cancer biomarkers. Med Res Rev. 2023;43(3):464–569.
2. Singh D. Nanotechnology-based assays for the detection of cancer through sputum. Curr Anal Chem. 2023;19(9):633–41.
3. Hsu CC, Wu Y. Recent advances in nanotechnology-enabled biosensors for detection of exosomes as new cancer liquid biopsy. Exp Biol Med. 2022;247(23):2152–72.
4. Barani M, Sabir F, Rahdar A, Arshad R, Kyzas GZ. Nanotreatment and nanodiagnosis of prostate cancer: recent updates. Nano. 2020;10(9):1696.
5. Yadav N, Dahiya T, Chhillar AK, Rana JS, Saini HM. Nanotechnology in cancer diagnostics and therapeutics: a review. Curr Pharm Biotechnol. 2022;23(13):1556–68.

6. Hajjafari A, Sadr S, Rahdar A, Bayat M, Lotfalizadeh N, Dianaty S, et al. Exploring the integration of nanotechnology in the development and application of biosensors for enhanced detection and monitoring of colorectal cancer. Inorg Chem Commun. 2024;112409.
7. Singh R. Nanotechnology based therapeutic application in cancer diagnosis and therapy 3 Biotech. 2019;9(11):415.
8. Kang BJ, Jeun M, Jang GH, Song SH, Jeong IG, Kim CS, et al. Diagnosis of prostate cancer via nanotechnological approach. Int J Nanomed. 2015;6555–69.
9. Tantray J, Patel A, Parveen H, Prajapati B, Prajapati J. Nanotechnology-based biomedical devices in the cancer diagnostics and therapy. Med Oncol. 2025;42(2):50.
10. Ramesh M, Janani R, Deepa C, Rajeshkumar L. Nanotechnology-enabled biosensors: a review of fundamentals, design principles, materials, and applications. Biosensors. 2023;13(1). Available from: https://www.mdpi.com/2079-6374/13/1/40
11. Nikolelis DP, Nikoleli GP. Nanotechnology and biosensors. Elsevier; 2018.
12. Shahat FM, Youssef DG, Sayed FE, Elbadry AMM, Fouad FA, Mohammed MS, et al. Fundamentals of biosensors. Handb nanosensors Mater Technol Appl. 2024;265–301.
13. Malhotra BD, Ali MA. Nanomaterials in biosensors: fundamentals and applications. Nanomater Biosens. 2017;1.
14. Ahmad R, Wolfbeis OS, Hahn YB, Alshareef HN, Torsi L, Salama KN. Deposition of nanomaterials: a crucial step in biosensor fabrication. Mater Today Commun. 2018;17:289–321.
15. Sha R, Badhulika S. Recent advancements in fabrication of nanomaterial based biosensors for diagnosis of ovarian cancer: a comprehensive review. Microchim Acta. 2020;187:1–15.
16. Putzbach W, Ronkainen NJ. Immobilization techniques in the fabrication of nanomaterial-based electrochemical biosensors: a review. Sensors. 2013;13(4):4811–40.
17. Malik S, Singh J, Goyat R, Saharan Y, Chaudhry V, Umar A, et al. Nanomaterials-based biosensor and their applications: a review. Heliyon. 2023;9(9).
18. Fonash SJ. Unique features of the nano-scale. J Nanopart Res. 2018;20(12):323.
19. Draz MS, Shafiee H. Applications of gold nanoparticles in virus detection. Theranostics. 2018;8(7):1985–2017.
20. Le LTP, Nguyen AHQ, Phan LMT, Ngo HTT, Wang X, Cunningham B, et al. Current smartphone-assisted point-of-care cancer detection: towards supporting personalized cancer monitoring. TrAC Trends Anal Chem. 2024;174:117681. Available from: https://www.sciencedirect.com/science/article/pii/S0165993624001638
21. Benhal P, Quashie D, Kim Y, Ali J. Insulator based dielectrophoresis: micro, nano, and molecular scale biological applications. Sensors. 2020;20(18). Available from: https://www.mdpi.com/1424-8220/20/18/5095
22. Abdelwahab SI, Elhassan Taha MM, Sahli KA, Salem Alqhtani HA, Farasani A, Khamjan NA, et al. Graphene-based biosensors for PSA. Clin Chim Acta. 2025;576:120406. Available from: https://www.sciencedirect.com/science/article/pii/S0009898125002852
23. Chen HMHYHHH, Zhang JJJJ, Huang R, Wang DDXDDD, Deng D, Zhang QQQQQQ, et al. Nanomaterial-based electrochemical sensors for the detection of pharmaceutical drugs. Schatten H, editor. Cancers (Basel). 2022;14(1):35. Available from: https://www.sciencedirect.com/science/article/pii/S0039914020305671
24. Medintz IL, Uyeda HT, Goldman ER, Mattoussi H. Quantum dot bioconjugates for imaging, labelling and sensing. Nat Mater. 2005;4(6):435–46. https://doi.org/10.1038/nmat1390.
25. Li S, Zhang H, Zhu M, Kuang Z, Li X, Xu F, et al. Electrochemical biosensors for whole blood analysis: recent progress, challenges, and future perspectives. Chem Rev. 2023;123(12):7953–8039. https://doi.org/10.1021/acs.chemrev.1c00759.
26. Sudha PN, Sangeetha K, Vijayalakshmi K, Barhoum A. Nanomaterials history, classification, unique properties, production and market. In: Emerging applications of nanoparticles and architecture nanostructures. Elsevier; 2018. p. 341–84.
27. Zhao D, Bai P, Zhou A, Meng HM, Li Z. Functionalized nanoscale metal oxides for biosensing, bioimaging and cancer therapy. TrAC Trends Anal Chem. 2024:117684.
28. Liu Z, Ji X, He D, Zhang R, Liu Q, Xin T. Nanoscale drug delivery systems in glioblastoma. Nanoscale Res Lett. 2022;17(1):27.

29. Li X, Aftab S, Mukhtar M, Kabir F, Khan MF, Hegazy HH, et al. Exploring nanoscale perovskite materials for next-generation photodetectors: a comprehensive review and future directions. Nano Micro Lett. 2025;17(1):28.
30. Jan N, Shah H, Khan S, Nasar F, Madni A, Badshah SF, et al. Old drug, new tricks: polymer-based nanoscale systems for effective cytarabine delivery. Naunyn Schmiedeberg's Arch Pharmacol. 2024;397(6):3565–84.
31. Mayer LD, Tardi P, Louie AC. CPX-351: a nanoscale liposomal co-formulation of daunorubicin and cytarabine with unique biodistribution and tumor cell uptake properties. Int J Nanomed. 2019;3819–30.
32. Víšová I, Houska M, Vaisocherová-Lísalová H. Biorecognition antifouling coatings in complex biological fluids: a review of functionalization aspects. Analyst. 2022;147(12):2597–614.
33. Ning W, Di Z, Yu Y, Zeng P, Di C, Chen D, et al. Imparting designer biorecognition functionality to metal–organic frameworks by a DNA-mediated surface engineering strategy. Small. 2018;14(11):1703812.
34. Costa D, Pereira-Silva P, Sousa P, Pinto V, Borges J, Vaz F, et al. Critical issues on the surface functionalization of plasmonic au-ag/TiO2 thin films with thiolated oligonucleotide-based biorecognition elements. Biosensors. 2024;14(4):159.
35. Ahmad F, Salem-Bekhit MM, Khan F, Alshehri S, Khan A, Ghoneim MM, et al. Unique properties of surface-functionalized nanoparticles for bio-application: functionalization mechanisms and importance in application. Nanomaterials. 2022;12(8):1333.
36. Abbasy L, Mohammadzadeh A, Hasanzadeh M, Ehsani M, Mokhtarzadeh A. Biosensing of prostate specific antigen (PSA) in human plasma samples using biomacromolecule encapsulation into KCC-1-npr-NH2: A new platform for prostate cancer detection. Int J Biol Macromol. 2020;154:584–95.
37. Ji S, Lee M, Kim D. Detection of early stage prostate cancer by using a simple carbon nanotube@ paper biosensor. Biosens Bioelectron. 2018;102:345–50.
38. Ouyang N, Hong L, Zhou Y, Zhang J, Shafi S, Pan J, et al. Application of fluorescent nano-biosensor for the detection of cancer bio-macromolecular markers. Polym Test. 2022;115:107746.
39. Lin M, Pei H, Yang F, Fan C, Zuo X. Applications of gold nanoparticles in the detection and identification of infectious diseases and biothreats. Adv Mater. 2013;25(25):3490–6. Available from: https://advanced.onlinelibrary.wiley.com/doi/abs/10.1002/adma.201301333
40. Schumacher D, Hackenberger CPR. More than add-on: chemoselective reactions for the synthesis of functional peptides and proteins. Curr Opin Chem Biol. 2014;22:62–9. Available from: https://www.sciencedirect.com/science/article/pii/S1367593114001276
41. Jiao M, Zhang P, Meng J, Li Y, Liu C, Luo X, et al. Recent advancements in biocompatible inorganic nanoparticles towards biomedical applications. Biomater Sci. 2018;6(4):726–45. https://doi.org/10.1039/C7BM01020F.
42. Lu N, Gao A, Zhou H, Wang Y, Yang X, Wang Y, et al. Progress in silicon nanowire-based field-effect transistor biosensors for label-free detection of DNA. Chinese J Chem. 2016;34(3):308–16. Available from: https://onlinelibrary.wiley.com/doi/abs/10.1002/cjoc.201500857
43. Akbari Jonous Z, Shayeh JS, Yazdian F, Yadegari A, Hashemi M, Omidi M. An electrochemical biosensor for prostate cancer biomarker detection using graphene oxide–gold nanostructures. Eng Life Sci. 2019;19(3):206–16.
44. Wu J, Liu H, Chen W, Ma B, Ju H. Device integration of electrochemical biosensors. Nat Rev Bioeng. 2023;1(5):346–60.
45. Singh A, Sharma A, Ahmed A, Sundramoorthy AK, Furukawa H, Arya S, et al. Recent advances in electrochemical biosensors: applications, challenges, and future scope. Biosensors. 2021;11(9):336.
46. Cesewski E, Johnson BN. Electrochemical biosensors for pathogen detection. Biosens Bioelectron. 2020;159:112214.
47. Mejía-Salazar JR, Oliveira ON Jr. Plasmonic biosensing: focus review. Chem Rev. 2018;118(20):10617–25.

48. Liu J, Jalali M, Mahshid S, Wachsmann-Hogiu S. Are plasmonic optical biosensors ready for use in point-of-need applications? Analyst. 2020;145(2):364–84.
49. Esfahani Monfared Y. Overview of recent advances in the design of plasmonic fiber-optic biosensors. Biosensors. 2020;10(7):77.
50. Liyanage T, Lai M, Slaughter G. Label-free tapered optical fiber plasmonic biosensor. Anal Chim Acta. 2021;1169:338629.
51. Balaban Hanoglu S, Harmanci D, Ucar N, Evran S, Timur S. Recent approaches in magnetic nanoparticle-based biosensors of miRNA detection. Magnetochemistry. 2023;9(1):23.
52. Gessner I, Fries JWU, Brune V, Mathur S. Magnetic nanoparticle-based amplification of microRNA detection in body fluids for early disease diagnosis. J Mater Chem B. 2021;9(1):9–22.
53. Wang Z, Liu A, Li X, Guan L, Xing H, He L, et al. Multifunctional nanoprobe for multi-mode imaging and diagnosis of metastatic prostate cancer. Talanta. 2023;256:124255.
54. Bidarra D, Constâncio V, Barros-Silva D, Ramalho-Carvalho J, Moreira-Barbosa C, Antunes L, et al. Circulating microRNAs as biomarkers for prostate cancer detection and metastasis development prediction. Front Oncol. 2019;9:900.
55. Toth R, Schiffmann H, Hube-Magg C, Büscheck F, Höflmayer D, Weidemann S, et al. Random forest-based modelling to detect biomarkers for prostate cancer progression. Clin Epigenetics. 2019;11(1):148. https://doi.org/10.1186/s13148-019-0736-8.
56. Choudhury AD, Werner L, Francini E, Wei XX, Ha G, Freeman SS, et al. Tumor fraction in cell-free DNA as a biomarker in prostate cancer. JCI Insight. 2018;3(21).
57. Song C, Chen H, Chen L, Ru G, Guo J, Ding Q. The potential of microRNAs as human prostate cancer biomarkers: a meta-analysis of related studies. J Cell Biochem. 2018;119(3):2763–86.
58. Tsang CF, Lai TCT, Lam W, Ho BSH, Ng ATL, Ma WK, et al. Is prostate specific antigen (PSA) density necessary in selecting prostate cancer patients for active surveillance and what should be the cutoff in the Asian population? Prostate Int. 2019;7(2):73–7.
59. Nan LB, Yin XT, Gao JP. Significant diagnostic value of free-serum PSA (FPSA)/prostate-specific antigen density (PSAD) and (F/T)/PSAD for prostate cancer of the Chinese population in a single institution. Med Sci Monit Int Med J Exp Clin Res. 2019;25:8345–51.
60. Narain TA, Sooriakumaran P. Beyond prostate specific antigen: new prostate cancer screening options. World J Mens Health. 2022;40(1):66–73.
61. Wang Y, Wang M, Yu H, Wang G, Ma P, Pang S, et al. Screening of peptide selectively recognizing prostate-specific antigen and its application in detecting total prostate-specific antigen. Sensors Actuators B Chem. 2022;367:132009. Available from: https://www.sciencedirect.com/science/article/pii/S0925400522006517
62. Ploussard G, de la Taille A. The role of prostate cancer antigen 3 (PCA3) in prostate cancer detection. Expert Rev Anticancer Ther. 2018;18(10):1013–20.
63. Lemos AEG, Matos A da R, Ferreira LB, Gimba ERP. The long non-coding RNA PCA3: an update of its functions and clinical applications as a biomarker in prostate cancer. Oncotarget. 2019;10(61):6589–603.
64. Chunhua L, Zhao H, Zhao H, Lu Y, Wu J, Gao Z, et al. Clinical significance of peripheral blood PCA3 gene expression in early diagnosis of prostate cancer. Transl Oncol. 2018;11(3):628–32. Available from: https://www.sciencedirect.com/science/article/pii/S1936523317304783
65. Ghafouri-Fard S, Khoshbakht T, Hussen BM, Baniahmad A, Taheri M, Rashnoo F. A review on the role of PCA3 lncRNA in carcinogenesis with an especial focus on prostate cancer. Pathol Res Pract. 2022;231:153800. Available from: https://www.sciencedirect.com/science/article/pii/S0344033822000437
66. Gao Y, Huo W, Zhang L, Lian J, Tao W, Song C, et al. Multiplex measurement of twelve tumor markers using a GMR multi-biomarker immunoassay biosensor. Biosens Bioelectron. 2019;123:204–10. Available from: https://www.sciencedirect.com/science/article/pii/S0956566318306699
67. Gil Rosa B, Akingbade OE, Guo X, Gonzalez-Macia L, Crone MA, Cameron LP, et al. Multiplexed immunosensors for point-of-care diagnostic applications. Biosens Bioelectron.

2022;203:114050. Available from: https://www.sciencedirect.com/science/article/pii/S0956566322000902
68. Chandrasekaran AR, MacIsaac M, Vilcapoma J, Hansen CH, Yang D, Wong WP, et al. DNA nanoswitch barcodes for multiplexed biomarker profiling. Nano Lett. 2021;21(1):469–75. https://doi.org/10.1021/acs.nanolett.0c03929.
69. Li Z, Guo M, Zhong W. Multiplex detection of biomarkers empowered by nanomaterials. Precis Chem. 2025. https://doi.org/10.1021/prechem.4c00096.
70. Van Gool A, Corrales F, Čolović M, Krstić D, Oliver-Martos B, Martínez-Cáceres E, et al. Analytical techniques for multiplex analysis of protein biomarkers. Expert Rev Proteomics. 2020;17(4):257–73.
71. Chen MY, Skewes J, Woodruff MA, Dasgupta P, Rukin NJ. Multi-colour extrusion fused deposition modelling: a low-cost 3D printing method for anatomical prostate cancer models. Sci Rep. 2020;10(1):10004. https://doi.org/10.1038/s41598-020-67082-7.
72. Shah S, Famta P, Kumar R, Sharma A, Vambhurkar G, Pandey G, et al. Quality by design fostered fabrication of cabazitaxel loaded pH-responsive improved nanotherapeutics against prostate cancer. Colloids Surfaces B Biointerfaces. 2024;234:113732. Available from: https://www.sciencedirect.com/science/article/pii/S0927776523006264
73. Rezaei Z, Alemzadeh I, Vossoughi M. Design and fabrication of an electrochemical-based nanofibrous immunosensor for detection of prostate cancer biomarker. PSMA Polym Adv Technol. 2022;33(6):1967–77.
74. Osuchowski M, Osuchowski F, Latos W, Kawczyk-Krupka A. The use of upconversion nanoparticles in prostate cancer photodynamic therapy. Life. 2021;11(4). Available from: https://www.mdpi.com/2075-1729/11/4/360
75. Barabadi H, Damavandi Kamali K, Jazayeri Shoushtari F, Tajani B, Mahjoub MA, Alizadeh A, et al. Emerging theranostic silver and gold nanomaterials to combat prostate cancer: a systematic review. J Clust Sci. 2019;30(6):1375–82. https://doi.org/10.1007/s10876-019-01588-7.
76. Emanet Ciofani M, Şen Ö, Çulha M. Hexagonal boron nitride nanoparticles for prostate cancer treatment. ACS Appl Nano Mater. 2020;3(3):2364–72. https://doi.org/10.1021/acsanm.9b02486.
77. Stolarczyk EU, Leś A, Łaszcz M, Kubiszewski M, Strzempek W, Menaszek E, et al. The ligand exchange of citrates to thioabiraterone on gold nanoparticles for prostate cancer therapy. Int J Pharm. 2020;583:119319. Available from: https://www.sciencedirect.com/science/article/pii/S0378517320303033
78. Zhuo Y, Wang Y, Gao R, Zhan C, Liu H, Liu Y, et al. Novel simultaneous separation and detection of CTCs and PSA on an integrated multistage microfluidic chip for early diagnosis of prostate cancer. Microchem J. 2025;212:113330. Available from: https://www.sciencedirect.com/science/article/pii/S0026265X2500685X.
79. Jiang L, Khawaja H, Tahsin S, Clarkson TA, Miranti CK, Zohar Y. Microfluidic-based human prostate-cancer-on-chip. Front Bioeng Biotechnol. 2024;12:1302223.
80. Padmyastuti A, Sarmiento MG, Dib M, Ehrhardt J, Schoon J, Somova M, et al. Microfluidic-based prostate cancer model for investigating the secretion of prostate-specific antigen and microRNAs in vitro. Sci Rep. 2023;13(1):11623. https://doi.org/10.1038/s41598-023-38834-y.
81. Gao R, Cheng Z, Wang X, Yu L, Guo Z, Zhao G, et al. Simultaneous immunoassays of dual prostate cancer markers using a SERS-based microdroplet channel. Biosens Bioelectron. 2018;119:126–33. Available from: https://www.sciencedirect.com/science/article/pii/S0956566318306031.
82. Jiang L, Ivich F, Tahsin S, Tran M, Frank SB, Miranti CK, et al. Human stroma and epithelium co-culture in a microfluidic model of a human prostate gland. Biomicrofluidics. 2019;13(6).
83. Kim CJ, Dong L, Amend SR, Cho YK, Pienta KJ. The role of liquid biopsies in prostate cancer management. Lab Chip. 2021;21(17):3263–88.
84. Gao R, Lv Z, Mao Y, Yu L, Bi X, Xu S, et al. SERS-based pump-free microfluidic chip for highly sensitive immunoassay of prostate-specific antigen biomarkers. ACS Sens. 2019;4(4):938–43.

85. Lu Y, Zhan C, Yu L, Yu Y, Jia H, Chen X, et al. Multifunctional nanocone array as solid immunoassay plate and SERS substrate for the early diagnosis of prostate cancer on microfluidic chip. Sensors Actuators B Chem. 2023;376:133046. Available from: https://www.sciencedirect.com/science/article/pii/S0925400522016896.
86. Numan A, Singh S, Zhan Y, Li L, Khalid M, Rilla K, et al. Advanced nanoengineered—customized point-of-care tools for prostate-specific antigen. Microchim Acta. 2021;189(1):27. https://doi.org/10.1007/s00604-021-05127-y.
87. Wang L, Ji Y, Wang L, Zheng S, Chen Y, Xu X, et al. Ratio fluorescence/colorimetric dual mode aptasensor and smartphones-assisted miniaturized device for early diagnosis of prostate cancer. Chem Eng J. 2024;485:150152. Available from: https://www.sciencedirect.com/science/article/pii/S1385894724016383
88. Ortega FG, Gómez GE, González-Martinez C, Valero T, Expósito-Hernández J, Puche I, et al. A novel, quick, and reliable smartphone-based method for serum PSA quantification: original design of a portable microfluidic immunosensor-based system. Cancers (Basel). 2022;14(18). Available from: https://www.mdpi.com/2072-6694/14/18/4483
89. Kim S, Park S, Cho YS, Kim Y, Tae JH, Il NT, et al. Electrical cartridge sensor enables reliable and direct identification of MicroRNAs in urine of patients. ACS Sens. 2021;6(3):833–41. https://doi.org/10.1021/acssensors.0c01870.
90. Bounoua N, Cetinkaya A, Piskin E, Kaya SI, Ozkan SA. The sensor applications for prostate and lung cancer biomarkers in terms of electrochemical analysis. Anal Bioanal Chem. 2024;416(9):2277–300. https://doi.org/10.1007/s00216-024-05134-x.
91. Ranjan P, Singhal A, Sadique MA, Yadav S, Parihar A, Khan R. Chapter 24 - Scope of biosensors, commercial aspects, and miniaturized devices for point-of-care testing from lab to clinics applications. In: Khan R, Parihar A, Sanghi SK, editors. Biosensor based advanced cancer diagnostics. Academic Press; 2022. p. 395–410. Available from: https://www.sciencedirect.com/science/article/pii/B9780128234242000041.
92. Deng M, Yang H, Zhang H, Li C, Chen J, Tang W, et al. Chapter 24 - Scope of biosensors, commercial aspects, and miniaturized devices for point-of-care testing from lab to clinics applications. Adv Healthc Mater. 2024;13(3):2302117.
93. Khondakar KR, Dey S, Wuethrich A, Sina AAI, Trau M. Toward personalized cancer treatment: from diagnostics to therapy monitoring in miniaturized electrohydrodynamic systems. Acc Chem Res. 2019;52(8):2113–23. https://doi.org/10.1021/acs.accounts.9b00192.
94. Dey S, Kinoshita M, Puttick S, Rose S, Trau M, Roberts MJ, et al. Cancer-on-chip and integrative tumor microenvironment sensor technologies for progressing precision radiotherapy. Adv Sensor Res. 2024;3(7):2300193.
95. Na W, Kang M, Jang D, Shin S. Miniaturized surface plasmon resonance biosensor with vacuum-driven hydrodynamic focusing. Sensors Actuators B Chem. 2018;254:64–71. Available from: https://www.sciencedirect.com/science/article/pii/S0925400517312492
96. Bhaiyya M, Pattnaik PK, Goel S. A brief review on miniaturized electrochemiluminescence devices: from fabrication to applications. Curr Opin Electrochem. 2021;30:100800. Available from: https://www.sciencedirect.com/science/article/pii/S2451910321001149
97. Inderjeeth AJ, Topp M, Sanij E, Castro E, Sandhu S. Clinical application of poly(ADP-ribose) polymerase (PARP) inhibitors in prostate cancer. Cancers (Basel). 2022;14(23). Available from: https://www.mdpi.com/2072-6694/14/23/5922
98. Fraguas-Sánchez AI, Torres-Suárez AI. Medical use of cannabinoids. Drugs. 2018;78(16):1665–703.
99. Phan T, Crook SM, Bryce AH, Maley CC, Kostelich EJ, Kuang Y. Review: mathematical modeling of prostate cancer and clinical application. Appl Sci. 2020;10(8). Available from: https://www.mdpi.com/2076-3417/10/8/2721
100. Aurilio G, Cimadamore A, Mazzucchelli R, Lopez-Beltran A, Verri E, Scarpelli M, et al. Androgen receptor signaling pathway in prostate cancer: from genetics to clinical applications. Cells. 2020;9(12). Available from: https://www.mdpi.com/2073-4409/9/12/2653

101. da Silva LM, Pereira EM, Salles PGO, Godrich R, Ceballos R, Kunz JD, et al. Independent real-world application of a clinical-grade automated prostate cancer detection system. J Pathol. 2021;254(2):147–58.
102. Perincheri S, Levi AW, Celli R, Gershkovich P, Rimm D, Morrow JS, et al. An independent assessment of an artificial intelligence system for prostate cancer detection shows strong diagnostic accuracy. Mod Pathol. 2021;34(8):1588–95. Available from: https://www.sciencedirect.com/science/article/pii/S0893395222005725
103. Alabousi M, Salameh J, Gusenbauer K, Samoilov L, Jafri A, Yu H, et al. Biparametric vs multiparametric prostate magnetic resonance imaging for the detection of prostate cancer in treatment-naïve patients: a diagnostic test accuracy systematic review and meta-analysis. BJU Int. 2019;124(2):209–20.
104. Sathianathen NJ, Omer A, Harriss E, Davies L, Kasivisvanathan V, Punwani S, et al. Negative predictive value of multiparametric magnetic resonance imaging in the detection of clinically significant prostate cancer in the prostate imaging reporting and data system era: a systematic review and meta-analysis. Eur Urol. 2020;78(3):402–14. Available from: https://www.sciencedirect.com/science/article/pii/S0302283820302232
105. Monaghan TF, Rahman SN, Agudelo CW, Wein AJ, Lazar JM, Everaert K, et al. Foundational statistical principles in medical research: sensitivity, specificity, positive predictive value, and negative predictive value. Medicina (B Aires). 2021;57(5). Available from: https://www.mdpi.com/1648-9144/57/5/503
106. Chen X, Zhou G, Song P, Wang J, Gao J, Lu J, et al. Ultrasensitive electrochemical detection of prostate-specific antigen by using antibodies anchored on a DNA nanostructural scaffold. Anal Chem. 2014;86(15):7337–42.
107. Shahbazi-Derakhshi P, Mahmoudi E, Majidi MM, Sohrabi H, Amini M, Majidi MR, et al. An ultrasensitive miRNA-based genosensor for detection of MicroRNA 21 in gastric cancer cells based on functional signal amplifier and synthesized perovskite-graphene oxide and AuNPs. Biosensors. 2023;13(2). Available from: https://www.mdpi.com/2079-6374/13/2/172
108. Kavosi B, Salimi A, Hallaj R, Moradi F. Ultrasensitive electrochemical immunosensor for PSA biomarker detection in prostate cancer cells using gold nanoparticles/PAMAM dendrimer loaded with enzyme linked aptamer as integrated triple signal amplification strategy. Biosens Bioelectron. 2015;74:915–23.
109. Deng M, Ren Z, Zhang H, Li Z, Xue C, Wang J, et al. Unamplified and real-time label-free miRNA-21 detection using solution-gated graphene transistors in prostate cancer diagnosis. Adv Sci (Weinheim, Baden-Wurttemberg, Ger. 2023;10(4):e2205886.
110. Kant K, Abalde-Cela S. Surface-enhanced Raman scattering spectroscopy and microfluidics: towards ultrasensitive label-free sensing. Biosensors. 2018;8(3). Available from: https://www.mdpi.com/2079-6374/8/3/62
111. Conteduca V, Hess J, Yamada Y, Ku SY, Beltran H. Epigenetics in prostate cancer: clinical implications. Transl Androl Urol. 2021;10(7):3104.
112. Mahal BA, Gerke T, Awasthi S, Soule HR, Simons JW, Miyahira A, et al. Prostate cancer racial disparities: a systematic review by the Prostate Cancer Foundation Panel. Eur Urol Oncol. 2022;5(1):18–29. Available from: https://www.sciencedirect.com/science/article/pii/S2588931121001462
113. Yan Y, Huang H. Interplay among PI3K/AKT, PTEN/FOXO and AR signaling in prostate cancer. In: Dehm SM, Tindall DJ, editors. Prostate cancer: cellular and genetic mechanisms of disease development and progression. Cham: Springer International Publishing; 2019. p. 319–31. https://doi.org/10.1007/978-3-030-32656-2_14.
114. Lamy PJ, Allory Y, Gauchez AS, Asselain B, Beuzeboc P, de Cremoux P, et al. Prognostic biomarkers used for localised prostate cancer management: a systematic review. Eur Urol Focus. 2018;4(6):790–803. Available from: https://www.sciencedirect.com/science/article/pii/S2405456917300652
115. Klein EA, Richards D, Cohn A, Tummala M, Lapham R, Cosgrove D, et al. Clinical validation of a targeted methylation-based multi-cancer early detection test using an independent validation set. Ann Oncol. 2021;32(9):1167–77.

116. Van Den Eeden SK, Lu R, Zhang N, Quesenberry CP, Shan J, Han JS, et al. A biopsy-based 17-gene genomic prostate score as a predictor of metastases and prostate cancer death in surgically treated men with clinically localized disease. Eur Urol. 2018;73(1):129–38. Available from: https://www.sciencedirect.com/science/article/pii/S0302283817307777
117. Min X, Li M, Dong D, Feng Z, Zhang P, Ke Z, et al. Multi-parametric MRI-based radiomics signature for discriminating between clinically significant and insignificant prostate cancer: cross-validation of a machine learning method. Eur J Radiol. 2019;115:16–21. Available from: https://www.sciencedirect.com/science/article/pii/S0720048X19301020
118. Hempelmann JA, Lockwood CM, Konnick EQ, Schweizer MT, Antonarakis ES, Lotan TL, et al. Microsatellite instability in prostate cancer by PCR or next-generation sequencing. J Immunother Cancer. 2018;6(1):29. https://doi.org/10.1186/s40425-018-0341-y.
119. Rausch S, Hennenlotter J, Wiesenreiter J, Hohneder A, Heinkele J, Schwentner C, et al. Assessment of a new point-of-care system for detection of prostate specific antigen. BMC Urol. 2016;16(1):4. https://doi.org/10.1186/s12894-016-0119-9.
120. Annese VF, Patil SB, Hu C, Giagkoulovits C, Al-Rawhani MA, Grant J, et al. A monolithic single-chip point-of-care platform for metabolomic prostate cancer detection. Microsyst Nanoeng. 2021;7(1):21.
121. Fan Y, Shi S, Ma J, Guo Y. Smartphone-based electrochemical system with multi-walled carbon nanotubes/thionine/gold nanoparticles modified screen-printed immunosensor for cancer antigen 125 detection. Microchem J. 2022;174:107044. Available from: https://www.sciencedirect.com/science/article/pii/S0026265X21011309
122. Zhou R, Bai G, Zhu D, Xu Q, Zhang X, Li T, et al. Pump-free SERS microfluidic chip based on an identification-competition strategy for ultrasensitive and efficient simultaneous detection of liver cancer-related microRNAs. Biomed Opt Express. 2024;15(11):6469–85.
123. Farahmandpour M, Kordrostami Z. Wearable MXene-enhanced organic Bio-FET paper patch for glucose detection in sweat with pH and temperature calibration. Sci Rep. 2025;15(1):16219. https://doi.org/10.1038/s41598-025-00533-1.
124. Sun D, Chen Z, Wu M, Zhang Y. Nanomaterial-based microfluidic chips for the capture and detection of circulating tumor cells. Nanotheranostics. 2017;1(4):389–402.
125. Khonyoung S, Mangkronkaew P, Klayprasert P, Puangpila C, Palanisami M, Arivazhagan M, et al. Point-of-care detection of carcinoembryonic antigen (CEA) using a smartphone-based, label-free electrochemical immunosensor with multilayer CuONPs/CNTs/GO on a disposable screen-printed electrode. Biosensors. 2024;14(12). Available from: https://www.mdpi.com/2079-6374/14/12/600
126. Srinivasan B, Nanus DM, Erickson D, Mehta S. Highly portable quantitative screening test for prostate-specific antigen at point of care. Curr Res Biotechnol. 2021;3:288–99.
127. Ying Z, Feng L, Ji D, Zhang Y, Chen W, Dai Y, et al. Phase-regulated sensing mechanism of MoS2 based nanohybrids toward point-of-care prostate cancer diagnosis. Small. 2020;16(18):2000307.
128. Rong Z, Bai Z, Li J, Tang H, Shen T, Wang Q, et al. Dual-color magnetic-quantum dot nanobeads as versatile fluorescent probes in test strip for simultaneous point-of-care detection of free and complexed prostate-specific antigen. Biosens Bioelectron. 2019;145:111719.
129. Shen MM, Abate-Shen C. Molecular genetics of prostate cancer: new prospects for old challenges. Genes Dev. 2010;24(18):1967–2000.
130. Sharma P, Zargar-Shoshtari K, Pow-Sang JM. Biomarkers for prostate cancer: present challenges and future opportunities. Futur Sci OA. 2016;2(1):FSO72.
131. Gururajan M, Posadas EM, Chung LWK. Future perspectives of prostate cancer therapy. Transl Androl Urol. 2012;1(1):19–32.
132. Wallace TJ, Torre T, Grob M, Yu J, Avital I, Brücher B, et al. Current approaches, challenges and future directions for monitoring treatment response in prostate cancer. J Cancer. 2014;5(1):3–24.
133. Sharma S, Zapatero-Rodriguez J, O'Kennedy R. Prostate cancer diagnostics: clinical challenges and the ongoing need for disruptive and effective diagnostic tools. Biotechnol Adv. 2017;35(2):135–49.

134. Shore ND, Morgans AK, El-Haddad G, Srinivas S, Abramowitz M. Addressing challenges and controversies in the management of prostate cancer with multidisciplinary teams. Target Oncol. 2022;17(6):709–25. https://doi.org/10.1007/s11523-022-00925-7.
135. Valerio M, Emberton M, Eggener SE, Ahmed HU. The challenging landscape of medical device approval in localized prostate cancer. Nat Rev Urol. 2016;13(2):91–8. https://doi.org/10.1038/nrurol.2015.289.
136. He J, Wu J, Li Z, Zhao Z, Qiu L, Zhu X, et al. Immunotherapy vaccines for prostate cancer treatment. Cancer Med. 2024;13(20):e70294.
137. Jiang Y, Wang C, Zu C, Rong X, Yu Q, Jiang J. Synergistic potential of nanomedicine in prostate cancer immunotherapy: breakthroughs and prospects. Int J Nanomed. 2024;9459–86.
138. Cavallo AU, Stanzione A, Ponsiglione A, Trotta R, Fanni SC, Ghezzo S, et al. Prostate cancer MRI methodological radiomics score: a EuSoMII radiomics auditing group initiative. Eur Radiol. 2025;35(3):1157–65. https://doi.org/10.1007/s00330-024-11299-x.
139. Feng DC, Zhu WZ, Wang J, Li DX, Shi X, Xiong Q, et al. The implications of single-cell RNA-seq analysis in prostate cancer: unraveling tumor heterogeneity, therapeutic implications and pathways towards personalized therapy. Mil Med Res. 2024;11(1):21. https://doi.org/10.1186/s40779-024-00526-7.
140. McDonald AC, Vira M, Walter V, Shen J, Raman JD, Sanda MG, et al. Circulating microRNAs in plasma among men with low-grade and high-grade prostate cancer at prostate biopsy. Prostate. 2019;79(9):961–8.
141. Elnour AAM, Ashammakhi N, Sallam EB. Opportunities for investing in Organ-on-a-Chip (OoC) technology, breast-on-a-Chip (BoC) as an example technology transfer into Islamic Development Bank Members Countries (IsDB-MCs). In: Elnour AAM, editor. Gum Arabic and breast cancer biology: biotechnology perspective. Singapore: Springer Nature Singapore; 2025. p. 239–81. https://doi.org/10.1007/978-981-97-8518-6_7.
142. Dachani SR, Kaleem M, Mujtaba MA, Mahajan N, Ali SA, Almutairy AF, et al. A comprehensive review of various therapeutic strategies for the management of skin cancer. ACS Omega. 2024;9(9):10030–48. https://doi.org/10.1021/acsomega.3c09780.
143. Dhiman S, Mukherjee G. Prospects of bacterial tannase catalyzed biotransformation of agro and industrial tannin waste to high value gallic acid. Biorefinery Prod Technol Chem Energy. 2020:129–43.
144. Gökırmaklı Ç, Bayram M. Utilization, methods for obtaining, and health benefits of wheat, rice, and their by-products. In: Food by-product based functional food powders. CRC Press; 2018. p. 131–50.
145. Raghavendra PB, Pullaiah T. Advances in cell and molecular diagnostics. Academic Press; 2018.
146. Talyshinskii A, Hameed BMZ, Ravinder PP, Naik N, Randhawa P, Shah M, et al. Catalyzing precision medicine: artificial intelligence advancements in prostate cancer diagnosis and management. Cancers (Basel). 2024;16(10). Available from: https://www.mdpi.com/2072-6694/16/10/1809
147. Alitto AR, Gatta R, Vanneste BGL, Vallati M, Meldolesi E, Damiani A, et al. PRODIGE: PRediction models in prOstate cancer for personalized meDIcine challenGE. Future Oncol. 2017;13(24):2171–81.
148. Ren S, Li J, Dorado J, Sierra A, González-Díaz H, Duardo A, et al. From molecular mechanisms of prostate cancer to translational applications: based on multi-omics fusion analysis and intelligent medicine. Heal Inf Sci Syst. 2023;12(1):6. https://doi.org/10.1007/s13755-023-00264-5.
149. Feretzakis G, Juliebø-Jones P, Tsaturyan A, Sener TE, Verykios VS, Karapiperis D, et al. Emerging trends in AI and radiomics for bladder, kidney, and prostate cancer: a critical review. Cancers (Basel). 2024;16(4). Available from: https://www.mdpi.com/2072-6694/16/4/810
150. Adir O, Poley M, Chen G, Froim S, Krinsky N, Shklover J, et al. Integrating artificial intelligence and nanotechnology for precision cancer medicine. Adv Mater. 2020;32(13):1901989.

Point-of-Care Testing for Prostate Cancer

8

Sakshi Patel, Adnan Khan, Molakpogu Ravindra Babu, Brijesh Kumar Sharma, and Aroop Mohanty

Abbreviations

POC	Point-of-care
PSA	Prostate-specific antigen
PCA3	Prostate cancer antigen 3
CTC	Circulating tumor cell
EV	Extracellular vesicle
miRNA	MicroRNA
TMPRSS2: ERG	Transmembrane protease serine 2: ETS-related gene fusion
AI	Artificial intelligence
CRISPR	Clustered regularly interspaced short palindromic repeats
RT-PCR	Reverse transcription polymerase chain reaction
SPR	Surface plasmon resonance
LAMP	Loop-mediated isothermal amplification
EMR	Electronic medical record

S. Patel
Department of Pharmaceutical Technology, Meerut Institute of Engineering & Technology, Meerut, Uttar Pradesh, India

A. Khan · M. Ravindra Babu
Department of Pharmacy, School of Medical and Allied Sciences, Galgotias University, Greater Noida, Uttar Pradesh, India

B. K. Sharma
Government Pharmacy College, B.R.D. Medical College Campus, Gorakhpur, Uttar Pradesh, India

A. Mohanty (✉)
Department of Microbiology, All India Institute of Medical Sciences, Gorakhpur, Uttar Pradesh, India

S. Srivastava et al. (eds.), *Biosensor Technologies for Prostate Cancer*, https://doi.org/10.1007/978-981-95-8644-8_8

LMICs	Low- and middle-income countries
PHI	Prostate Health Index
LFAs	Lateral flow assays
AR-V7	Androgen receptor variant 7

8.1 Introduction

The healthcare industry has undergone major progress through point-of-care (POC) testing by delivering quick accurate results from decentralized medical stations [1]. The detection of prostate cancer proves vital due to its wide occurrence among men worldwide since it stands as one of the major cancer types affecting them [2]. The traditional diagnostic process that depends primarily on centralized laboratory tests and biopsies, in addition to medical imaging methods, struggles with several important drawbacks, which create challenges in time-consuming steps, high costs, and the absence of accessibility in low-resource areas [3]. POC technologies allow on-site testing at patient locations such as bedsides and outpatient clinics and in homes, which results in earlier treatments leading to better patient results [4].

8.1.1 Definition of POC Testing in Oncology

In oncology, POC testing refers to the rapid analysis of biomarkers or clinical parameters at or near the site of patient care, without the need for complex laboratory infrastructure (see Fig. 8.1 for a comparison of diagnostic pathways) [5]. Prostate cancer tests require analysis of prostate-specific antigen (PSA), prostate cancer antigen 3 (PCA3), and TMPRSS2: ERG gene fusion, circulating tumor cells

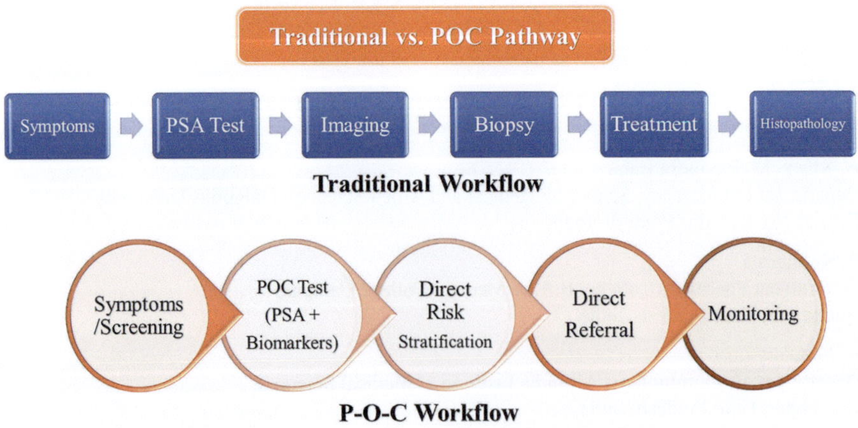

Fig. 8.1 Diagnostic workflow comparison—traditional vs. POC pathway

(CTCs) and exosomes, and emerging microRNA (miRNA) patterns in blood, urine, and seminal fluid [6]. Contemporary diagnostic equipment aims to produce results within short durations of up to several hours, thus enabling medical practitioners to perform prompt patient care choices.

POC testing devices exhibit small sizes that accompany simple operation requirements and need small amounts of sample processing [7]. Because of microfluidics and other advancements such as nanotechnology and biosensor development and digital health improvements, modern POC technology offers much higher sensitivity together with specificity and multi-analyte assessment potential, which is essential for prostate cancer diagnosis.

8.1.2 Importance of Early Detection in Prostate Cancer

As prostate cancer evolves, there are two main clinical outcomes that span from harmless tumors leading to no symptoms to aggressive cancers that need swift medical attention. There are no early warning signs for prostate cancer in the initial stages because patients usually lack any symptoms during this time that doctors can easily detect [8]. This fact leads them to discover prostate cancer during later advanced stages, in which treatment options create less success with better survival rates. The correct and early detection of cancer represents an essential necessity because it enables clinicians to first discover dangerous conditions early while preventing the need to treat slow-growing tumors, which remains a current issue when using PSA testing [9]. The widespread traditional PSA test usage faces limitations because PSA level increases affect both prostate cancer patients and those with BPH or prostatitis, as well as other non-cancerous conditions [10]. There is now significant research directed toward developing POC systems that do single biomarker testing to provide better risk evaluation and prevent unneeded biopsies. POC tests present hope to disperse prostate cancer screening capabilities along with diagnostic capacity through primary care facilities and rural centers and developing nations that need better diagnostic laboratory services [11]. The rapid diagnostic process can help patients decrease their anxious feelings, along with redirecting their care efficiently and enabling physicians to decide treatment options right away [12].

8.1.3 POC Versus Traditional Diagnostic Methods

Standard prostate cancer diagnostics require multiple steps, including PSA testing, after which health professionals conduct digital rectal examinations and multiparametric MRI studies to confirm diagnosis with prostate biopsies [13]. Multiple sequential healthcare steps can cause delays and increase risk exposures, as well as expenditures, which may affect the overall quality of patient care. The current screening and diagnostic approaches prove ineffective when implemented for continuous large-scale tests due to existing facility limitations (see Table 8.1 for a

Table 8.1 Comparative analysis of conventional vs. POC-based prostate cancer diagnostic approaches

Parameter	Conventional lab-based testing	POC testing	References
Turnaround time	2–7 days	Minutes to 1 hour	[16]
Infrastructure requirement	Centralized labs, trained personnel	Portable, minimal setup	[17]
Sample volume	3–5 mL blood	≤100 μL blood/urine	[18]
Patient accessibility	Hospital/clinic dependent	Remote, rural, or home-based	[7]
Biomarker scope	Mainly PSA	Multiplexed: PSA, PCA3, miRNAs, etc.	[19]
Diagnostic specificity	Moderate (PSA alone)	High (multi-marker capability)	[20]
Cost per test	$60–$150	$5–$40 (prototype estimates)	[21]

comparative overview) [14]. POC testing technologies function to overcome dilemmas in healthcare through their following features [15]:

Speed: The results produced by POC testing methods return within a few hours to several minutes, while standard laboratory tests take several days.

Accessibility: The testing platform requires minimal dependence on both centralized laboratories and highly trained personnel.

Cost-effectiveness: Healthcare expenses decrease substantially through this technology because it decreases the number of useless medical procedures and reduces patient hospital attendance.

Patient-centered care: POC testing enables healthcare providers to give patients quick results, which lets them instantly talk about what should be done next.

SMs with POC devices coupled to patient electronic records let patients perform remote health monitoring from their own homes, according to digital health trends [22].

8.1.4 Current Landscape and Future Promise

Research on POC devices dedicated to prostate cancer diagnosis remains a developing scientific field. Current prototype and commercial systems show success in detecting both PSA and various related biomarkers with high sensitivity as well as specificity results [23]. New biosensing technology based on Clustered Regularly Interspaced Short Palindromic Repeats (CRISPR), as well as nanomaterials platforms and artificial intelligence (AI) analytical systems, will advance POC testing by leading to prediction and personalization in addition to speed and accuracy [24]. Field development aims toward building a real-time diagnostic profile, which gives multi-dimensional guidance for screening, detection, and therapeutic monitoring, besides diagnosis and prognosis [25]. The next phase of prostate cancer management will approach precision medicine ideals because the advances will fit treatments to the distinct disease biology of each patient.

8.2 Biomarkers for POC Testing in Prostate Cancer

The success of POC testing in prostate cancer hinges critically on the selection and detection of highly specific and sensitive biomarkers (refer to Table 8.2 for key biomarker targets) [26]. Medical definitions of biomarkers indicate that they should provide reliable indicators of disease states and their trends, as well as predictive outcomes. POC platforms benefit strongly from combining three marker types, including genomic markers and proteomic markers, with exosomal markers into an advanced analytical system that brings better accuracy and speed to testing [27].

8.2.1 PSA and Its Limitations

PSA functions as the primary tool in prostate cancer examination since its discovery for screening purposes. PSA functions as a serine protease that originates from prostatic epithelial cells, which appear in higher amounts in the bloodstream during tumor development [28]. The diagnostic properties of PSA demonstrate shortcomings because it detects most cases yet fails to provide specific results. Benign prostatic hyperplasia (BPH) and prostatitis, along with other benign conditions, raise PSA levels, which trigger unnecessary biopsy procedures [29]. Research has explored various derivatives and modified versions of PSA as potential solutions to its identified shortcomings. *Free PSA (fPSA)*: Using the fPSA measurement along with the free to total PSA ratio proves beneficial for

Table 8.2 Key prostate cancer biomarkers used in POC biosensing platforms

Biomarker	Type	Diagnostic role	Detection challenges	POC sensor types used	References
PSA	Protein	General screening	Low specificity	Electrochemical, optical	[33]
PCA3	lncRNA	High specificity	RNA instability	RT-PCR-integrated biosensors	[34]
TMPRSS2:ERG	Fusion gene	Aggressive PCa	Requires nucleic acid amplification	Nucleic acid biosensors	[35]
miR-141, miR-21	miRNAs	Progression, metastasis	Low abundance	qPCR, microfluidic chips	[36]
Sarcosine	Metabolite	Prognostic marker	Matrix interference	Paper-based sensors	[37]

identifying specific cases while detecting prostate cancer among patients with PSA levels between 4 and 10 ng/mL. *[−2]pro PSA*: The [−2]pro PSA protein behaves as a PSA variant, which shows higher prostate cancer linkages to be included in the Prostate Health Index (PHI) analysis. *PSA Density and PSA Velocity*: Doctors use PSA Density along with PSA Velocity as metrics that merge PSA readings with prostate dimensions and PSA alteration rates. The diagnostic capabilities of PSA have improved through refinement work, but further biomarkers remain essential to boost accuracy in all situations, particularly those situations requiring prompt POC decisions [30].

8.2.2 Circulating Tumor Cells

Primary tumor cells, known as CTCs, detach from their original location before entering the circulation through the bloodstream. Study of CTCs provides instant monitoring of tumor severity in addition to its growth characteristics [31]. The POC platforms utilize two technologies, namely, microfluidic chips and immunomagnetic separation systems, for both CTC isolation and analysis. Protocol CTC analysis detects more than mere presence, as it demonstrates the potential to reveal androgen receptor mutations and both gene expression patterns and therapy resistance mechanisms associated with androgen deprivation therapy [32].

8.2.3 Exosomes and Extracellular Vesicles

The human body generates exosomes as nano-scale vesicles from cells, which contain proteins, lipids, and nucleic acids that mirror their cell of origin. Prostasomes represent an attractive non-invasive biomarker source, as they are detectable in urine, blood, and semen samples. Exosomal markers under investigation include the following: *PCA3 RNA*: overexpressed in prostate cancer tissues; *TMPRSS2*: ERG fusion RNA: a gene fusion highly specific to prostate cancer; and *exosomal PSA and* prostate-specific membrane antigen proteins. Modern nano-biosensing technologies allow POC devices to detect exosomes at high sensitivity through sensitive analysis of these exosome samples.

8.2.4 MicroRNAs

Numerous studies indicate that miRNAs function as short non-coding RNA molecules that manage gene expression after transcription occurs. The development of prostate cancer strongly correlates with abnormal patterns of miRNA expression [38]. Key prostate cancer-associated miRNAs include miR-141, miR-21, miR-375, and miR-221. Different POC platforms with electrochemical and optical biosensing capabilities are now advancing to detect miRNAs directly from bodily fluids in a specific manner, utilizing simplified sample preparation processes [39].

8.2.5 Genomic and Epigenomic Markers

Multiple DNA mutations and several epigenetic alterations in prostate cancer serve as key elements for early detection through genomic analysis [40]. *DNA methylation markers*: The epigenetic change known as hypermethylation of GSTP1 stands among the most dependable DNA methylation markers in prostate cancer. *Somatic mutations*: Genes BRCA1/2, TP53, and PTEN, along with other cancer-related genes, undergo somatic mutations, which benefit patient risk evaluation and treatment planning. *Androgen receptor variants*: Particularly, androgen receptor variant 7 (AR-V7) variants demonstrate the strongest association with biological resistance toward particular hormone-based treatments. The fast and on-site genetic alteration detection is enabled by current developments in both microfluidics devices and CRISPR-based biosensors [41].

8.2.6 Multiplexed Biomarker Panels: The Future of POC Testing

Prostate cancer requires multiple biomarkers for complete evaluation because any one biomarker alone does not fully represent the disease. Medical research now focuses on developing combined biomarker testing systems within multiplexed panels, which generate a combined risk indication from multiple biomarkers [42]. Examples of multi-analyte tests include the following:

PHI: Incorporates total PSA, fPSA, and [−2]proPSA. *The 4Kscore Test*: Uses total PSA alongside fPSA and intact PSA, along with hK2, to calculate aggressive prostate cancer risk assessment. *ExoDx Prostate IntelliScore*: Functions as a urinary test that utilizes exosomes to assess three distinct genes. Driven by developments in microfluidics, nanoparticle labeling, and machine learning (ML) algorithms for data interpretation, incorporating such multiplexed techniques into POC devices remains technically difficult but is being actively pursued [43].

8.3 Biosensor Technologies for POC Applications

Prostate cancer biomarker detection becomes possible through POC diagnostics because of innovative biosensor technologies, which deliver fast and user-friendly sensitive detections [20]. A biosensor functions through a combination of its main elements, which include a biorecognition element matched with a transducer that detects biological events and then transforms them into detectable signals. Technological integration between miniature electronic devices and microfluidic systems with advanced biosensing platforms has made it possible to develop handheld testing devices for early diagnosis of prostate cancer [44].

8.3.1 Electrochemical Biosensors

The development of electrochemical biosensors is one of the most promising approaches for prostate cancer POC diagnostic tools. The sensor system produces electrical responses through target molecule bindings that can result in current alterations or voltages or changes in impedance [45]. The electrochemical diagnostic method stands out for POC applications because it brings together high sensitivity with simplified operation and economical costs and miniature capabilities. Innovations in materials science using gold nanoparticles, carbon nanotubes, and graphene-based electrodes have raised electrochemical biosensor detection limits to picomolar and femtomolar levels for PSA and other biomarker identification [46]. The creation of multiplexed electrochemical biosensors allows medical practitioners to detect multiple prostate cancer markers simultaneously during POC diagnosis [47].

8.3.2 Optical Biosensors

Biosensors based on optics function through modifications in optical characteristics, including fluorescence and absorbance, together with luminescence and refractive index, for biomolecular interaction detection [48]. The platforms function with premium detection abilities, together with specificity that enables them to identify rare biomarkers such as circulating tumor DNA (ctDNA) and exosomal RNA specific to prostate cancer detection [49]. Compact optical detection equipment, used in conjunction with smartphones and handheld readers, enables the implementation of fluorescence resonance energy transfer (FRET)-based assays alongside surface plasmon resonance (SPR)-based sensors for POC diagnostics. By using nanomaterials, particularly quantum dots and plasmonic nanoparticles, signal amplification in optical biosensors has advanced to new levels, enabling the quick and accurate identification of prostate cancer biomarkers with less sample processing required [50].

8.3.3 Microfluidic and Lab-on-a-Chip Systems

The field of POC diagnostics received a breakthrough from microfluidic technology, which scientists refer to as lab-on-a-chip technology, because of its capability to work with tiny fluid volumes in tiny channels [51]. Multiple experimental functions, including biomarker extraction and signal detection, are combined into a single portable device through these platforms [52]. Research groups created microfluidic technology to extract CTCs combined with exosomes by processing blood or urine directly through their systems [53]. Microfluidic chips employ three technologies to enrich cancer-derived rare elements through size-based filtration, immunocapture selection, and dielectrophoretic sorting protocols. The use of lab-on-a-chip devices decreases assay durations while decreasing reagent usage and opens possibilities for automatic and user-friendly diagnostic systems for prostate cancer outside conventional laboratories [54].

8.3.4 Paper-Based and Wearable Biosensors

Paper-based biosensors provide a good solution for POC diagnostics because they are affordable and portable, which benefits resource-constrained environments [55]. The most popular detection format, called lateral flow assays (LFAs), enables prostate cancer marker detection along with PSA measurements through visual observations or smartphone-based readings [56]. Modern improvements involving nanomaterials, along with enzyme-linked amplification, as well as microfluidic paper analytical devices, have made paper-based tests much more sensitive and specific [57]. Wearable biosensors are currently in early development phases to monitor oncology patients, despite ongoing research. Healthcare professionals will eventually monitor prostate cancer and treatment responses through smart patches and flexible sensor platforms, which collect biomarkers from sweat and interstitial fluid, and blood micro-samples for non-stop, real-time assessment [58].

8.3.5 Smartphone-Integrated Diagnostic Platforms

Mobile health solutions and biosensor technology converge as the main drivers that affect the development trajectory of POC diagnostics [59]. Smartphones serve as perfect devices to implement biosensors because they contain excellent resolution cameras, as well as strong processors and embedded wireless capabilities [60]. A single mobile-based POC system for prostate cancer diagnosis includes functions for image acquisition and data processing as well as signal analysis and remote clinical support [61]. Multiple tests using biosensors connected to smartphones have demonstrated that PSA testing, combined with biomarker detection through multiplexing, is feasible. Extended patient tracking, telemedicine services, and AI processing to improve diagnostic accuracy are all made possible by the cloud connection system [62].

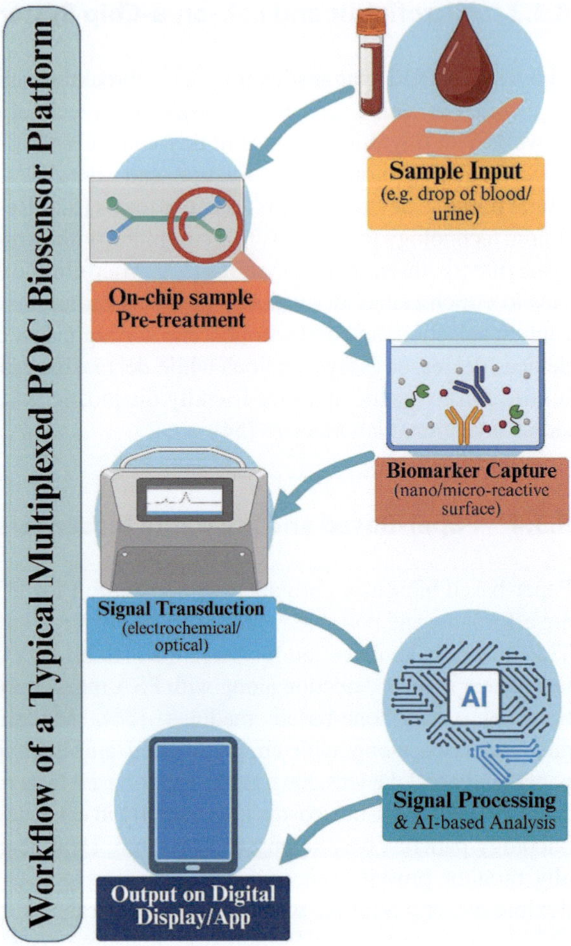

Fig. 8.2 Workflow of a typical multiplexed POC biosensor platform

8.4 Recent Advances and Innovative Approaches

POC testing for prostate cancer has witnessed significant advancements with the use of modern technologies that integrate with innovative biosensing methods. Testing for PSA utilizes a broad yet limited methodology that healthcare professionals have criticized because it leads to low detection precision [63]. Numerous researchers now direct their attention toward complex biosensing platforms, microfluidic systems, and nanomaterial-based sensing strategies because these methods present improved analytical capabilities and faster operations with parallel biomarker detecting potential [64]. By implementing ML and AI algorithms by providing clinical decision support systems, personal risk assessments, and real-time data interpretation services, POC Diagnostics advances (see Fig. 8.2 for the internal process of a POC biosensor system) [65]. New innovations extend prostate cancer screening services outside centralized labs into settings that are accessible and serve individual patients. Precision oncology, alongside decentralized healthcare centers, is emerging with the assistance of POC testing, which brings stronger accuracy and faster speed to clinical testing [66].

8.4.1 CRISPR-Based Biosensing Technologies

CRISPR technology revolutionized molecular diagnostics while transforming POC testing for prostate cancer at present. The CRISPR/Cas system specifically uses Cas12 and Cas13 components to develop sensitive detectors for nucleic acid analysis [35]. Systems based on collateral cleavage generate measurable signals after detecting their designated target DNA or RNA sequences. Prostate cancer diagnosis now relies on CRISPR-based biosensors that identify oncogenic fusions like TMPRSS2: ERG together with mutations present in ctDNA, which indicates disease advancement [67]. The technology has enabled its integration into paper-based tests along with microfluidic systems, which facilitate affordable and quick DNA-based molecular testing without central laboratory requirements. CRISPR-based detection platforms show great potential for future decentralized prostate cancer screening because of their high specificity and fast operation times [68].

8.4.2 AI and ML Integration

AI and ML technology continue to penetrate POC diagnostics because they boost both clinical decision-making abilities and prediction precision. Medical interpretation of different biomarker patterns becomes necessary for diagnosing prostate cancer because such profiles exhibit distinct variations across patients [69]. The applicability of deep learning methods and ensemble learning approaches allows researchers to gather and utilize big datasets that merge clinical findings with biological signs and imaging results and genetic information [70]. These models operating with biosensing systems make it possible to detect patterns that standard evaluation methods fail to reveal. AI-based electrochemical biosensors use improved technology for detecting rare biomarkers, but predictive models help medical staff determine aggressive disease risks for patients. AI applications united with POC testing allow healthcare providers to create better specific and adaptable solutions for prostate cancer management [71].

8.4.3 Nanotechnology-Enhanced Biosensors

Highly sensitive and multiplexed POC diagnostic devices continue to develop through the transformational features of nanotechnology. Engineered nanomaterials composed of gold nanoparticles, carbon nanotubes, quantum dots, and magnetic nanoparticles show unique optical, electrical, and catalytic behavior, which intensifies biosensor signals [72]. The sensitivity of SPR and fluorescence-based sensors reaches new heights when plasmonic nanoparticles are added into the detection process of PSA and exosomal RNA and ctDNA [73]. Magnetic nanoparticles isolate biomarkers through simple blood and urinary testing, which optimizes tests by making them faster while enhancing their capability to identify specific targets. The application of nanomaterials with multiple functions enables the detection of various biomarkers at once, which helps tackle prostate cancer's biological diversity to perform complete POC diagnosis systems [74].

8.4.4 3D Printing in Biosensor Development

The implementation of 3D printing brings revolutionary fabrication techniques for customized POC medical devices at low cost and integration level [75]. Using 3D printers allows the precise manufacturing of complex microfluidic systems, test cartridges, and sensor compartments [76]. Laboratory professionals have adopted 3D-printed microfluidic chips for prostate cancer diagnosis through integrated features that support automated sample automation and biomarker collection and combined detection capabilities [77]. The platform enables speedy development cycles for product design, which speeds up the time needed to move from research experiments to medical product deployment [78]. 3D-printed devices will enable detection systems with multiple analytes and user-friendly interfaces to advance available POC diagnostic options for healthcare environments of different kinds.

8.4.5 Wearable and Continuous Monitoring Devices

The medical field demonstrates growing interest in automatic prostate cancer biomarker detection utilizing wearable devices that preserve patient comfort [79]. Scientists create biosensor patches and implantable microdevices together with flexible electronics to detect PSA and lactate dehydrogenase with inflammatory cytokines from minimal blood volumes and interstitial fluid and sweat [80]. The technology of wearable systems gives medical teams access to real-time data about disease progression as well as therapeutic responsiveness and indicate new disease outbreaks. POC devices connected through wireless systems and cloud data storage networks supply immediate health data to medical professionals and patients, which enables proactive healthcare approaches [81]. Despite being in the early stages of research, wearable biosensors for prostate cancer offer a very promising path for future diagnostic paradigms.

8.4.6 Sample-to-Answer and Automation Innovations

The main obstacle in POC testing involves reducing the requirement for complicated specimen processing. Salt test system development features automated machines that unify the steps of cell disruption and nucleic acid retrieval alongside amplicon generation and signal processing [82]. Molecular testing can be performed portably with the help of isothermal amplification methods like loop-mediated isothermal amplification, which eliminates thermal cycling requirements. Microfluidic chip-based automation combined with lyophilized reagent cartridges reduces operator involvement, improving assay consistency [83]. Prostate cancer POC tests depend on these technological advancements because they ensure that the instruments deliver fast and dependable results in all healthcare settings [84]. Model diagnostic approaches for prostate cancer at the POC are undergoing transformation through quick developments in CRISPR technology, alongside AI and nanomaterials, 3D printing, and wearable electronics [85]. These diagnostic developments shift beyond PSA screening by creating specific patient diagnostic systems that provide real-time multi-parametric tests [86]. With technological advancements and regulatory standards development in progress, these vision-sharing and precise decentralized prostate cancer diagnostics systems will eventually become a clinical reality for worldwide medical benefits [87].

8.5 Clinical Applications and Case Studies

The application of POC diagnostic tools for prostate cancer has moved past experimental phases to real clinical use, which improves patient care procedures [88]. This section analyzes POC devices in the market that detect prostate cancer while exploring case studies about their achievements and restrictions and examines how these technologies meet various clinical implementation needs [89].

8.5.1 Current Commercial POC Devices for Prostate Cancer

Numerous POC diagnostic systems for prostate cancer exist in the market today to offer fast accessible detection alternatives to well-established laboratory tests [90]. PSA remains the dominant subject of widespread diagnostic tests, yet researchers are working to develop multi-marker tests that utilize liquid biopsy techniques (see Table 8.3 for commercial and experimental examples) [91]. The *Abaxis Piccolo Xpress Chemistry Analyzer* serves as an illustrative case, as this medical instrument began its development for comprehensive laboratory chemical analysis before healthcare providers used its adapted function to measure PSA levels together with other biomarkers at the patient site [92]. This diagnostic device provides laboratory-standard results immediately from small blood tests, making it highly beneficial for patient care in outpatient clinics [93].

The *OPKO Health 4Kscore® Test* quantifies four kallikrein proteins together with PSA for calculating patient risk of prostate cancer [97]. Laboratory testing of these multiplex biomarker panels usually occurs in centralized facilities, yet researchers strive to develop near-patient testing solutions similar to these platforms. The rapid PSA test kit, *On Site PSA Rapid Test*, has become popular in areas with restricted laboratory facilities through the LFA technology. The

Table 8.3 Selected commercial and experimental POC devices for prostate cancer

Device name	Developer	Biomarker(s)	Format	Status	Unique feature	References
PSAcheck	Abbott	PSA	Lateral flow strip	Commercial	CLIA-waived	[94]
uCheck POC	Johns Hopkins	PCA3	Microfluidic	Prototype	Urine-based RNA test	[95]
ONCO-POC	MIT spin-off	PSA + miR-141	Smartphone-integrated chip	In development	Dual biomarker detection	[60]
Prosta-Sense	Indian Institute of Technology	PSA	Electro-chemical strip	Pilot phase	Designed for rural clinics	[96]
eNanoLab	EU project	PCA3 + TMPRSS2: ERG	Lab-on-a-chip	Preclinical	Fully automated	[87]

testing devices provide diagnostic information after 15–20 min, giving primary care medical personnel a helpful screening capability [98]. The immunoassay analyzer *FREND*™ System from *NanoEntek* brings POC PSA detection capabilities along with a short preparation time to help physicians make quicker decisions. The POC molecular systems owned by *Cepheid* are currently being evaluated for incorporation of prostate cancer-specific nucleic acid assays by the company, but require further clinical validation [99]. The development of an autonomous multiplexed POC medical device that assesses comprehensive prostate cancer biomarkers awaits completion, but remains in the developmental stage instead of reaching commercial markets.

8.5.2 Case Studies: Success Stories and Limitations

Medical investigations demonstrate that POC prostate cancer detections bring advantages and potential challenges to diagnostics. Rapid PSA tests introduced at healthcare facilities throughout sub-Saharan Africa achieved notable success due to their minimal requirements for laboratory facilities. Medical staff used POC PSA tests to speed up the referral process of patients at high risk, so more prostate cancer cases were found at early stages [100]. The achievement demonstrates why rapid testing systems that operate with limited resources play an essential part in enhancing cancer treatment fairness across the world. The results of a multicenter clinical trial demonstrated some clear downsides regarding the evaluation of a novel microfluidic POC device for CTC detection [101]. The device proved its ability to identify prostate cancer specifically above 90%, but it rated below the projected level in sensitively detecting early-stage prostate cancer because CTCs are uncommon within peripheral blood [102]. The trial confirmed the technical constraints of detecting infrequent biomarkers in direct patient settings as well as the need to improve the test before implementing it systematically for clinical use. Patient response and physician satisfaction reached high marks during a POC PSA testing pilot project, which integrated screenings into standard evaluations at U.S. city medical clinics. The demonstration revealed workplace integration complications because healthcare professionals had difficulty interpreting marginal PSA results simultaneously with standard follow-up treatment procedures. The success of POC devices depends entirely on choosing appropriate biomarkers and conducting technical validations with simultaneous incorporation into complete clinical work processes [103].

8.5.3 Real-World Implementation Challenges

The extensive adoption of POC diagnostics for prostate cancer diagnosis faces multiple substantial obstacles that stand in the way of widespread implementation. The main barrier currently exists at the level of *regulatory approval* [104]. Food and drug administration (FDA) clearance and conformité européenne (CE) marking demands thorough clinical testing procedures for proving both safety performance, along with effectiveness and reproducibility, but especially so for new biomarkers and complex assay solutions [105]. *Reimbursement and cost-effectiveness* present additional hurdles. Reimbursement systems of multiple healthcare organizations base their payment models on centralized laboratory testing, so they discourage healthcare providers from implementing decentralized diagnostics. The lack of specific reimbursement routes makes it difficult for technologically advanced POC devices to gain market penetration [106]. *Technical issues* persist, which mainly affect assay stability, together with batch-to-batch consistency and unpredictable user-operated variations. The devices should operate accurately in unpredictable settings, and new users should manage them without extensive training, particularly in remote and primary care facilities [107]. Implementation of POC devices depends heavily on the successful integration of their testing process within existing *clinical workflows*. POC test implementations require results to provide action steps to clinical processes, yet avoid making the overall system more complicated [108]. The adoption of POC testing depends heavily on three essential elements, which include electronic medical record compatibility with automated result reporting and clear clinical decision algorithms. *Patient education*, combined with *acceptance*, needs to be the last essential aspect. Patients need a complete understanding of POC diagnostic tests in their medical evaluation process and must have confidence in testing accuracy to properly follow medical advice [109]. Addressing these everyday problems remains crucial for achieving the complete benefits offered by POC diagnosis in prostate cancer care advancement.

8.6 Challenges and Limitations in POC Testing for Prostate Cancer

POC prostate cancer tests have shown promise, yet multiple essential difficulties prevent their widespread clinical acceptance and accurate implementation [110]. The next part discusses vital technical and regulatory limitations in addition to socio-economic challenges, which need resolution to migrate innovative POC biosensing foundations into general clinical usage [111].

8.6.1 Analytical Sensitivity and Specificity

The creation of POC tests for prostate cancer encounters significant hurdles because of maintaining proper analytical sensitivity and specificity. The detection of PSA proves inadequate for distinguishing BPH from prostatitis and malignant tumors when the PSA levels remain low [112]. The result of false positives requires physicians to perform unnecessary biopsies, while false negatives delay effective medical diagnosis. Current biosensors that examine PCA3 RNA along with exosomal miRNAs and the TMPRSS2: ERG fusion transcripts show promise in advancing testing, but they need to demonstrate stable performance across numerous patient populations [113]. The assessment of test reproducibility faces challenges because blood and urine differential effects interfere with results, while the test quantity range remains narrow across different laboratory conditions. Combined with changing humidity and temperature, this impacts testing accuracy in non-laboratory settings [114]. The majority of POC platforms currently do not feature internal control systems or multiple marker redundancy systems that help decrease errors and enhance diagnostic certainty [115].

8.6.2 Regulatory and Standardization Hurdles

The regulatory process for POC prostate cancer diagnostic tests continues to evolve while remaining complex. Payment of Attention devices need to fulfill three mandatory requirements, including analytical validity criteria and clinical performance standards alongside manufacturing quality benchmarks [116]. The benchmark instability regarding biomarkers, as well as assay operations and result interpretation, makes systematic evaluation between systems difficult, thus extending regulatory review periods. Regulators face challenges in understanding the new technologies POC devices use because they do not synchronize with existing regulatory guidelines [117]. The process of device validation requires builders to wait longer than expected and face uncertain regulatory requirements, especially when developing products for use in homes and decentralized clinical settings. The global deployment of medical equipment becomes complicated due to differing regulatory systems throughout the world, such as the FDA in the United States, the CE marking in Europe, and the central drugs standard control organization (CDSCO) in India, until performance standards and clinical benchmarks receive international harmonization [118].

8.6.3 Sample Collection and Pre-processing Issues

The process of attaining regulatory approval for POC prostate cancer diagnostics remains intricate yet fluid because of ongoing evolution. Payment of Attention devices need to fulfill three mandatory requirements, including analytical validity criteria and clinical performance standards alongside manufacturing quality benchmarks [119]. The benchmark instability regarding biomarkers, as well as assay operations and result interpretation, makes systematic evaluation between systems difficult, thus extending regulatory review periods. Many POC devices use cutting-edge technologies, including microfluidics and nanomaterials, combined with AI-enhanced interpretation engines, which present legal issues since they do not follow standardized rules [120]. The process of device validation requires builders to wait longer than expected and face uncertain regulatory requirements, especially when developing products for use in homes and decentralized clinical settings [121]. The deployment of POC devices worldwide becomes problematic due to different regulatory frameworks, such as the FDA in the United States, the CE marking in Europe, and the CDSCO in India, unless standard performance measures and clinical evaluation criteria receive international harmonization [122].

8.6.4 Cost, Accessibility, and User Compliance

The promise of affordable and accessible testing through POC tests does not translate precisely into the actual situation. Current manufacturing rates for various advanced biosensor systems that use nanotechnology, microfluidics, or multiplex platforms make them expensive to produce at larger volumes [123]. The current infrastructure and production costs make it difficult to deploy these testing systems where clinical early prostate cancer diagnosis needs are most pressing. Relatively inexpensive devices may prove unaffordable in practice because of costs that remain hidden from the purchase price, such as equipment maintenance costs, supply costs, and requirements for calibration and connection infrastructure to include smartphone integration or cloud data storage [124]. The level of accessibility depends on multiple factors, including user compliance combined with their trust in the testing products. Patients who undergo self-tests must thoroughly understand both the meaning and the necessary next steps following their test outcomes [125]. Programs offering POC testing experience reduced value toward public health because user compliance decreases when people misinterpret test results or exhibit concerns about cancer diagnosis or data privacy. Healthcare provider education, together with community education and sensitivity in design development, led to better adoption rates and extended positive results [126].

8.7 Future Perspectives

POC testing for prostate cancer continues to evolve toward the creation of individualized healthcare services that connect patients to decentralized services [127]. The present devices have initiated workflow changes, but future developments will establish precise healthcare where population-level remote care and predictive assessments occur (see Table 8.4 for a strategic advancement roadmap) [128]. The next section studies where analytical POC testing for prostate cancer will evolve by identifying upcoming technological advancements [129].

Table 8.4 Roadmap for future development of POC biosensors for prostate cancer

Focus area	Short-term goal (1–3 years)	Long-term goal (5–10 years)	References
Biomarker panel	Integrate PSA + PCA3	Develop multi-omics panels	[130]
Device design	Improve portability and battery life	Fully disposable smart devices	[76]
AI integration	Real-time test interpretation	Predictive analytics + risk scoring	[89]
Regulatory pathways	Pilot region-specific trials	Harmonized global approval	[105]
Global access	Subsidized distribution in LMICs	Universal prostate screening tools	[81]

8.7.1 Toward Personalized Medicine and Home-Based POC Testing

The next vital step in prostate cancer POC diagnostics will be the development of customized diagnosis tools instead of standard screening technology [131]. Future diagnostic devices will merge multi-analyte biosensor technologies to inspect genomic, transcriptomic, proteomic, and metabolomic indicators as an alternative to PSA levels and isolated marker detection. The new platforms create the means for healthcare providers to build modified patient analysis systems that give precise risk assessment tools and customized treatment strategies [132]. The future of POC devices includes disease monitoring capabilities, which allow real-time assessment of patients both during active surveillance and post-therapy follow-up phase [133]. Extended home testing becomes possible because wearable technology pairs with non-invasive sampling methods, which utilize saliva or urine or even detect biomarkers in sweat. Full self-administered POC test kits with AI interpretation capabilities will exist to enable home-based regular testing [134]. Self-conducted diagnoses through the upcoming POC devices are vital tools that specifically benefit two major groups—seniors and people residing in underserved areas with travel limitations.

8.7.2 Integration of Biosensors with Telemedicine Platforms

Healthcare delivery toward remote and virtual care needs POC biosensors to integrate fully with telemedicine and digital health platforms for their operation. Medical practices around the world have sped up their implementation of remote care through virtual consultations, remote diagnostics, and decentralized clinical trials because of the COVID-19 pandemic [135]. Prostate cancer diagnosis will receive added benefits through cloud-connected biosensor devices, which allow patients to share results immediately with their healthcare providers [136]. The integrated system enables continuous care feedback where patients conduct their tests at home before their smartphone application transmits the data to receive either automated responses or clinical feedback within hours [137]. By using this model, healthcare becomes more convenient, and healthcare providers achieve improved longitudinal observation while detecting early recurrence cases and conducting more regular risk evaluations. ML together with AI will make healthcare decisions better through the analysis of biosensor information merged with patient data and imaging outcomes, as well as genomic information [138]. Such platforms track minimal biomarker changes that occur before patients start showing clinical symptoms, thus enabling therapy before symptoms appear. Portable diagnostic hubs with biosensor-enabled devices and telehealth capabilities could act as decentralized cancer screening centers in rural or low-resource areas, therefore closing disparities in infrastructure and specialist availability.

8.7.3 Vision for Next-Generation POC Diagnostics

The upcoming generation of POC prostate cancer diagnostics will harness characteristics including automated operation, together with multiplexing capabilities, reduced size, and enhanced intelligence capabilities [139]. Devices will become small and strong systems that need simplified operation from users to deliver professional test results in under a minute. Nanotechnology innovations combined with lab-on-chip architectures supported by AI analysis tools will drive the evolution of prostate cancer POC diagnostics. Next-generation POC systems will bring together biosensing components with microfluidic processors and digital readers, wireless connection systems in either disposable or reusable units [140]. The intelligent analysis systems will interpret healthcare signatures directly on location and change diagnostic criteria in real-time for individual patients rather than applying standard population benchmarks. A combination of interdisciplinary innovation will create seamless integration with robots and augmented reality displays and voice command functionalities, which will enable all demographic groups to access POC testing [141]. The devices connect to electronic health records, which allows health professionals to document clinical data while acquiring population health analytical information. A sustainable next-generation POC diagnostic framework needs to focus on producing devices at affordable costs using environmentally friendly materials that demonstrate large-scale manufacturing potential to promote worldwide healthcare equality. POC testing, combined with precision medicine, advances the possibility of prostate cancer management to become more efficient, along with delivering a more humane outcome for patient populations and equitable care to all patients [142].

8.8 Conclusion

Current medical practices in prostate cancer detection and management experience transformation through POC diagnostic tests. The deployment of biosensor-based POC platforms for prostate cancer diagnosis requires analysis of technological elements and recent innovations alongside clinical applications and system-level implementation obstacles.

The chapter started with a rationale explaining why POC testing holds merit for prostate cancer, yet spots the urgent requirement for fast decentralized diagnostic solutions that overlap the diagnostic gap from suspicion to final confirmation. Standard clinical diagnostic procedures achieve success in medical clinics, but they inefficiently manage unnecessary diagnostic errors, creating long delays and operational complications that affect marginalized populations. Our investigation encompassed various biosensor techniques, including electrochemical detection, optical, piezoelectric, and microfluidic system measurements. The new innovations enable the detection of prostate cancer biomarkers, such as PSA and PCA3, miRNAs, and fusion transcripts, with high sensitivity in real-time measurements. Combining multiple assays or physical chips provides medical experts with better simultaneous diagnosis results, reducing misdiagnosis. The integration of smartphone-based interfaces combined with miniaturized electronics systems drives POC tools toward developing user-friendly home-based products. The clinical section introduced existing commercial tools and provided technology demonstrations alongside practical assessments that mirrored healthcare opportunities and boundaries. Research advances are visible, but the implementation of POC devices faces ongoing obstacles due to analytical weaknesses, standardized standards, sample management requirements, economic challenges, and user compliance issues. A direct evaluation of these items was conducted in the section on challenges and limitations to identify the key issues standing in the way of success. The development of POC testing for prostate cancer will succeed based on advancements in personalized medicine while consolidating with digital health solutions. Smart diagnostics will exist as part of wearable and portable devices that apply AI technologies for delivering personalized data-based information. This technology will serve two roles by diagnosing conditions and then tracking disease evolution while evaluating risk levels and selecting appropriate treatments from within the patient's living space. Healthcare providers can implement telemedicine systems to unite diagnostic results with medical interpretation and live care services. Advancement of this field requires a detailed multi-approach strategic plan. This includes the following: the medical field should progress toward creating standardized biomarkers which discern aggressive conditions from non-aggressive cases; the development of scalable manufacturing together with design innovations must focus on producing cheap POC devices which fulfill requirements of high durability and easy user operations; the implementation of collaborative efforts between bioengineers and clinicians and regulators and health economists will achieve practical alignment for healthcare innovation; the development of POC diagnostics with flexible characteristics enables better equity worldwide for patients in various infrastructure conditions and cultural environments; and the development of powerful regulatory systems and validation systems remains essential especially for both AI-integrated and home-use diagnostic tools. The clinical adoption phase, together with early developmental stages of POC prostate cancer tests, demonstrates strong potential despite existing limitations. POC and mobile urology continue to revolutionize medical detection because they deliver swift diagnosis services at affordable costs with improved diagnostic accuracy. Strategic remedy of existing challenges combined with cross-specialty teamwork will advance POC biosensor technologies to their status as a global foundation for individualized prostate cancer healthcare.

8.9 Summary

The revolutionary role of POC diagnostics in the identification and treatment of prostate cancer, one of the most common cancers affecting men globally, is examined in this chapter. Conventional diagnostic methods, such as PSA testing and biopsies, have poor specificity, are expensive, and are unavailable in environments with limited resources. POC technologies, which provide multi-biomarker, low-cost, decentralized, and real-time diagnostic capabilities, are becoming essential solutions. In addition to highlighting cutting-edge biosensing platforms, such as electrochemical, optical, microfluidic, and wearable biosensors, the chapter describes several biomarkers used in the diagnosis of prostate cancer, including PSA, PCA3, TMPRSS2: ERG, and miRNAs. The accuracy and usability of POC tools are improved by recent advancements in nanotechnology, CRISPR-based detection, smartphone integration, and AI-assisted interpretation. Additionally, it introduces both commercial and experimental proof-of-concept devices, discusses their unique qualities and drawbacks, and evaluates practical implementation issues such as user compliance, regulatory barriers, and analytical sensitivity. In order to promote fair and effective prostate cancer care globally, the chapter ends with a strategic roadmap for developing global access, personalized diagnostics, and harmonized regulations.

Glossary

Biosensor An analytical device combining a biological component with a physicochemical detector to identify biomolecules.

Biomarker A measurable indicator of a biological condition or disease, used for diagnosis or prognosis.

POC Medical diagnostic testing performed at or near the site of patient care, rather than in centralized laboratories.

PSA A protein produced by the prostate gland, elevated levels of which can indicate prostate cancer or other conditions.

Microfluidics Technology that manipulates fluids at a microscale level to conduct biochemical assays efficiently.

CRISPR A genome-editing technology that can also be used in biosensors for specific and sensitive molecular detection.

Wearable Biosensor A body-worn sensor that continuously monitors biomarkers or physiological parameters.

Multiplexing The ability of a diagnostic device to simultaneously detect multiple biomarkers in a single test.

Exosomes Small extracellular vesicles released by cells that carry proteins and RNA, often used as non-invasive biomarkers.

Telemedicine The remote diagnosis and treatment of patients through telecommunications technology.

References

1. Meyer AR, Gorin MA. First point-of-care PSA test for prostate cancer detection. Nat Rev Urol. 2019;16(6):331–2. https://doi.org/10.1038/s41585-019-0179-1.
2. Annese VF, Patil SB, Hu C, Giagkoulovits C, Al-Rawhani MA, Grant J, et al. A monolithic single-chip point-of-care platform for metabolomic prostate cancer detection. Microsyst Nanoeng. 2021;7(1):21.
3. Yamani HZ, Safwat N, Mahmoud AM, Ayad MF, Abdel-Ghany MF, Gomaa MM. Point-of-care diagnostics for rapid determination of prostate cancer biomarker sarcosine: application of disposable potentiometric sensor based on oxide-conductive polymer nanocomposite. Anal Bioanal Chem. 2023;415(22):5451–62. https://doi.org/10.1007/s00216-023-04818-0.
4. Martin FL, Morais CLM, Dickinson AW, Saba T, Bongers T, Singh MN, et al. Point-of-Care disease screening in primary care using saliva: a biospectroscopy approach for lung Cancer and prostate cancer. J Pers Med. 2023;13(11). Available from: https://www.mdpi.com/2075-4426/13/11/1533.
5. Srinivasan B, Nanus DM, Erickson D, Mehta S. Highly portable quantitative screening test for prostate-specific antigen at point of care. Curr Res Biotechnol. 2021;3:288–99.
6. Hazra RS, Hasan Khan MR, Kale N, Tanha T, Khandare J, Ganai S, et al. Bioinspired materials for wearable devices and point-of-care testing of Cancer. ACS Biomater Sci Eng. 2023;9(5):2103–28. https://doi.org/10.1021/acsbiomaterials.1c01208.
7. Maj-Hes A, Sevcenco S, Szarvas T, Kramer G. Claros system: a rapid microfluidics-based point-of-Care system for quantitative prostate specific antigen analysis from finger-stick blood. Adv Ther. 2019;36(4):916–22.
8. Van Poppel H, Roobol MJ, Chapple CR, Catto JWF, N'Dow J, Sønksen J, et al. Prostate-specific antigen testing as part of a risk-adapted early detection strategy for prostate Cancer: European Association of Urology Position and Recommendations for 2021. Eur Urol. 2021;80(6):703–11.
9. Van Poppel H, Hogenhout R, Albers P, van den Bergh RCN, Barentsz JO, Roobol MJ. A European model for an organised risk-stratified early detection programme for prostate cancer. Eur Urol Oncol. 2021;4(5):731–9.
10. Merriel SWD, Funston G, Hamilton W. Prostate cancer in primary care. Adv Ther. 2018;35(9):1285–94. https://doi.org/10.1007/s12325-018-0766-1.
11. Costello AJ. Considering the role of radical prostatectomy in 21st century prostate cancer care. Nat Rev Urol. 2020;17(3):177–88.
12. Sathianathen NJ, Konety BR, Crook J, Saad F, Lawrentschuk N. Landmarks in prostate cancer. Nat Rev Urol. 2018;15(10):627–42.
13. Bezdekova J, Plevova M, Nejdl L, Macka M, Masarik M, Pacik D, et al. Prostate cancer diagnosed and staged using UV-irradiated urine samples and a paper-based analytical device. Sensors Actuators B Chem. 2024;403:135146.
14. Pellerin O, Déan C, Reb P, Chaix C, Floch F, Tierny D, et al. Prostate artery chemoembolization in prostate cancer: A proof of concept study in spontaneous prostate cancer in a canine model. Diagn Interv Imaging. 2021;102(12):709–15.
15. Winkel DJ, Wetterauer C, Matthias MO, Lou B, Shi B, Kamen A, et al. Autonomous detection and classification of PI-RADS lesions in an MRI screening population incorporating

multicenter-labeled deep learning and Biparametric imaging: proof of concept. Diagnostics. 2020;10(11):951.
16. Lawrentschuk N. PSA testing and early management of test-detected prostate cancer- consensus at last. BJU Int. 2016;117(S4):5–6. Available from: https://bjui-journals.onlinelibrary.wiley.com/doi/abs/10.1111/bju.13481.
17. Pan LH, Pang ST, Fang PY, Chuang CK, Yang HW. Label-free biochips for accurate detection of prostate cancer in the clinic: dual biomarkers and circulating tumor cells. Theranostics. 2017;7(17):4289–300.
18. Sheydaei O, Khajehsharifi H, Rajabi HR. Rapid and selective diagnose of sarcosine in urine samples as prostate cancer biomarker by mesoporous imprinted polymeric nanobeads modified electrode. Sensors Actuators B Chem. 2020;309:127559. Available from: https://www.sciencedirect.com/science/article/pii/S0925400519317587.
19. Ferraro S, Biganzoli D, Rossi RS, Palmisano F, Bussetti M, Verzotti E, et al. Individual risk prediction of high grade prostate cancer based on the combination between total prostate-specific antigen (PSA) and free to total PSA ratio. Clin Chem Lab Med. 2023;61(7):1327–34. https://doi.org/10.1515/cclm-2023-0008.
20. Dou Y, Li Z, Su J, Song S. A portable biosensor based on Au nanoflower interface combined with electrochemical immunochromatography for POC detection of prostate-specific antigen. Biosensors. 2022;12(5):259.
21. Lee B, Park JH, Byun JY, Kim JH, Kim MG. An optical fiber-based LSPR aptasensor for simple and rapid in-situ detection of ochratoxin A. Biosens Bioelectron. 2018;102:504–9. Available from: https://www.sciencedirect.com/science/article/pii/S0956566317307923.
22. Krausewitz P, Kluemper N, Richter AP, Büttner T, Kristiansen G, Ritter M, et al. Early dynamics of quantitative SEPT9 and SHOX2 methylation in circulating cell-free plasma DNA during prostate biopsy for prostate Cancer diagnosis. Cancers (Basel). 2022;14(18):4355.
23. Gillette CM, Yette GA, Cramer SD, Graham LS. Management of advanced prostate cancer in the precision oncology era. Cancers (Basel). 2023;15(9):2552.
24. Christenson M, Song CS, Liu YG, Chatterjee B. Precision targets for intercepting the lethal progression of prostate cancer: potential avenues for personalized therapy. Cancers (Basel). 2022;14(4):892.
25. Shore ND. Current and future management of locally advanced and metastatic prostate cancer. Rev Urol. 2020;22(3):110–23.
26. Narayan VM. A critical appraisal of biomarkers in prostate cancer. World J Urol. 2020;38:547–54.
27. Meehan J, Gray M, Martínez-Pérez C, Kay C, McLaren D, Turnbull AK. Tissue-and liquid-based biomarkers in prostate cancer precision medicine. J Pers Med. 2021;11(7):664.
28. Nordström T, Akre O, Aly M, Grönberg H, Eklund M. Prostate-specific antigen (PSA) density in the diagnostic algorithm of prostate cancer. Prostate Cancer Prostatic Dis. 2018;21(1):57–63.
29. Narain TA, Sooriakumaran P. Beyond prostate specific antigen: new prostate Cancer screening options. World J Mens Health. 2022;40(1):66–73.
30. Ferraro S, Bussetti M, Bassani N, Rossi RS, Incarbone GP, Bianchi F, et al. Definition of outcome-based prostate-specific antigen (PSA) thresholds for advanced prostate cancer risk prediction. Cancers (Basel). 2021;13(14):3381.
31. Enikeev D, Morozov A, Babaevskaya D, Bazarkin A, Malavaud B. A systematic review of circulating tumor cells clinical application in prostate Cancer diagnosis. Cancers (Basel). 2022;14(15). Available from: https://www.mdpi.com/2072-6694/14/15/3802.
32. Cieślikowski WA, Antczak A, Nowicki M, Zabel M, Budna-Tukan J. Clinical relevance of circulating tumor cells in prostate Cancer management. Biomedicine. 2021;9(9). Available from: https://www.mdpi.com/2227-9059/9/9/1179.
33. Soongsong J, Arivazhagan M, Banet P, Aubert PH, Jakmunee J. Microfluidic paper-based electrochemical Immunosensor for the detection of prostate-specific antigen (PSA) based on modified flexible screen-printed carbon electrodes. ACS Omega. 2025; https://doi.org/10.1021/acsomega.5c04238.

34. Tonry CL, Leacy E, Raso C, Finn SP, Armstrong J, Pennington SR. The role of proteomics in biomarker development for improved patient diagnosis and clinical decision making in prostate cancer. Diagnostics. 2016;6(3). Available from: https://www.mdpi.com/2075-4418/6/3/27.
35. Chen W, Wu S, Li G, Duan X, Sun X, Li S, et al. Accurate diagnosis of prostate cancer with CRISPR-based nucleic acid test strip by simultaneously identifying PCA3 and KLK3 genes. Biosens Bioelectron. 2023;220:114854.
36. Akkilic N, Geschwindner S, Höök F. Single-molecule biosensors: recent advances and applications. Biosens Bioelectron. 2020;151:111944. Available from: https://www.sciencedirect.com/science/article/pii/S095656631931022X.
37. Mokni M, Fourati N, Zerrouki C, Othmane A, Omezzine A, Bouslama A. Review on recent advances in urinary biomarkers based electrochemical sensors for prostate cancer detection. In: Kanoun O, Derbel N, editors. Advanced sensors for biomedical applications. Cham: Springer International Publishing; 2021. p. 123–36. https://doi.org/10.1007/978-3-030-71225-9_8.
38. Lorenc T, Klimczyk K, Michalczewska I, Słomka M, Kubiak-Tomaszewska G, Olejarz W. Exosomes in prostate cancer diagnosis, prognosis and therapy. Int J Mol Sci. 2020;21(6). Available from: https://www.mdpi.com/1422-0067/21/6/2118.
39. Vlaeminck-Guillem V. Exosomes and prostate cancer management. Semin Cancer Biol. 2022;86:101–11. Available from: https://www.sciencedirect.com/science/article/pii/S1044579X21002169
40. Conteduca V, Hess J, Yamada Y, Ku SY, Beltran H. Epigenetics in prostate cancer: clinical implications. Transl Androl Urol. 2021;10(7):3104.
41. Houlahan KE, Shiah YJ, Gusev A, Yuan J, Ahmed M, Shetty A, et al. Genome-wide germline correlates of the epigenetic landscape of prostate cancer. Nat Med. 2019;25(10):1615–26.
42. Gil Rosa B, Akingbade OE, Guo X, Gonzalez-Macia L, Crone MA, Cameron LP, et al. Multiplexed immunosensors for point-of-care diagnostic applications. Biosens Bioelectron. 2022;203:114050. Available from: https://www.sciencedirect.com/science/article/pii/S0956566322000902.
43. Mitchell KR, Esene JE, Woolley AT. Advances in multiplex electrical and optical detection of biomarkers using microfluidic devices. Anal Bioanal Chem. 2022;414(1):167–80.
44. Hwang IM, Cantu CM, Chawla R, Kamei DT. Biosensor-based point-of-Care devices: detection of infectious diseases and cancer. In: Borse V, Chandra P, Srivastava R, editors. BioSensing, theranostics, and medical devices: from laboratory to point-of-Care testing. Singapore: Springer Singapore; 2022. p. 105–32. https://doi.org/10.1007/978-981-16-2782-8_5.
45. Akbari Jonous Z, Shayeh JS, Yazdian F, Yadegari A, Hashemi M, Omidi M. An electrochemical biosensor for prostate cancer biomarker detection using graphene oxide–gold nanostructures. Eng Life Sci. 2019;19(3):206–16.
46. Hasan MR, Ahommed MS, Daizy M, Bacchu MS, Ali MR, Al-Mamun MR, et al. Recent development in electrochemical biosensors for cancer biomarkers detection. Biosens Bioelectron X. 2021;8:100075.
47. Abedi R, Raoof JB, Hashkavayi AB, Asghary M. Highly sensitive and label-free electrochemical biosensor based on gold nanostructures for studying the interaction of prostate cancer gene sequence with epirubicin anti-cancer drug. Microchem J. 2021;170:106668.
48. Azab MY, Hameed MFO, Obayya SSA. Overview of optical biosensors for early cancer detection: fundamentals, applications and future perspectives. Biology (Basel). 2023;12(2). Available from: https://www.mdpi.com/2079-7737/12/2/232.
49. Son MH, Park SW, Sagong HY, Jung YK. Recent advances in electrochemical and optical biosensors for cancer biomarker detection. Biochip J. 2023;17(1):44–67. https://doi.org/10.1007/s13206-022-00089-6.
50. Tai J, Fan S, Ding S, Ren L. Gold nanoparticles based optical biosensors for cancer biomarker proteins: a review of the current practices. Front Bioeng Biotechnol. 2022;10:877193.
51. García-Hernández LA, Martínez-Martínez E, Pazos-Solís D, Aguado-Preciado J, Dutt A, Chávez-Ramírez AU, et al. Optical detection of cancer cells using lab-on-a-chip. Biosensors. 2023;13(4):439.

52. Guo Q-R, Zhang L-L, Liu J-F, Li Z, Li J-J, Zhou W-M, et al. Multifunctional microfluidic chip for cancer diagnosis and treatment. Nanotheranostics. 2021;5(1):73.
53. Maciel Braga LA, Mota FB. Early cancer diagnosis using lab-on-a-chip devices: A bibliometric and network analysis. COLLNET J Sci Inf Manag. 2021;15(1):163–96.
54. Carvalho Â, Ferreira G, Seixas D, Guimaraes-Teixeira C, Henrique R, Monteiro FJ, et al. Emerging lab-on-a-chip approaches for liquid biopsy in lung cancer: status in CTCs and ctDNA research and clinical validation. Cancers (Basel). 2021;13(9):2101.
55. Suntornsuk W, Suntornsuk L. Recent applications of paper-based point-of-care devices for biomarker detection. Electrophoresis. 2020;41(5–6):287–305.
56. Dukle A, Nathanael AJ, Panchapakesan B, Oh TH. Role of paper-based sensors in fight against cancer for the developing world. Biosensors. 2022;12(9):737.
57. Kummari S, Panicker LR, Rao Bommi J, Karingula S, Sunil Kumar V, Mahato K, et al. Trends in paper-based sensing devices for clinical and environmental monitoring. Biosensors. 2023;13(4):420.
58. Linh VTN, Lee MY, Mun J, Kim Y, Kim H, Han IW, et al. 3D plasmonic coral nanoarchitecture paper for label-free human urine sensing and deep learning-assisted cancer screening. Biosens Bioelectron. 2023;224:115076.
59. Asci Erkocyigit B, Ozufuklar O, Yardim A, Guler Celik E, Timur S. Biomarker detection in early diagnosis of cancer: recent achievements in point-of-Care devices based on paper microfluidics. Biosensors. 2023;13(3). Available from: https://www.mdpi.com/2079-6374/13/3/387.
60. Beduk T, Beduk D, Hasan MR, Guler Celik E, Kosel J, Narang J, et al. Smartphone-based multiplexed biosensing tools for health monitoring. Biosensors. 2022;12(8). Available from: https://www.mdpi.com/2079-6374/12/8/583.
61. Kanchi S, Sabela MI, Mdluli PS, Inamuddin BK. Smartphone based bioanalytical and diagnosis applications: a review. Biosens Bioelectron. 2018;102:136–49.
62. Bui TH, Thangavel B, Sharipov M, Chen K, Shin JH. Smartphone-based portable bio-chemical sensors: exploring recent advancements. Chemosensors. 2023;11(9):468.
63. Capuozzo M, Santorsola M, Ianniello M, Ferrara F, Zovi A, Petrillo N, et al. Innovative drug modalities for the treatment of advanced prostate Cancer. Diseases. 2024;12(5). Available from: https://www.mdpi.com/2079-9721/12/5/87.
64. Pucci C, Martinelli C, Ciofani G. Innovative approaches for cancer treatment: current perspectives and new challenges. Ecancermedicalscience. 2019;13:961.
65. Gao P, Li T, Zhang K, Luo G. Recent advances in the molecular targeted drugs for prostate cancer. Int Urol Nephrol. 2023;55(4):777–89.
66. Le TK, Duong QH, Baylot V, Fargette C, Baboudjian M, Colleaux L, et al. Castration-resistant prostate cancer: from uncovered resistance mechanisms to current treatments. Cancers (Basel). 2023;15(20):5047.
67. Teng P, Gao Z, Quan Q, He G, Song Q, Zhang X, et al. SERS-based CRISPR/Cas12a assays for protein biomarker prostate-specific antigen detection. Anal Bioanal Chem. 2025;417(3):573–82.
68. Zavvar TS, Khoshbin Z, Ramezani M, Alibolandi M, Abnous K, Taghdisi SM. CRISPR/Cas-engineered technology: innovative approach for biosensor development. Biosens Bioelectron. 2022;214:114501.
69. Chen H, Liu J, Chen Y, Song Z, Shao J, Shi B, et al. Multienzyme isothermal rapid amplification combined with CRISPR/Cas12a for sensitive prostate cancer screening using urine collected without digital rectal examination. Microchem J. 2025;212:113218.
70. Gong S, Zhang S, Lu F, Pan W, Li N, Tang B. CRISPR/Cas-based in vitro diagnostic platforms for Cancer biomarker detection. Anal Chem. 2021;93(35):11899–909.
71. Wang J, Yang X, Wang X, Wang W. Recent advances in CRISPR/Cas-based biosensors for protein detection. Bioengineering. 2022;9(10):512.
72. Shrestha B, Tang L, Hood RL. Nanotechnology for personalized medicine. In: Gu N, editor. Nanomedicine. Singapore: Springer Nature Singapore; 2023. p. 555–603.

73. Wang Y, Li B, Tian T, Liu Y, Zhang J, Qian K. Advanced on-site and in vitro signal amplification biosensors for biomolecule analysis. TrAC Trends Anal Chem. 2022;149:116565.
74. Yang Y, Huang Q, Xiao Z, Liu M, Zhu Y, Chen Q, et al. Nanomaterial-based biosensor developing as a route toward in vitro diagnosis of early ovarian cancer. Mater Today Bio. 2022;13:100218.
75. Kothawade S, Padwal V. Cutting-edge 3D printing in immunosensor design for early cancer detection. Microchim Acta. 2024;192(1):42.
76. Remaggi G, Zaccarelli A, Elviri L. 3D printing technologies in biosensors production: recent developments. Chemosensors. 2022;10(2):65.
77. Sharafeldin M, Jones A, Rusling JF. 3D-printed biosensor arrays for medical diagnostics. Micromachines. 2018;9(8):394.
78. Zhang Y. 3D printing for Cancer diagnosis: what unique advantages are gained? ACS Mater Au. 2023;3(6):620–35.
79. Huang Y, Upadhyay U, Dhar E, Kuo LJ, Syed-Abdul S. A scoping review to assess adherence to and clinical outcomes of wearable devices in the cancer population. Cancers (Basel). 2022;14(18):4437.
80. Peeke P, Billes SK, Vetter A, Naghavi N, Le D, Smith M, et al. Feasibility of a novel wearable thermal device for management of bothersome hot flashes in patients with prostate cancer. Prostate Cancer Prostatic Dis. 2024;27(4):736–42.
81. Feng G, Parthipan M, Breunis H, Timilshina N, Soto-Perez-de-Celis E, Mina DS, et al. Daily physical activity monitoring in older adults with metastatic prostate cancer on active treatment: feasibility and associations with toxicity. J Geriatr Oncol. 2023;14(7):101576.
82. Koo KM, Dey S, Trau M. A sample-to-targeted gene analysis biochip for Nanofluidic manipulation of solid-phase circulating tumor nucleic acid amplification in liquid biopsies. ACS Sens. 2018;3(12):2597–603.
83. Ye X, Li Y, Wang L, Fang X, Kong J. All-in-one microfluidic nucleic acid diagnosis system for multiplex detection of sexually transmitted pathogens directly from genitourinary secretions. Talanta. 2021;221:121462.
84. Silva MLS. Microfluidic devices for glycobiomarker detection in cancer. Clin Chim Acta. 2021;521:229–43.
85. Cheng HP, Yang TH, Wang JC, Chuang HS. Recent trends and innovations in bead-based biosensors for cancer detection. Sensors. 2024;24(9):2904.
86. Rey Gomez LM, Hirani R, Care A, Inglis DW, Wang Y. Emerging microfluidic devices for sample preparation of undiluted whole blood to enable the detection of biomarkers. ACS Sens. 2023;8(4):1404–21.
87. Primiceri E, Chiriacò MS, Notarangelo FM, Crocamo A, Ardissino D, Cereda M, et al. Key enabling technologies for point-of-care diagnostics. Sensors. 2018;18(11):3607.
88. Aurilio G, Cimadamore A, Mazzucchelli R, Lopez-Beltran A, Verri E, Scarpelli M, et al. Androgen receptor signaling pathway in prostate cancer: from genetics to clinical applications. Cells. 2020;9(12). Available from: https://www.mdpi.com/2073-4409/9/12/2653.
89. Cuocolo R, Cipullo MB, Stanzione A, Ugga L, Romeo V, Radice L, et al. Machine learning applications in prostate cancer magnetic resonance imaging. Eur Radiol Exp. 2019;3(1):35. https://doi.org/10.1186/s41747-019-0109-2.
90. Ćwikła JB, Roslan M, Skoneczna I, Kempińska-Wróbel M, Maurin M, Rogowski W, et al. Initial experience of clinical use of [99mTc]Tc-PSMA-T4 in patients with prostate cancer. A pilot study. Pharmaceuticals. 2021;14(11):1107.
91. Fraguas-Sánchez AI, Torres-Suárez AI. Medical use of cannabinoids. Drugs. 2018;78(16):1665–703.
92. Spengler JR, Welch SR, Genzer SC, Coleman-McCray J, Harmon JR, Nichol ST, et al. Suboptimal handling of piccolo samples or reagent discs for consideration in Ebola response. Emerg Infect Dis. 2019;25:1238–40.
93. Fleishhacker ZJ, Rastogi P, Davis SR, Aman DR, Morris CS, Dyson RL, et al. Impact of interfacing near point of Care clinical chemistry and hematology analyzers at urgent Care clinics at an academic health system. J Pathol Inform. 2022;13:100006.

94. Lao TD, Nguyen TN, Le TAH. Promoter Hypermethylation of tumor suppressor genes located on short arm of the chromosome 3 as potential biomarker for the diagnosis of nasopharyngeal carcinoma. Diagnostics. 2021;11(8). Available from: https://www.mdpi.com/2075-4418/11/8/1404.
95. Bardhan NM, Radisic M, Nurunnabi M. Bioinspired materials for wearable diagnostics and biosensors. ACS Biomater Sci Eng. 2023;9(5):2015–9. https://doi.org/10.1021/acsbiomaterials.3c00348.
96. Lin JT, Chung YP, Wu TL, Lin WC, Sriram B, Wang SF, et al. Empowering early detection of prostate cancer: a point-of-care biosensing perspective. Microchem J. 2025;215:114538. Available from: https://www.sciencedirect.com/science/article/pii/S0026265X25018922.
97. Haese A, Tin AL, Carlsson SV, Sjoberg DD, Pehrke D, Steuber T, et al. A pre-specified model based on four kallikrein markers in blood improves predictions of adverse pathology and biochemical recurrence after radical prostatectomy. Br J Cancer. 2020;123(4):604–9.
98. Vertosick EA, Zappala S, Punnen S, Hugosson J, Boorjian SA, Haese A, et al. Individual patient data Meta-analysis of discrimination of the four Kallikrein panel associated with the inclusion of prostate volume. Urology. 2021;157:102–6.
99. Bhattu AS, Zappala SM, Parekh DJ, Punnen S. A 4Kscore cut-off of 7.5% for prostate biopsy decisions provides high sensitivity and negative predictive value for significant prostate cancer. Urology. 2021;148:53–8.
100. Vandekerkhove G, Struss WJ, Annala M, Kallio HML, Khalaf D, Warner EW, et al. Circulating tumor DNA abundance and potential utility in De novo metastatic prostate cancer. Eur Urol. 2019;75(4):667–75.
101. Linkon AHM, Labib MM, Hasan T, Hossain M, Jannat ME. Deep learning in prostate cancer diagnosis and Gleason grading in histopathology images: an extensive study. Inform Med Unlocked. 2021;24:100582.
102. Zhong X, Cao R, Shakeri S, Scalzo F, Lee Y, Enzmann DR, et al. Deep transfer learning-based prostate cancer classification using 3 Tesla multi parametric MRI. Abdom Radiol. 2019;44(6):2030–9.
103. Venderink W, Bomers JG, Overduin CG, Padhani AR, de Lauw GR, Sedelaar MJ, et al. Multiparametric magnetic resonance imaging for the detection of clinically significant prostate Cancer: what urologists need to know. Part 3: targeted biopsy. Eur Urol. 2020;77(4):481–90.
104. Beckmann K, Garmo H, Franck Lissbrant I, Stattin P. The value of real-world data in understanding prostate cancer risk and improving clinical care: examples from Swedish registries. Cancers (Basel). 2021;13(4):875.
105. Liu Y, Uemura H, Ye D, Lee JY, Chiong E, Pu YS, et al. Prostate cancer in Asia: design of a patient registry to inform real-world treatments, outcomes, and quality of life. Prostate Int. 2019;7(3):108–13.
106. Magnani CJ, Bievre N, Baker LC, Brooks JD, Blayney DW, Hernandez-Boussard T. Real-world evidence to estimate prostate Cancer costs for first-line treatment or active surveillance. Eur Urol Open Sci. 2021;23:20–9.
107. George DJ, Sartor O, Miller K, Saad F, Tombal B, Kalinovský J, et al. Treatment patterns and outcomes in patients with metastatic castration-resistant prostate cancer in a real-world clinical practice setting in the United States. Clin Genitourin Cancer. 2020;18(4):284–94.
108. Murtojärvi M, Halkola AS, Airola A, Laajala TD, Mirtti T, Aittokallio T, et al. Cost-effective survival prediction for patients with advanced prostate cancer using clinical trial and real-world hospital registry datasets. Int J Med Inform. 2020;133:104014.
109. Pereira-Salgado A, Kwan EM, Tran B, Gibbs P, De Bono J, IJzerman M. Systematic review of efficacy and health economic implications of real-world treatment sequencing in prostate Cancer: where do the newer agents enzalutamide and Abiraterone fit in? Eur Urol Focus. 2021;7(4):752–63.
110. Yeasmin S, Ammanath G, Onder A, Yan E, Yildiz UH, Palaniappan A, et al. Current trends and challenges in point-of-care urinalysis of biomarkers in trace amounts. TrAC Trends Anal Chem. 2022;157:116786.

111. Knaul FM, Doubova SV, Gonzalez Robledo MC, Durstine A, Pages GS, Casanova F, et al. Self-identity, lived experiences, and challenges of breast, cervical, and prostate cancer survivorship in Mexico: a qualitative study. BMC Cancer. 2020;20(1):577.
112. Rodríguez SVM, García-Perdomo HA. Diagnostic accuracy of prostate cancer antigen 3 (PCA3) prior to first prostate biopsy: A systematic review and meta-analysis. Can Urol Assoc J = J l'Association des Urol du Canada. 2020;14(5):E214–9.
113. Perera M, Papa N, Roberts M, Williams M, Udovicich C, Vela I, et al. Gallium-68 prostate-specific membrane antigen positron emission tomography in advanced prostate cancer—updated diagnostic utility, sensitivity, specificity, and distribution of prostate-specific membrane antigen-avid lesions: a systematic review and meta-analysis. Eur Urol. 2020;77(4):403–17. Available from: https://www.sciencedirect.com/science/article/pii/S0302283819300958
114. Descotes JL. Diagnosis of prostate cancer. Asian J Urol. 2019;6(2):129–36.
115. Bass EJ, Pantovic A, Connor M, Gabe R, Padhani AR, Rockall A, et al. A systematic review and meta-analysis of the diagnostic accuracy of biparametric prostate MRI for prostate cancer in men at risk. Prostate Cancer Prostatic Dis. 2021;24(3):596–611.
116. Shore ND, Morgans AK, El-Haddad G, Srinivas S, Abramowitz M. Addressing challenges and controversies in the management of prostate cancer with multidisciplinary teams. Target Oncol. 2022;17(6):709–25. https://doi.org/10.1007/s11523-022-00925-7.
117. Tsaur I, Brandt MP, Juengel E, Manceau C, Ploussard G. Immunotherapy in prostate cancer: new horizon of hurdles and hopes. World J Urol. 2021;39(5):1387–403.
118. Mahmoud AM, Kostrzewa M, Marolda V, Cerasuolo M, Maccarinelli F, Coltrini D, et al. Cannabidiol alters mitochondrial bioenergetics via VDAC1 and triggers cell death in hormone-refractory prostate cancer. Pharmacol Res. 2023;189:106683.
119. Salama WM, Aly MH. Prostate cancer detection based on deep convolutional neural networks and support vector machines: a novel concern level analysis. Multimed Tools Appl. 2021;80(16):24995–5007.
120. Nakai H, Suman G, Adamo DA, Navin PJ, Bookwalter CA, LeGout JD, et al. Natural language processing pipeline to extract prostate cancer-related information from clinical notes. Eur Radiol. 2024;34(12):7878–91.
121. Salvi M, Molinari F, Acharya UR, Molinaro L, Meiburger KM. Impact of stain normalization and patch selection on the performance of convolutional neural networks in histological breast and prostate cancer classification. Comput Methods Programs Biomed Update. 2021;1:100004.
122. Sowmya D, Bhavani SA, Sasank VVS, Rao TS. Prostate cancer classification using adaptive swarm Intelligence based deep attention neural network. Biomed Signal Process Control. 2024;96:106654.
123. Terjung A, Kummer S, Friedrich M. Simultaneous 24 h-infusion of high-dose 5-fluorouracil and sodium-folinate as alternative to capecitabine in advanced breast cancer. Anticancer Res. 2014;34(12):7233–8.
124. Agochukwu NQ, Skolarus TA, Wittmann D. Telemedicine and prostate cancer survivorship: a narrative review. mHealth. 2018;4:45.
125. Rai KS, Mann U, Harasemiw O, Tangri N, Eng A, Patel P, et al. A prospective evaluation of patient perspectives and financial considerations during prostate cancer treatment decision-making. Can Urol Assoc J = J l'Association des Urol du Canada. 2023;17(9):E244–51.
126. Yang SM, Lv S, Zhang W, Cui Y. Microfluidic Point-of-Care (POC) devices in early diagnosis: a review of opportunities and challenges. Sensors. 2022;22(4). Available from: https://www.mdpi.com/1424-8220/22/4/1620.
127. Heidt B, Siqueira WF, Eersels K, Diliën H, van Grinsven B, Fujiwara RT, et al. Point of care diagnostics in resource-limited settings: a review of the present and future of PoC in its most needed environment. Biosensors. 2020;10(10):133.
128. Gubala V, Harris LF, Ricco AJ, Tan MX, Williams DE. Point of Care diagnostics: status and future. Anal Chem. 2012;84(2):487–515.

129. Hayes B, Murphy C, Crawley A, O'Kennedy R. Developments in point-of-care diagnostic technology for cancer detection. Diagnostics. 2018;8(2). Available from: https://www.mdpi.com/2075-4418/8/2/39.
130. Constâncio V, Lobo J, Sequeira JP, Henrique R, Jerónimo C. Prostate cancer epigenetics – from pathophysiology to clinical application. Nat Rev Urol. 2025;22(7):447–69. https://doi.org/10.1038/s41585-024-00991-8.
131. Tasoglu S. Toilet-based continuous health monitoring using urine. Nat Rev Urol. 2022;19(4):219–30.
132. Trinh L, Kramer AF, Rowland K, Strom DA, Wong JN, McAuley E. A pilot feasibility randomized controlled trial adding behavioral counseling to supervised physical activity in prostate cancer survivors: behavior change in prostate cancer survivors trial (BOOST). J Behav Med. 2021;44(2):172–86.
133. Smokovski I, Steinle N, Behnke A, Bhaskar SMM, Grech G, Richter K, et al. Digital biomarkers: 3PM approach revolutionizing chronic disease management – EPMA 2024 position. EPMA J. 2024;15(2):149–62.
134. Bangma CH, Loeb S, Busstra M, Zhu X, El Bouazzaoui S, Refos J, et al. Outcomes of a bladder cancer screening program using home hematuria testing and molecular markers. Eur Urol. 2013;64(1):41–7.
135. Hemdan M, Ali MA, Doghish AS, Mageed SSA, Elazab IM, Khalil MM, et al. Innovations in biosensor technologies for healthcare diagnostics and therapeutic drug monitoring: applications, recent progress, and future research challenges. Sensors (Basel). 2024;24(16):5143.
136. Umme S, Siciliano G, Primiceri E, Turco A, Tarantini I, Ferrara F, et al. Electrochemical sensors for liquid biopsy and their integration into lab-on-Chip platforms: revolutionizing the approach to diseases. Chemosensors. 2023;11(10). Available from: https://www.mdpi.com/2227-9040/11/10/517.
137. Le LTP, Nguyen AHQ, Phan LMT, Ngo HTT, Wang X, Cunningham B, et al. Current smartphone-assisted point-of-care cancer detection: towards supporting personalized cancer monitoring. TrAC Trends Anal Chem. 2024;174:117681. Available from: https://www.sciencedirect.com/science/article/pii/S0165993624001638.
138. Georgescu I, Dricu A, Artene SA, Vrăjitoru NR, Barcan E, Tache DE, et al. Digital-focused approaches in cancer patients' management in the Post-COVID era: challenges and solutions. Appl Sci. 2024;14(18)
139. Pang B, Zhu Y, Ni J, Thompson J, Malouf D, Bucci J, et al. Extracellular vesicles: the next generation of biomarkers for liquid biopsy-based prostate cancer diagnosis. Theranostics. 2020;10(5):2309.
140. Koo KM. Unifying next-generation biomarkers and Nanodiagnostic platforms for precision prostate cancer management. In: Advancing gene fusion detection towards personalized cancer nanodiagnostics. Cham: Springer International Publishing; 2019. p. 1–29.
141. Ramirez-Garrastacho M, Bajo-Santos C, Line A, Martens-Uzunova ES, de la Fuente JM, Moros M, et al. Extracellular vesicles as a source of prostate cancer biomarkers in liquid biopsies: a decade of research. Br J Cancer. 2022;126(3):331–50.
142. Han GR, Goncharov A, Eryilmaz M, Ye S, Palanisamy B, Ghosh R, et al. Machine learning in point-of-care testing: innovations, challenges, and opportunities. Nat Commun. 2025;16(1):3165.

Multiplex Biosensing for Prostate Cancer

9

Molakpogu Ravindra Babu, Arya Tripathi, Shriyansh Srivastava, and Rahul Kumar

Abbreviations

AI	artificial intelligence
DNA	deoxyribonucleic acid
EC	electrochemical
ELISA	enzyme-linked immunosorbent assay
FDA	Food and Drug Administration
LoC	lab-on-a-chip
LOD	limit of detection
LSPR	localized surface plasmon resonance
ML	machine learning
POC	point-of-carc
PSA	prostate-specific antigen
RNA	ribonucleic acid
SPR	surface plasmon resonance

9.1 Introduction

Prostate cancer exists as both a major worldwide diagnosis among men and a significant reason for cancer-related deaths. The disease follows multiple paths, which range from gradual tumor development around the prostate zone to aggressive

M. Ravindra Babu · A. Tripathi · S. Srivastava
Department of Pharmacy, School of Medical and Allied Sciences, Galgotias University, Greater Noida, Uttar Pradesh, India

R. Kumar (✉)
Faculty of Pharmacy, Vidya University, Meerut, Uttar Pradesh, India

S. Srivastava et al. (eds.), *Biosensor Technologies for Prostate Cancer*,
https://doi.org/10.1007/978-981-95-8644-8_9

tissue spread throughout the body [1]. The prostate-specific antigen (PSA) testing, along with digital rectal examination and biopsy procedures, has significant drawbacks because it produces few positive results correctly, yet many false alarms create unnecessary operations and cause patient distress. The crucial requirement for cancer diagnosis involves developing sophisticated diagnostic instruments that enhance precision levels, while minimizing medical procedures and enabling continuous monitoring [2]. New biosensing technologies serve as effective cancer diagnostic instruments, excelling at identifying specific biomarkers associated with diseases. Biosensors combine bioreceptors (which include antibodies, nucleic acids, and aptamers) with transducers (electrochemical, optical, and piezoelectric) to measure biological signals that develop through receptor reactions. The simultaneous integration of multiple biomarker detection systems represents a significant improvement over single-analyte examinations, as it enhances diagnostic accuracy while reducing false results [3]. The platforms enable rapid screening processes with improved detection capacity for healthcare applications that help clinical environments, along with individualized patient care programs. Early and accurate detection of prostate cancer significantly improves patient outcomes by enabling timely intervention and personalized treatment strategies. Multiplex biosensing platforms allow for the simultaneous detection of multiple prostate cancer biomarkers, such as PSA, circulating tumor cells (CTCs), exosomes, and microRNAs (miRNAs), leading to improved specificity and reliability [4]. The integration of cutting-edge technologies, such as nanomaterials, microfluidics, and artificial intelligence (AI), has further enhanced the analytical performance of these biosensors, paving the way for rapid, cost-effective, and non-invasive diagnostic solutions. This chapter explores the fundamentals of biosensing platforms, their application in prostate cancer detection, key biomarkers, and recent technological advancements. Additionally, challenges such as reproducibility, regulatory approval, and clinical translation will be discussed. By the end of this chapter, readers will gain insights into how multiplex biosensing platforms are revolutionizing prostate cancer diagnosis and shaping the future of precision oncology [5].

9.2 Fundamentals of Multiplex Biosensing Technologies

Modern biosensing operations have established themselves as essential technological approaches for detecting diseases early and maintaining constant medical observation while creating patient-specific treatment methods. Every platform in this system allows users to detect biological markers through precise and specific measures [6]. Prostate cancer diagnosis and monitoring benefit significantly from biosensors, which enable efficient quantitative assessments of disease biomarkers, including PSA, CTCs, and exosomal RNA. The use of tissue biopsies alongside imaging procedures represents a diagnostic method that is time-consuming, costly, and invasive. Easily accessible body fluids, such as blood, urine, and saliva, can be successfully diagnosed for prostate cancer biomarkers using quick and minimally invasive biosensors at a low cost [7]. The diagnostic precision of biosensing platforms increases when they monitor multiple biomarkers simultaneously, thereby reducing incorrect positive and negative test results. The section explores the fundamental principles of biosensors, including essential components and their benefits for multiplex diagnostic testing of prostate cancer.

9.2.1 Principles of Biosensors

An analytical device known as a biosensor combines biological recognition elements with transduction components to detect particular biological molecules through its system (Fig. 9.1). These devices act as essential instruments for disease diagnosis, together with environmental quality assessment and food security assessment, as well as biomedical investigations [8]. The diagnostic testing for prostate cancer gets enhanced by biosensors, which provide quick biomarker detection with high sensitivity and do not require invasive procedures. A biosensor functions through a three-step process, which represents its fundamental [9].

9.2.1.1 Biorecognition

A biosensor operates through biorecognition, which serves as its central step because it brings the biological sensing element into contact with the target analyte [10]. The biosensor obtains its ability to detect the proper biomarker accurately through the specificity assessment of this phase, while maintaining low sensitivity

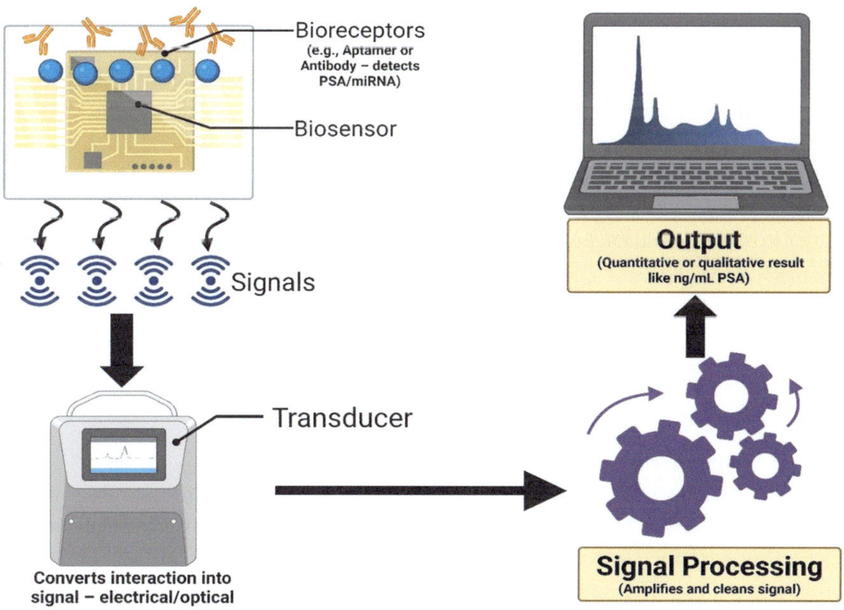

Fig. 9.1 Structural components of a multiplex biosensor

Table 9.1 List of biorecognition elements for biosensing

Element type	Target analyte	Stability	Cost	Application example	References
Antibodies	PSA, proteins	Medium	High	Immunosensors	[12]
Aptamers	miRNAs, PSA	High	Low	Electrochemical	[12]
Enzymes	Glucose, PSA	Moderate	Medium	Colorimetric	[12]
DNA probes	miRNA, ctDNA	High	Medium	Hybridization	[12]
Whole cells	Drugs, toxins	Low	High	Toxicity testing	[12]

to alternative molecules [10]. A list of essential features defines the role of biorecognition in biosensors. Software-based identification methods require biorecognition components that bind tightly with target materials in order to produce accurate tests [8]. Under diverse physical and biological settings, the biological recognition component must function actively as designed. The biosensor needs to repeat the precise detection of target molecules throughout all testing cycles [11]. *Types of Biorecognition Elements*: The selection of bioreceptor components relies on both the analytical target substance and intended biosensor usage purposes. Common biorecognition elements include the following (Table 9.1) [12].

Antibodies The detection of specific protein biomarkers, including PSA, relies on either monoclonal or polyclonal antibodies as bioreceptors. The high specific recognition capacity of these elements needs chemical stabilization procedures before they can function properly in biosensor applications [13]. *Aptamers*: DNA or RNA molecules that function as short single-stranded units possess strong binding capabilities for target molecules. Engineers have successfully developed them for continuous use as recognition elements in biosensing applications due to their enhanced stability [14]. Enzymes: These compounds act as catalysts for biochemical reactions, producing signals that are suitable for detection. Glucose oxidase-based biosensors serve as one of the primary devices for diabetes monitoring applications [15]. *Nucleic Acid Probes (DNA/RNA Probes)*: The detection mechanism of hybridization-based biosensors operates by recognizing prostate cancer genetic mutations and miRNAs or circulating tumor DNA (ctDNA) [16]. *Cell-Based Receptors*: Avoiding whole-cell systems, some biosensors detect external stimulus responses from cell-based detection systems, particularly for drug testing and toxicity evaluation. Signal transduction occurs when the biorecognition element binds to the target analyte, converting it into a detectable signal [17].

9.2.1.2 Signal Transduction

A biosensor must transform the biorecognition outcome into measurable signals following binding recognition events. A transducer functions as a crucial component in this step since it converts biological signals into detectable physical or chemical changes [18]. The selection of transduction principles for biosensors depends on the biomarker being detected. *Electrochemical Biosensors*: These biosensors use electronic variations such as current and voltage shifts, as well as impedance changes, to indicate target molecule affinities [19]. The amperometric biosensing mechanism measures electrical current changes resulting from reactions that facilitate electron transfer. Staff members measure voltage shifts that result from electrostatic events within these biosensors [20]. The surface impedance detects resistance fluctuations that occur when biomarkers bind to the device [8]. The technique of electrochemical biosensing has become prevalent among laboratories that conduct PSA level screening for prostate cancer diagnosis [19].

Optical Biosensors The detection methods of optical biosensors include fluorescence in combination with absorbance and surface plasmon resonance (SPR) [21]. This biosensor technology utilizes fluorescent detection through antibodies or aptamers that signal upon detecting the target molecule. SPR measures changing light reflections as biomarkers attach to the sensor [22]. Colorimetric biosensors identify changes within coloring territories after enzymatic reactions take place [20].

Advantages of Optical Biosensors The advantages include label-free detection (especially SPR-based biosensors); real-time monitoring of biomolecular interactions; and high sensitivity and specificity. Due to their light-based operating principle, optical biosensors find extensive application in research facilities for investigating biomolecular bonding, as well as DNA hybridization processes and clinical test evaluation [23].

Piezoelectric Biosensors Biosensor devices base their detection method on acoustic wave propagation for measuring mass changes. The Quartz Crystal Microbalance (QCM) sensors represent a widespread detection method among biosensors due to their capacity to detect changes in resonant frequency resulting from biomolecular attachments on the sensor surface [24]. The device performs label-free CTC and exosome detection in prostate cancer patients [25].

Thermal Biosensors The change in heat released during biomolecular reactions provides data for analysis to thermal biosensors. The interpretation of metabolic changes in cancer cells benefits from these detectors, although they occur irregularly in prostate cancer examinations [26]. When the transduction mechanism produces a signal, the biosensor progresses to interpreting and processing the signal [27].

9.2.1.3 Signal Processing and Interpretation

Finally, biosensing systems need signal analysis to translate measured signals into essential clinical data output [28]. The signal processing systems function at two levels: first, to maintain high detection precision and, second, to reduce noise interference and enable quantitative biomarker detection [29].

Signal Amplification Modern biosensors depend on nanomaterials, including gold nanoparticles (AuNPs) and carbon nanotubes (CNTs), for the purpose of signal amplification and sensitivity improvement [30]. Signal amplification, conducted through enzymatic processes, is utilized in both optical sensors and electrochemical devices.

Noise Reduction and Background Signal Filtering Modern biosensors utilize machine learning (ML) technology to start noise removal procedures, which enhances their detection precision levels [31]. Biosensors that use AI technology succeed in distinguishing cancerous from non-cancerous biomarker patterns.

Data Interpretation and Digital Integration The device transforms its detected output data into a specific numeric measurement, such as PSA concentration expressed in ng/mL [32]. Medical biosensors now work in conjunction with smartphone software and cloud computing systems, which provide remote disease screening services alongside continuous patient health assessment capabilities.

Clinical Relevance of Signal Interpretation in Prostate Cancer The PSA biosensor system should trigger additional clinical exams when PSA levels reach >4 ng/mL. A biosensor system that measures PSA, prostate cancer antigen 3 (PCA3), and miRNAs simultaneously yields better outcomes for prostate cancer risk measurement [33]. Healthcare predictions about disease development are derived from extended sensor-generated information through ML systems.

9.2.2 Key Components: Bioreceptors, Transducers, and Signal Processing

A biosensor system requires the combined functions of bioreceptors and transducers, along with signal processing units, to effectively and accurately identify prostate cancer biomarkers. Specialized biological elements known as bioreceptors exhibit high specificity when they bind to target molecules, including PSA, PCA3, miRNAs, and CTCs [34]. Bioreceptors consist of antibodies, aptamers, enzymes, and nucleic acids (DNA/RNA probes), with whole-cell receptors being most frequently utilized. The high specificity of antibodies makes them the preferred bioreceptor choice in immunosensor PSA detection; however, aptamers present themselves as a cost-saving and stable alternative [35]. Prostate cancer subtype detection relies heavily on nucleic acids, which serve as essential elements for hybrid-based biosensor systems. The biological recognition process leads to transducer-generated detectable signals. Biosensor sensitivity and reliability depend on different transducer types available in detection processes. Electrochemical transducers produce electrical signals when binding targets occur, thus making them ideal for point-of-care (POC) diagnostics because they offer both fast results through rapid detection and cost-efficient operations [36]. The optical transducing methods of fluorescence and SPR sensors deliver precise and direct detection that does not require labeling. Molecular interactions can be detected by mass-based transducers through their measurement of mass variations at the same time they detect CTCs [37]. The use of thermal transducers remains relatively rare because they detect temperature variations from biomolecular reactions to observe metabolic changes in cancer cells. The signals become diagnostic data following the conclusion of signal transduction. Nanomaterial-based components, such as CNTs and AuNPs, reinforced through laboratory methods, improve the detection of scarce prostate cancer biomarkers. Reference electrodes, together with optical filtering elements, process chemical measurements by identifying background noise, which leads to improved measurement precision [38]. Data interpretation from biosensors has reached new levels because of AI and ML advancements that allow automatic diagnosis and personalized medicine approaches. Real-time disease tracking abilities, together with cancer versus health conditions differentiation, fall under the range of capabilities offered by AI-based biosensors. Young technologies combine microfluidics platforms with cloud platforms for biosensors, enabling them to acquire enhanced functionalities that support remote medical services.

9.2.3 Advantages of Multiplex Biosensing

The diagnostic field advanced through multiplex biosensing because it provides simultaneous analysis of multiple biomarkers through a unified testing method [39]. A single multiplex biosensing system directs the detection of both PSA and PCA3 together with miRNAs and CTCs simultaneously as prostate cancer biomarkers [40]. Multitarget detection methods enhance both diagnostic accuracy and test efficiency, as well as test reliability, thereby functioning effectively for early detection, disease monitoring, and treatment planning purposes (Table 9.2). Multiplex biosensing transforms prostate cancer diagnostics through its utility in clinical and POC applications because it delivers superior capabilities compared to traditional approaches [41].

Higher Sensitivity and Specificity Single biomarker detection currently results in incorrect prostate cancer determinations because it generates too many false positive and negative results during diagnosis. PSA measurements alone do not provide reliable results, as they cannot distinguish between cancerous conditions and non-cancerous situations, such as prostatitis or benign prostatic hyperplasia (BPH) [48].

Table 9.2 Advantages of multiplex biosensing

Feature	Description	References
Sensitivity and specificity	Detects multiple biomarkers, reducing false positives/negatives	[42]
High throughput	Analyzes many samples simultaneously	[43]
Low sample volume	Needs minimal blood/saliva	[44]
Portability	Useful in POC settings	[45]
Cost effectiveness	Fewer reagents, faster results, less clinical follow-up	[46]
Digital integration	Cloud, smartphone, and AI-compatible	[47]

Multiplex biosensors address this issue by detecting multiple biomarkers simultaneously, which enhances their ability to identify actual positives and eliminate potential false positives. Multiplex biosensors construct diagnostic profiles that incorporate PSA, together with PCA3 and miRNAs, to perform precise risk assessments of prostate cancer patients [49].

Rapid and High-Throughput Analysis The standard diagnostic practices for prostate cancer, including biopsies and immunoassays, demand extended periods of time and numerous sessions at medical facilities. The multiplex biosensing diagnostic technique performs biomarker detection operations through one test, which eliminates the requirement for successive or repetitive medical examinations [50]. Patients benefit from reduced analysis time, as well as quicker clinical decision-making and more appropriate treatment delivery, due to these features. Multiplex biosensors enable integration in automated laboratory work environments with high-throughput screening platforms, which helps healthcare workers analyze large numbers of samples fast and boosts clinical diagnostic operations [51].

Minimal Sample Volume Requirement Multiplex biosensing has a key advantage because it needs only minimal biological samples to perform complete biomarker detection. The diagnostic approaches of earlier times needed various blood collections and tissue biopsy procedures that brought painful experiences along with invasive procedures to patients [52]. Multiplex biosensors reduce the volume of biological samples required to test prostate cancer markers in blood, urine samples, and saliva. Such a method provides alternative diagnostic procedures that enhance patient comfort throughout both medical screening tests and examinations, as well as the treatment of elderly patients. Reducing sample volume offers advantages to low-resource healthcare facilities because such institutions lack both advanced diagnostic tools and complete laboratory access [53].

POC and Portable Usability Modern multiplex biosensors with POC applications enable real-time prostate cancer diagnostics to take place outside standard laboratory facilities. The combination of portable and miniaturized biosensors, including lab-on-a-chip (LOC) devices and microfluidic platforms, enables testing to occur directly at remote or resource-limited healthcare environments and homes [54]. Point-of-need patients, particularly those living in rural regions and those who cannot easily access cancer specialty centers, gain significant benefits from this technology. Immediate on-the-spot testing enables faster patient results, which promotes both early medical intervention and continuous disease checkup processes, as well as personalized treatment modifications [55].

Integration With Digital Health Technologies Digital health technology advancements propelled medical diagnostics so quickly that multiplex biosensors merged into successful smartphone and wearable device and cloud-based healthcare system markets [56]. Biosensors that incorporate intelligent capabilities enable wireless data transfers between blockchain and Wi-Fi and near field communication (NFC) systems, automatically sending patient information for virtual patient treatment to healthcare professionals. Biosensor data, interpreted through AI algorithms, enables the modern analysis of biological information to discover disease-evolution patterns and assess treatments [57]. Healthcare professionals achieve personalized services through real-time biosensor data because they can produce exact treatment solutions for specific patient groups.

Cost-Effectiveness Every testing process of multiplex biosensing proves more efficient in terms of expense than traditional procedures for prostate cancer diagnostics. Healthcare expenses decrease because one multiplex biosensor device generates all necessary biomarker results within a single laboratory assay, which reduces both reagent and laboratory expenses and overall healthcare costs [58]. Large-scale prostate cancer screening operations benefit most from multiplex biosensing technology, as financial restrictions typically limit access to diagnostic resources. The implementation of multiplex biosensors leads to decreased hospital stays because they substitute for biopsies in diagnosis, resulting in reduced health expenses for patients. The advancement of biosensing technology, along with the development of inexpensive, disposable, portable multiplex biosensors, will result in accessible early prostate cancer detection for diverse communities [59].

9.3 Biomarkers for Prostate Cancer Detection

The role of additional biomarkers remains essential to perform prostate cancer screening duties, together with diagnostics and disease surveillance tasks. Medical applications of PSA tests encounter important disadvantages because the tests have a weak ability to identify specific conditions and lack distinction between cancerous and benign tumors [60]. Researchers within medical science investigate new biomarkers using CTCs and exosomes together with miRNAs because these markers improve detection methods with non-invasive testing procedures [61]. Determining multiple biomarkers (Table 9.3) through multiplexing methods produces precise diagnostic information, which helps doctors create better patient groups and specific treatment strategies [62]. The glycoprotein PSA originates from prostate epithelial cells to serve as a biomarker for prostate cancer screening tests. PSA testing remains vital for prostate abnormality detection, yet produces many inaccuracies because it generates false-positive results among patients with BPH or prostatitis and fails to detect some aggressive prostate cancers correctly [63]. PSA-based screening resulted in two significant adverse effects, which include the discovery of non-threatening prostate tumors leading to both potentially unnecessary invasive biopsies and unwarranted medical treatments [64]. Scientists introduced PSA velocity, PSA density, and the free-to-bound PSA ratio as enhanced screening tests; however, these refinements lack the necessary accuracy to distinguish cancer from benign tumors. Research into specific and reliable biomarkers continues because PSA

Table 9.3 Emerging prostate cancer biomarkers and their diagnostic potential

Biomarker	Type	Role in prostate cancer	Clinical relevance	References
PSA	Protein	Gold standard but limited specificity	Useful for initial screening	[68]
PCA3	Non-coding RNA	Overexpressed in prostate cancer	Improves specificity over PSA	[68]
miRNAs (e.g., miR-141 and miR-375)	Small RNA molecules	Regulate cancer-related genes	Potential for early-stage detection	[68]
Exosomes	Extracellular vesicles	Carry tumor-specific RNA and proteins	Useful for non-invasive liquid biopsy	[68]
CTCs	Tumor-derived cells	Reflect metastatic potential	Helps in monitoring disease progression	[68]

testing has shown its limitations in the field [65]. Through liquid biopsy, the analysis of CTCs in the bloodstream becomes a powerful tool for both early detection of cancer and accurate disease assessment and continuous disease tracking. The detection of these rare biomarkers becomes increasingly difficult during early cancer stages since their quantity remains low, so scientists must develop improved microfluidic techniques with immunoaffinity enrichment mechanisms [66]. The cancer-specific expression patterns combined with high stability in bodily fluids make miRNA small non-coding RNAs (miRNAs) promising biomarkers. The different expression patterns of miR-141 together with miR-21, miR-34a, and miR-143 in prostate cancer allow doctors to distinguish malignant from benign conditions. The analysis of exosomes stands as a new promising biomarker because these small extracellular vesicles transfer tumor-derived proteins and DNA and RNAs between cells. Exosomal biomarkers provide several benefits because practitioners can easily obtain them through non-intrusive sample collection from urine or blood, alongside saliva, and they deliver vital molecular information to assess cancer development and tumor aggressiveness [37, 67].

The problems with current PSA diagnostic testing have encouraged specialists to create innovative diagnostic methods that examine PSA with CTCs and multiple miRNAs and exosomes to identify advanced prostate cancer [69]. Multiplex biosensing devices enhance diagnostic outcomes because multiple biomarkers are analyzed together under the same measurement procedure to decrease the probability of false readings produced from single-agent tests [70]. A single biosensing assay provides fast and precise detection of advanced prostate cancer subtypes by testing numerous cancer-related molecules. The efficient cooperation between electrochemical platforms and microfluidic biosensors and nanomaterial-based biosensing devices enhances biomarker analysis for multiple targets, which improves screening processes, allows monitoring treatment response, and enables custom treatment [71].

9.4 Types of Multiplex Biosensing Platforms for Prostate Cancer

Prostate cancer diagnostics has increased in efficiency because modern multiplex biosensing platforms now perform multiple biomarker tests simultaneously in each assay. The three diagnostic tools, enzyme-linked immunosorbent assay (ELISA), polymerase chain reaction (PCR), and histopathological evaluation, need different biomarker-specific tests, which lengthens diagnostic times through increased costs and procedural complexity [72]. Multiplex biosensors optimize detection workflows by combining multiple tests into one platform, which achieves high sensitivity and specificity and manages to work with small test materials and reagent requirements. Advanced biosensing platforms combine different transduction methods through optical, electrochemical, and microfluidic and nanomaterial-based platforms for optimized prostate cancer screening practice [73]. The section demonstrates different biosensing platforms used for multiplex analysis in prostate cancer (Table 9.4) diagnostics, along with their operational principles and their diagnostic applications [74].

9.4.1 Optical Biosensors

The detection of biomolecular interactions through optical biosensors happens by tracking variations in light characteristics, including absorbance, fluorescence, and refractive index. The biosensors provide label-free detection with real-time analysis and high specificity, so they become very effective tools for complicated prostate cancer diagnostics [81]. The biomedical field of diagnostics made use of optical biosensors to revolutionize the optical sensitivity of real-time, highly sensitive, label-free detection of cancer biomarkers. The current biosensors are based on the light interaction with biological molecules, the fluorescence, absorbance, or refractive index changes are due to the presence of a specific biomarker [82]. Largely because of their capacity for quickly and accurately producing data, optical biosensors are readily used in the diagnosis of cancer, particularly prostate cancer. In optical biosensors, there are several methods based on fluorescence, absorbance measurement, and SPR, which have their own advantages to be applied for multiplex biosensing platforms [83].

9.4.1.1 SPR Biosensors

SPR is a label-free optical sensing method based on the detection of changes in the refractive index at a metal-dielectric interface. The prostate cancer diagnostic version of an SPR biosensor is based on a thin metal (usually gold) film on which biomolecules (Fig. 9.2), that is, antibodies or aptamers, are usually immobilized. When cancer biomarkers interact with the bioreceptor, the refractive index of the surface is changed, altering the SPR signal that can be measured [84].

SPR biosensors are due to their use in real-time monitoring of biomolecular interactions without external labels. They are highly specific, sensitive, and rapid detection. Moreover, SPR technology is compatible with microfluidic systems and,

Table 9.4 Comparative overview of biosensor types for prostate cancer detection

Biosensor type	Detection mechanism	Key advantages	Major limitations	Example applications	References
Electrochemical biosensors	Measures electrical signals (current, voltage, impedance)	High sensitivity, cost-effective, rapid response, portable, and compatible with miniaturization	Requires precise calibration, potential interference from biological fluids	PSA detection using amperometric biosensors, multiplex detection of miRNAs in prostate cancer	[75]
Optical biosensors	Measures changes in light properties (SPR, fluorescence, SERS)	Label-free detection, real-time analysis, high specificity, and multiplexing capabilities	Requires sophisticated and expensive instrumentation, signal variations due to sample composition	miRNA detection using fluorescence-based biosensors, exosome detection in liquid biopsy	[76]
Mass-based (piezoelectric) biosensors	Measures frequency shifts due to biomolecular interactions and mass binding	High accuracy, no labeling required, real-time monitoring, and excellent sensitivity	Susceptible to environmental factors (e.g., temperature and humidity), requires stable surface functionalization	CTC detection using QCM, exosome-based cancer diagnostics	[77]
Thermal biosensors	Measures temperature changes due to biomolecular interactions	No need for external labels, simple design, and suitable for metabolic monitoring	Less commonly used for prostate cancer detection, with relatively lower specificity	Detection of metabolic changes in cancer cells, thermal enzyme biosensors for biomarker quantification	[78]
Microfluidic-based biosensors	Integrates biosensing components into a miniaturized LOC system	Low sample volume requirement, rapid analysis, high-throughput, and automation potential	Fabrication complexity, requires microfluidic expertise for design optimization	POC prostate cancer diagnostics, multiplex biomarker detection in blood and urine samples	[79]
Nanomaterial-enhanced biosensors	Uses nanomaterials (AuNPs, CNTs, and QDs) for enhanced signal transduction	Ultra-sensitive detection, enhanced stability, improved biocompatibility, and possibility for wearable integration	Costly synthesis and functionalization of nanomaterials, potential toxicity concerns	Femtomolar-level PSA detection, nanoplasmonic sensors for miRNA and protein biomarker detection	[80]

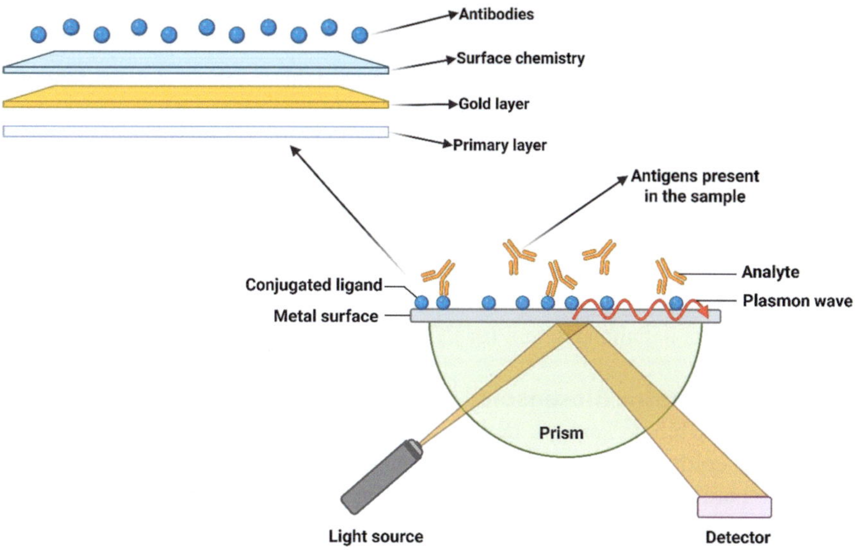

Fig. 9.2 Working principle of the SPR biosensor

therefore, constitutes a useful tool for multiplex detection of prostate cancer biomarkers [85]. Yet, low performance is associated with SPR-based biosensors as they demand precise instrumentation and controlled experimental conditions. SPR measures changing light reflections as biomarkers attach to the sensor. Clinical and research practitioners use SPR biosensors because they allow unambiguous detection of weak biomolecular signals without the need for labeling solutions. The detection mechanism of this sensor depends on refractive index changes that occur when target biomarkers attach to bioreceptor molecules bound to the biosensor surface [86]. SPR platforms detect several biomarkers, including PSA, PCA3, and miRNAs, to generate a complete picture of prostate cancer stage through multiplex prostate cancer diagnosis. SPR biosensors can perform high-speed unmarked detection of biomolecular events for prostate cancer screening operations because of their direct time-based refractive index measurements [87].

9.4.1.2 Fluorescence-Based Biosensors

Biosensors that use fluorescence identify biomarker reactions through fluorescent dye detection and quantum dot (QD) measurements in addition to fluorescence resonance energy transfer (FRET) processes. These biosensors deliver high sensitivity for detecting multiple types of nucleic acids together with proteins alongside metabolites that indicate prostate cancer development progress [88]. The detection platform operates through fluorescence microarrays, which analyze miRNAs, ctDNA, and exosomal markers from patient samples by presenting high specificity with minimal false positives. These biosensors provide optimal performance for high-throughput prostate cancer diagnostic tools because they allow the distinction of multiple biomarkers through different fluorophore labeling capabilities [89].

9.4.1.3 Surface-Enhanced Raman Spectroscopy Biosensors

Biosensors with surface-enhanced Raman spectroscopy (SERS) functionality utilize metal nanostructured surfaces comprised of gold or silver nanoparticles for intensifying biomolecule Raman scattering signals. These biosensors demonstrate outstanding detection capability through which they manage to identify cancer biomarkers of low concentration that exist in blood, urine, or saliva testing materials [90]. The combination of SERS-based biosensors proves useful in diagnosing cancer through the identification of CTCs and exosomal biomarkers, as well as prostate cancer-associated protein markers, to enable both cancer monitoring systems in real time. SERS technology operates without labels, so it effectively enhances its capacity to function as a diagnostic tool for POC systems [91].

9.4.1.4 Colorimetric Biosensors

Prostate cancer biomarkers are detected by colorimetric biosensors that measure changes in color following enzymatic or nanoparticle-mediated reaction [92]. Biosensors are simple, inexpensive, and can be readily integrated into POC diagnostic platforms. For example, there are AuNP-based colorimetric biosensors that detect biomarkers and cause the aggregation of the AuNPs to have a visible color change that is quantifiable with a spectrophotometer or the naked eye [93]. Similarly, color shifts are used in an enzyme-linked colorimetric assay, including ELISA-based biosensors, in order to indicate when the enzyme-linked immunoassay of enzymatically hydrolyzed prostate cancer markers is present [94]. Any biosensors that can be obtained in whole colorimetric form convey a significant advantage and can be applied in high-speed, low-cost, and portable cancer screening, especially in resource-limited scenarios [95]. Nevertheless, the sensitivity of fluorescence- or SPR-based biosensors that they may lack renders them ideally suited for initial screenings rather than definitive diagnostics. Colorimetric biosensors identify changes within coloring territories after enzymatic reactions take place.

Advantages of Optical Biosensors The advantages include label-free detection (especially SPR-based biosensors); real-time monitoring of biomolecular interactions; and high sensitivity and specificity. Due to their light-based operating principle, optical biosensors find extensive application in research facilities for investigating biomolecular bonding, as well as DNA hybridization processes and clinical test evaluation [96].

9.4.2 Electrochemical Biosensors

The detection mechanism of electrochemical biosensors relies on evaluating electrical signals through changes in current, voltage, or impedance measurements. Multiplex platforms use the widely preferred electrochemical biosensors for prostate cancer detection because of their high sensitivity alongside quick response, affordability, and mobility features [97].

9.4.2.1 Amperometric Biosensors

The detection method in amperometric biosensors determines electrical current variations that occur during biomolecule reduction or oxidation processes. Producers utilize biosensors linked with electrodes featuring enzyme or nanomaterial components such as graphene and AuNPs to achieve superior sensing capabilities [98]. Scientists have created multiplexed amperometric biosensors for parallel detection of PSA, PCA3, and miRNA, enabling the quantitative analysis of prostate cancer disease evolution. Biosensors operate through rapid on-site assessments, which ensure their compatibility with POC testing environments.

9.4.2.2 Impedimetric Biosensors

Biosensors employing the impedimetric approach measure variations in electrical impedance triggered by the attachment of biomarkers. The sensors detect biomarkers label-free within highly sensitive measurements since they function optimally in multiplex prostate cancer diagnosis [99]. Impedimetric biosensors built from graphene material enable precise detection of early-stage prostate cancer by identifying both prostate-specific exosomal biomarkers and CTCs.

9.4.2.3 Potentiometric Biosensors

The potential change observed at electrode surfaces constitutes a measurement method for potentiometric biosensors through biomarker interactions. Biosensors offer an optimal solution to develop fast, portable testing tools that diagnose multiple biomarkers directly through patient blood, urine, or saliva samples [100].

9.4.3 Microfluidic and LOC Systems

Miniature biosensing systems, such as microfluidic and LOC platforms, serve as testing methods for the simultaneous analysis of multiple biomarkers within a single microdevice. The platforms need minimal sample materials alongside automatic, quick analysis that allows integration with electrochemical and optical, and nanomaterial based biosensing methods [101]. Biosensors within microfluidic systems control biological materials through their small fluidic networks. The designed systems utilize cost-optimizing features that simultaneously boost detection speeds and boost assay functionality [102]. A combination of biosensors operating in multiple microfluidic chambers detects prostate cancer biomarkers with high sensitivity through measurements of miRNAs, along with ctDNA and protein markers. The LOC platform combines many biosensing technology components into one compact device system, which enables on-site testing and real-time test results monitoring [103]. LOC platforms operate advantageously in remote regions and areas with scarce resources by delivering early-stage prostate cancer screening that remains both accessible and affordable.

9.4.4 Nanomaterial-Based Biosensors

The implementation of nanotechnology has enhanced biosensors by improving both sensitivity and specificity, as well as introducing features for multiplexing capability. The multiplex biosensing applications depend heavily on nanomaterials, which include AuNPs, CNTs, graphene, and quantum dots (QDs) [104].

9.4.4.1 AuNP-Based Biosensors

AuNP-based biosensors enhance signal transduction through SPR, fluorescence, and electrochemical biosensors, resulting in high effectiveness in the multiplex detection of PSA, miRNAs, and ctDNA. Biosensor applications benefit from the use of graphene and CNT technologies in their development [105]. The excellent biomolecular binding capabilities, together with the high electrical conductivity of graphene and CNTs, strengthen the sensitivity of electrochemical biosensors. The nanomaterials show excellent performance when detecting scarce biomarkers, including CTCs as well as exosomal markers.

9.4.4.2 QD-Based Biosensors

QDs combine potent fluorescence strength with adjustable signal characteristics, which makes them perfectly suitable for running multiplex detection applications [106]. The biosensor technology enables the simultaneous observation of multiple DNA, RNA, and protein biomarkers in prostate cancer investigations.

9.5 Recent Advances in Multiplex Biosensing Platforms

The modern multiplex biosensing field demonstrated significant advancement through the alignment of POC devices together with AI and ML, wearable biosensors, and wireless technologies [107]. Medical screening methods today deliver rapid, painless diagnoses of prostate cancer because they provide reliable verification of this condition. Acute testing procedures for prostate cancer detection are performed alongside smart digital tools and data analytics, and real-time monitoring systems, which result in improved clinical choices concerning prostate cancer diagnosis [108].

9.5.1 Integration of AI and ML

New multiplex biosensing platforms are enhanced through the use of AI and ML algorithms, as these algorithms help platforms identify biomarkers while producing more accurate predictive models through advanced data analysis [109]. Single biosensing methods often yield excessively complicated biological results that require refined analytical equipment for precise measurements. AI-powered biosensors analyze multiple parameters better than conventional sensors to verify samples for cancer and non-cancer factors with increased accuracy [110]. The training of deep learning algorithms is conducted using large clinical prostate cancer biomarker datasets that contain PSA, along with miRNAs, CTCs, and exosomes, to enhance diagnostic precision. The combination of multiple biomarkers becomes detectable through AI models, while human experts would not achieve this degree of analysis, leading to earlier diagnostic possibilities [111]. Decision tree and neural network models achieve accurate diagnoses through unification of biomolecular data from various sources, which lowers false and inaccurate results. Researchers are developing AI-based biosensors to perform real-time risk assessments, which categorize prostate cancer patients into three risk levels to enhance their treatment plans. The use of ML algorithms in automated data interpretation enables the efficient processing of results from electrochemical, optical, and microfluidic biosensors, leading to improved reliability and usability in clinical settings [112]. Current research reveals that biosensors utilizing AI perform better than traditional single-marker screening tests by providing individualized patient testing and continuous monitoring of medical conditions. POC multiplex biosensors enhanced by AI enable faster and more accurate prostate cancer diagnostics, potentially making invasive biopsies unnecessary [113].

9.5.2 POC and Wearable Biosensors

With POC biosensors, doctors can now screen for prostate cancer, as they can use the biosensors to detect biomarkers at patients' offices, even without complete laboratory equipment. Gadgets that provide convenient operation allow for speedy analysis results with minimal maintenance costs and extended testing capabilities that work well for resource-limited areas [114]. Microfluidic-based POC technology evaluates multiple biomarkers from small blood, urine, and saliva samples because it simplifies both specimen extraction and the required laboratory assessment [37]. Several LOC technology-based instruments produce tiny diagnostic devices that unite every analysis process by integrating specimen processing with simultaneous biomarker detection and signal analysis within a single system unit. These LOC biosensors maintain superior sensitivity, so they can diagnose cancer at initial stages through minimal sample analysis [115]. Prostate cancer biomarker observation exists now due to the combination of wearable biosensors with nanosensor elements and flexible electronics. The combination of smartwatch systems with patches that contain sensors for saliva and sweat provides continuous biomarker observation without destroying tissue, allowing for real-time measurements. A POC biosensor system integrated with cloud-based data storage enables remote result transmission for healthcare providers, thus improving telemedicine practice alongside patient care management [116]. The performance equivalence of paper-based and electrochemical POC biosensors toward laboratory tests has been demonstrated by scientific evidence in terms of sensitivity and specificity. Scientists have proven that biosensor wearables integrate with graphene nanomaterials alongside plasmonic technology detection systems to enhance early-stage prostate cancer detection abilities [117].

9.5.2.1 Wireless and Smartphone-Based Biosensing Systems

Cellular biosensors with built-in smartphone functions allow prostate cancer tests to reach directly into patients' hands [118]. The platforms implement mobile health technologies through mHealth to link remote testing with real-time data transfers, including AI-based analytics [109]. Portable PSA and additional cancer biomarker identification are achieved through smartphone-based electrochemical biosensors utilizing chip-based devices with precise detection capabilities. User interfaces on mobile platforms present results that help patients and doctors track disease development in a real-time manner [119]. Wireless biosensors equipped with Bluetooth technology and NFC components establish uninterrupted connectivity channels, enabling oncologists to receive instant updates on biomarker test results stored in hospital databases. Smartphone camera-connected biosensors based on nanotechnology-enabled paper allow simple, low-cost detection of biomarker presence through colorimetric changes that the camera can assess [120]. Biosensing platforms connected to the cloud enable patients to conduct home tests independently, which reduces their need to visit hospitals frequently. The implementation of blockchain encryption with data protection security features enhances patient privacy protection in wireless biosensing systems. Investigators demonstrate in current publications how smartphone biosensors effectively screen prostate cancer biomarkers simultaneously. Scientific evidence demonstrates that electrochemical biosensors integrated with smartphones, due to their low detection limit of 1 pg/mL, surpass traditional ELISA test levels [121]. The combination of 5G technology and internet of things (IoT)-based biosensing devices will bring a revolutionary change to the field by delivering rapid, decentralized prostate cancer diagnostics, working with high efficiency [122].

9.6 Current Challenges and Emerging Directions in Multiplex Biosensing for Prostate Cancer

Recent biosensing multiplex technologies have become vital investigative instruments for performing precise early detection of minimally invasive prostate cancer. The evaluation of multiple biomarkers at once through these systems better defines diagnoses and cuts down on improper test results, as well as enabling continuous disease surveillance [123]. The full adoption of multiplex biosensing systems for routine medical practice faces various substantial scientific, technical, regulatory, and clinical barriers [124]. The pathway toward utilizing biosensing in personalized medicine needs to resolve difficulties (Table 9.5) in sensitivity, along with specificity, reproducibility, regulatory approval matters, and future development plans.

9.6.1 Sensitivity, Specificity, and Reproducibility Issues

Reliable multiplex biosensor development faces the main challenge of delivering both high sensitivity and specific detection capabilities. Prostate cancer biomarker detection relies on sensor sensitivity to measure minute biomarker amounts and also depends on

Table 9.5 Challenges and future perspectives in multiplex biosensing

Challenge	Description	Potential solution	References
Sensitivity and specificity issues	Difficulty in distinguishing between benign and malignant cases	Integration of AI and ML for data refinement	[125]
Reproducibility concerns	Variation in sensor performance across different samples	Standardized fabrication and validation protocols	[125]
Regulatory and clinical validation	Complex approval process for biosensor-based diagnostics	Collaboration with regulatory agencies for streamlined approval	[125]
Cost and accessibility	High production costs limit widespread use	Development of affordable, POC biosensors	[125]
Integration with digital health	Need for real-time monitoring and data sharing	Wireless, cloud-based biosensors for remote patient tracking	[125]

its ability to identify target biomolecules specifically, without reacting to unrelated biological substances [126]. In prostate cancer detection, there exist biomarkers that include PSA as well as CTCs, along with miRNAs and exosomes, which naturally occur at minimal levels in blood, urine, and saliva samples. To measure scarce molecules, researchers require extremely sensitive bioreceptor and transducer systems that eliminate unwanted signals and prevent responses from adjacent molecules [127]. Sensor malfunctions occur due to variations in biological samples, as well as protein cross-reactivity and the nonspecific attraction of molecules to the detection surface. The occurrence of unpredictable results becomes more severe when multiple biomarkers are evaluated simultaneously through multiplex analysis due to component interactions [128]. Reproducibility is another major issue. Testing biosensors for laboratory success must be accompanied by evaluating their ability to produce equivalent results across different clinical locations and patient groups in multiple environmental settings [129]. Various elements affect reproducibility because of the following reasons: inconsistencies that happen during biosensor creation at the manufacturing stage result in detection performance variation; biosensor stability and signal accuracy are affected when placed in environments that include temperature, pH, and humidity conditions; the detection process is affected when different patient samples contain compounds that act as inhibitors or contaminants during analyses; and long-term materials reliability suffers when biosensors have restrictions related to storage and shelf-life duration. The combination of intensive surface chemistry research, optimized nanomaterial properties for durable signals, and sample and noise correction through ML allows the accomplishment of these hurdles.

9.6.2 Clinical Validation and Regulatory Approvals

Medical professionals must subject multiplex biosensors to strict clinical tests before their adoption in clinical medicine to prove their accuracy and application validity, and performance reliability [130]. Researchers need to conduct extensive clinical tests, which should analyze how well biosensor systems function compared to typical diagnostic measures such as ELISA tests, PCR, and tissue biopsies.

Heterogeneity of Prostate Cancer Biomarkers The multiple types present in prostate cancer result in unsatisfying biomarker performance since no biomarker stands alone for definitive diagnosis. The multiplex biosensing system must accommodate the variations that exist among different patient subgroups and various stages of cancer.

Standardization of Sample Collection and Handling Standardized procedures must be implemented with biosensors because they require proper functioning with blood, urine, and saliva samples, without degradation or contamination damage.

Comparison With Existing Diagnostic Standards The accuracy standards set by regulatory agencies for new biosensors must be higher than or equivalent to those of gold-standard biopsy and MRI imaging, yet must overcome discrepancy thresholds.

Validation Across Diverse Patient Populations Clinical evaluations must incorporate diverse study participants to validate that biosensors operate properly in different ethnic groups, genetic backgrounds, and environmental settings. Medical biosensors must meet rigorous regulatory requirements before manufacturers can market and apply them for clinical purposes. The U.S. Food and Drug Administration tests biosensors to ensure their safety, as well as assess their efficacy and reproducibility for market release [131]. Biosensors available in European markets need to demonstrate regulatory compliance through the Conformité Européenne marking system. Regulatory pathways include laboratory-based validation (preclinical testing on patient samples) and clinical trials (testing in real-world settings). To guarantee biosensor production quality control, the implementation of Good Manufacturing Practice standards is necessary. The regulatory approval process is time-consuming and costly, requiring universities to collaborate with medical institutions and industrial businesses to generate sufficient validation data.

9.6.3 Future Trends in Personalized Medicine and Biosensing Technologies

Multiplex biosensing technology has created a direct connection between next-level personalized medicine development and AI applications and digital healthcare system integration, according to recent trends [132]. Several novel biosensing developments are expected to emerge from current trends, enabling the following advancements.

AI-Driven Data Interpretation and Digital Health Integration The diagnosis of biosensor signals and signal processing operate better through ML alignment with

AI [133]. AI-powered biosensors can identify aggressive prostate cancer in its advanced stages and indolent forms, which are not dangerous. The system analyzes both subtle changes in protein levels and small genetic mutations. This system makes automated diagnosis testing more efficient, encouraging healthcare services without reliance on laboratories. AI biosensors serve as comprehensive components of cloud-based healthcare platforms with EHR capabilities, enabling doctors to track disease progression for more effective treatment adaptations.

9.6.3.1 POC and Wearable Biosensors

Medical practitioners aim to develop POC and wearable biosensors for prostate cancer diagnostics, as they require portable, real-time diagnostic tools that are non-invasive [134]. Advanced technology platforms support two operational features that provide remote medical care to providers within restricted healthcare areas, as well as home testing capabilities for patients. Potential future developments include the following: biosensors inserted into wearable technology devices analyze cancer biomarkers through the assessment of blood and saliva specimens and sweat fluid testing; modern smartphones come equipped with cell phone sensors that help users access fast diagnostic outcomes through medical Health applications named mHealth [135]; and the evolution of 3D printer technology during decades resulted in the development of biosensor microfluidic chips which use hospital patient areas for ultra-sensitive biomarker detection.

9.6.3.2 Nanotechnology for Ultra-Sensitive Detection

For the detection of prostate cancer using ultra-sensitive biosensors, nanotechnology has emerged as a game-changing approach. Although conventional biosensors have been effective, they suffer from low detection limits, instability of the signal, and poor miniaturization that limits their clinical use. On the other hand, the biosensors based on nanomaterials take advantage of the peculiar physicochemical properties of nanoparticles, because they exhibit higher sensitivity, higher selectivity, and shorter response times [136]. Due to exceptional electrical, optical, and biochemical properties that characterize nanomaterials such as graphene, CNTs, AuNPs, and QDs, these nanomaterials are broadly used in multiplex biosensing platforms. For example, such isometric graphene-based biosensors possess a large surface area and electrical conductivity and therefore are highly suited for electrochemical detection of cancer biomarkers [137]. Through a similar rapid electron transfer mechanism, CNTs are also utilized for highly sensitive amperometric and impedimetric biosensing applications. The strong biocompatibility and optical properties of AuNPs have drawn much interest in using them in SPR and colorimetric biosensors to improve sensitivity in detection. The unique fluorescence properties of QDs make them very suitable for optical biosensing in a highly specific and multiplexed fashion [138]. These nanomaterials have therefore enabled the integration of biosensors with detection specificity at femtomolar levels of prostate cancer biomarkers, resulting in a significant improvement in capabilities for early diagnosis. Also, nanostructured biosensors provide feature size reduction, which fits the requirements for POC usage, thereby allowing rapid as well as cost-effective cancer screening [139]. In addition, their clever role in signal transduction and stability has created better, more reliable, and more reproducible biosensing platforms. Advancement of nanotechnology in biosensing will continue in prostate cancer diagnostics to meet traditional assays' limitations and allow early detection with minimal sample volumes.

9.6.3.3 Biosensing for Precision Oncology

Precision oncology is at the heart of biosensing technologies, and will be the future for biosensing [technology] in a way that the diagnostic tools that guide personalized treatment strategies based on an individual's molecular and genetic profile. Traditional cancer treatments typically work in a general manner and thus exhibit variation in treatment responses. Assuming that the biosensors can be integrated with precision oncology techniques, then biosensors can provide real-time, patient-specific information to clinicians for making informed therapeutic decisions [139]. The integration of biosensors with liquid biopsy techniques is one of the most significant advancements in this area. Biosensors for liquid biopsy based on the detection of ctDNA, CTCs, and extracellular vesicles like exosomes allow for monitoring of tumor progression, metastasis, and drug resistance by means without tissue destruction [140]. Biosensors track these biomarkers continuously, allowing us to dynamically and adaptively adjust treatment strategies to enhance patient outcomes and reduce reliance on unnecessary interventions. AI-assisted biosensor platforms enhance precision oncology by automating data analysis and identifying subtle biomarker patterns that are not detectable by conventional diagnostic methods. Biosensing systems driven by AI can process large datasets faster to provide actionable data, such as diagnostic accuracy, and predict treatment response modeling. Furthermore, biosensors incorporated with wearable and cell phone-based devices enable continuous monitoring of biomarker fluctuations, enabling novel levels of comfort in managing a cancer [141]. With the continued evolution of biosensing technologies, biosensing will become increasingly important in determining which cancer treatments are tailored to a given case. In the time scale of minutes to hours, it will allow the real-time monitoring of therapy effectiveness and subsequent proactive adjustments of treatment plans to minimize the adverse effects and increase the therapeutic benefit [81]. Having biosensing, AI, and liquid biopsy work together is a paradigm and the beginning of a new era of highly personalized, data-driven oncology for prostate cancer management.

9.7 Conclusion

Despite this, prostate cancer is one of the most prevalent malignancies throughout the globe, and early and accurate detection is crucial to enhance patient prognosis. Historically, the PSAs and biopsies are great cancer diagnostics, but often false positives, invasive, and not specific. Prostate cancer diagnostics have been revolutionized by emerging biosensing technologies, which enable sensitive, rapid, and minimally invasive methods of detection. Multiplex biosensing platforms, which detect multiple biomarkers all at once, have been shown to possess better diagnostic capabilities than any of these by eliminating diagnostic errors and, in turn, rallying this level of accuracy. Biosensing technologies for the detection of prostate cancer biomarkers have excellent sensitivity based on well-defined principles of bioreceptors, transducers, and signal processing units. Such biosensors as SPR, fluorescence-based sensors, and SERS have shown great promise in label-free, real-time detection of cancer markers. Similarly, electrochemical biosensors, such as amperometric, impedimetric, and potentiometric platforms, have become prevalent, which are portable, are inexpensive, and can be engineered to coexist with digital health technologies. Microfluidic and lab on a chip-systems have taken biosensing even further by the development of high-throughput screening with few sample requirements, making them applicable to POC systems. Furthermore, by using graphene, CNTs, AuNPs, and QDs as nanomaterials to construct biosensors, the signal transduction has been vastly improved in the biosensors, and thus the biomarker detection is enlarged at ultra-low concentrations. Advancing the biosensor technology has been based heavily on the identification of prostate cancer biomarkers. Currently, PSA is still a widely used marker, but its limitations have pushed researchers to explore more complete information of tumor biology with the emerging biomarkers, such as CTCs, miRNAs, and exosomes. Multiplexing these biomarkers is a breakthrough in prostate cancer diagnostics because your ability to do a more holistic, more precise assessment of the disease status gets us closer to personalized medicine. With the latest advances in AI and ML, these platforms have evolved into the field of biosensing, as they now feature automated data interpretation, reduced human error, and predictive modeling for disease progression. Another avenue that has been opened due to the integration of wearable and smartphone-based biosensing systems has been in the real-time remote monitoring of cancer biomarker, which has increased the ease of early detection and time to treatment. By virtue of being wireless and POC biosensors, these sensors remove cancer screening and monitoring from centralized laboratories and bring it to the communities in resource-limited settings. While these groundbreaking innovations have opened amazing, exciting possibilities for multiplex biosensors, they also present several outstanding challenges in their clinical translation. To provide valuable clinical insights, biosensors to measure tumor viability and glucose have problems with sensitivity, specificity, and reproducibility. Furthermore, clinical validation and regulatory approval are major hurdles, as extensive testing and validation are still needed before these biosensors can be broadly introduced in clinical practice. Challenges to be overcome include the complexities of integration between scientists, engineers, clinicians, and regulators. This is true for the future of biosensor technologies embedded in the context of personalized medicine, where the diagnostics and treatment plan are tailored to your genetics and molecular profile. In later advancement, biosensors will be embedded in the methods of liquid biopsy to gain real-time monitoring of cancer, allowing for real-time detection of tumor evolution, drug resistance, and treatment efficacy. Precision oncology will continue to move a bit farther as nanotechnology, AI-driven analytics, and digital health solutions all begin to converge for prostate cancer to be more proactive, data-driven, and patient-centric. Based on the above, multiplex biosensing technologies have the potential for future prostate cancer detection that is not reactive, but proactive for disease management. Thus, their ability to allow fast, precise, personalized diagnostic general information assured that the patient has the best informed and exact remedy at the right time, improving survival rates and the quality of life. These innovative platforms will enable the future advancement of the field of biomedical sensing research and development in the increasingly important and global war on prostate cancer, as well as in the evolving field of cancer diagnosis.

9.8 Summary

This chapter provides an extensive review of multiplex biosensing technologies, with a focus on their applications in prostate cancer monitoring and detection. An overview of prostate cancer and the limitations of existing diagnostic techniques is provided at the outset, emphasizing the need for sophisticated biosensing platforms. The principles, essential elements, and special benefits of multiplex biosensors are covered in the discussion of the foundations of biosensing technologies. A thorough analysis of prostate cancer biomarkers reveals how important they are for prognosis and early diagnosis. The design and operation of several multiplex biosensing platform types, including optical, electrochemical, microfluidic, and nanomaterial-based platforms, are then examined. The integration of AI, POC testing, and smartphone-based biosensing systems is among the recent developments in the field that are reviewed in this chapter. Finally, future developments in personalized medicine and biosensing innovation are explored, along with contemporary issues such as sensitivity, reproducibility, and regulatory barriers. The potential of multiplex biosensing to revolutionize prostate cancer diagnosis and patient care is reaffirmed in the chapter's conclusion.

Glossary

Biosensor An analytical device that combines a biological component with a physicochemical detector to identify and measure substances.

Multiplexing A technique that allows simultaneous detection of multiple targets (e.g., biomarkers) in a single assay.

Bioreceptor A biological molecule (e.g., antibody, enzyme, and aptamer) that recognizes the analyte in a biosensor system.

Transducer A component that converts the biorecognition event into a measurable signal.

PSA A protein biomarker commonly used in the diagnosis of prostate cancer.

Microfluidics A technology involving the precise control and manipulation of fluids at the microscale, often used in LOC devices.

Nanomaterials Materials with structures at the nanometer scale that offer unique optical, electrical, or chemical properties.

POC Diagnostic testing conducted at or near the site of patient care.

AI Computer systems able to perform tasks that typically require human intelligence, such as pattern recognition and decision-making.

ML A subset of AI focused on algorithms that improve automatically through experience.

References

1. Dunn MW, Kazer MW. Prostate cancer overview. In: Seminars in oncology nursing. Elsevier; 2011. p. 241–50.
2. Schatten H. Brief overview of prostate cancer statistics, grading, diagnosis and treatment strategies. In: Schatten H, editor. Cell {\&} molecular biology of prostate cancer: updates, insights and new frontiers [Internet]. Cham: Springer International Publishing; 2018. p. 1–14. Available from: https://doi.org/10.1007/978-3-319-95693-0_1.
3. Schröder FH. Prostate cancer around the world. An overview. In: Urologic oncology: seminars and original investigations. Elsevier; 2010. p. 663–7.
4. Uhr A, Glick L, Gomella LG. An overview of biomarkers in the diagnosis and management of prostate cancer. Can J Urol. 2020;27(S3):24–7.
5. Rawla P. Epidemiology of prostate cancer. World J Oncol. 2019;10(2):63.
6. Sarkar S, Gogoi M, Mahato M, Joshi AB, Baruah AJ, Kodgire P, et al. Biosensors for detection of prostate cancer: a review. Biomed Microdevices [Internet]. 2022;24(4):32. Available from: https://doi.org/10.1007/s10544-022-00631-1.
7. Sohrabi N, Valizadeh A, Farkhani SM, Akbarzadeh A. Basics of DNA biosensors and cancer diagnosis. Artif Cells, Nanomedicine, Biotechnol. 2016;44(2):654–63.
8. Takita S, Nabok A, Mussa M, Kitchen M, Lishchuk A, Smith D. Ultrasensitive prostate cancer marker PCA3 detection with impedimetric biosensor based on specific label-free aptamers. Biosens Bioelectron X [Internet]. 2024;18:100462. Available from: https://www.sciencedirect.com/science/article/pii/S2590137024000268.
9. Funari R, Chu KY, Shen AQ. Multiplexed opto-microfluidic biosensing: advanced platform for prostate cancer detection. ACS Sensors [Internet]. 2024;9(5):2596–604. Available from: https://doi.org/10.1021/acssensors.4c00312.
10. Purohit A, Jain S, Panda PK. Chapter 5 - Biosensors used for anticancer therapeutics. In: Hasnain MS, Nayak AK, Aminabhavi TM, editors. Applications of biosensors in healthcare [Internet]. Academic Press; 2025. p. 73–91. Available from: https://www.sciencedirect.com/science/article/pii/B9780443215926000239.
11. Broomfield J, Kalofonou M, Bevan CL, Georgiou P. Recent electrochemical advancements for liquid biopsy nucleic acid detection for point-of-care prostate cancer diagnostics and prognostics. Biosensors [Internet]. 2024;14(9). Available from: https://www.mdpi.com/2079-6374/14/9/443.
12. Li K, Wang Q, Tang X, Akakuru OU, Li R, Wang Y, et al. Advances in prostate cancer bio markers and probes. Cyborg Bionic Syst. 2024;5:129.
13. Anil İU, Sezgintürk MK. MIP-based sensing strategies for the diagnosis of prostate and lung cancers. Talanta Open. 2025:100432.
14. Zhong J, Liu D, Yang Q, Ding J, Chen X. A novel DNA Aptamer probe recognizing castration resistant prostate cancer in vitro and in vivo based on cell-SELEX. Drug Des Devel Ther. 2024:859–70.
15. Zhou Y, Zeng F, Richards GO, Wang N. ENO2, a glycolytic enzyme, contributes to prostate cancer metastasis: a systematic review of literature. Cancers (Basel). 2024;16(14):2503.
16. Barman SC, Ali M, Hasan EA, Wehbe N, Alshareef HN, Alsulaiman D. Smartphone-interfaced electrochemical biosensor for microRNA detection based on laser-induced graphene with π–π stacked peptide nucleic acid probes. ACS Mater Lett. 2024;6(3):837–46.

17. Luddy KA, West J, Robertson-Tessi M, Desai B, Bursell TM, Barrett S, et al. Evolutionary double-bind treatment using radiotherapy and NK cell-based immunotherapy in prostate cancer. bioRxiv. 2024:2003–24.
18. Zhang S, Ji X, Liu Z, Xie Z, Wang Y, Wang H, et al. Bimetallic nanoplatforms for prostate cancer treatment by interfering cellular communication. J Am Chem Soc. 2024;146(32):22530–40.
19. Lim S, Tan M, Tan E. Development of an aptamer-based electrochemical biosensor for early detection of prostate cancer markers. J Biomed Techno Nanomater. 2024;1(4):126–96.
20. Venugopal Iyer V, Rajendran R, Selvaraj S. Colorimetric and electrochemical sensors for the detection of sarcosine, a potential biomarker for prostate cancer: a review. Curr Anal Chem. 2024;20(1):2–13.
21. Moorthy DN, Dhinasekaran D, Rebecca PNB, Rajendran AR. Optical biosensors for detection of cancer biomarkers: current and future perspectives. J Biophotonics. 2024;17(12):e202400243.
22. Wang J, Deng M, Niu K, Wang C, Wang N, Li J, et al. Ultra-sensitive optical fiber spr biosensor for precise prostate cancer diagnosis by label-free detection of Mirna-21. Anal Chim Acta. 2026;1384:344985. Available SSRN 5115027.
23. Rasheed S, Kanwal T, Ahmad N, Fatima B, Najam-ul-Haq M, Hussain D. Advances and challenges in portable optical biosensors for onsite detection and point-of-care diagnostics. TrAC Trends Anal Chem [Internet]. 2024;173:117640. Available from: https://www.sciencedirect.com/science/article/pii/S0165993624001225.
24. Pohanka M. Piezoelectric chemosensors and biosensors in medical diagnostics. Biosensors. 2025;15(3):197.
25. Tripathi P, Dubey AK. Role of piezoelectricity in disease diagnosis and treatment: a review. ACS Biomater Sci Eng. 2024;10(10):6061–77.
26. Li F, Jiang Y, Wang X, Gao Y, Lo CS, Su S, et al. Titanium nitride meta-biosensors targeting extracellular vesicles for high-sensitivity prostate cancer detection. Biosens Bioelectron. 2025;277:117288.
27. Chen C, Wu B, Li X, Jin Y, Zhang H, Liu B, et al. Integrated device for cancer nucleic acid biomarker detection at body temperature. Micromachines. 2025;16(2):192.
28. Corso R, Stefano A, Salvaggio G, Comelli A. Shearlet transform applied to a prostate cancer radiomics analysis on MR images. Mathematics. 2024;12(9):1296.
29. Luo K, Zheng B, Lv S, Tao J, Wei Q. Enhanced cascade prostate cancer classifier in mp-MRI utilizing recall feedback adaptive loss and prior knowledge-based feature extraction. arXiv Prepr arXiv240809746. 2024;
30. Vafadar A, AlaviManesh S, Maddahi ME, Alizadeh M, Movahedpour A, Savardashtaki A. Exosome biosensors for detection of prostate cancer. Clin Chim Acta [Internet]. 2025;571:120243. Available from: https://www.sciencedirect.com/science/article/pii/S0009898125001226.
31. Haque M, Bhattacharyya K. Speech background noise removal using different linear filtering techniques. In: Advanced computational and communication paradigms: Proceedings of International Conference on ICACCP 2017, vol. 1. Springer; 2018. p. 297–307.
32. Prudhomme C, Homburg T, Ponciano JJ, Boochs F, Cruz C, Roxin AM. Interpretation and automatic integration of geospatial data into the Semantic Web: towards a process of automatic geospatial data interpretation, classification and integration using semantic technologies. Computing. 2020;102:365–91.
33. Singh AK, Srivastava VK. Improved filtering approach for identification of protein-coding regions in eukaryotes by background noise reduction using S–G filter. Netw Model Anal Heal Informatics Bioinforma. 2021;10(1):19.
34. Sobiepanek A, Kobiela T. Application of biosensors in cancer research. Adv Biomed Res Top. 2018:9.
35. Aleixandre M, Horrillo MC. Recent advances in SAW sensors for detection of cancer biomarkers. Biosensors. 2025;15(2):88.
36. Alharthi SD, Bijukumar D, Prasad S, Khan AM, Mathew MT. Evolution in biosensors for cancers biomarkers detection: a review. J Bio-and Tribo-Corrosion. 2021;7:1–17.

37. Adir O, Poley M, Chen GGG, Froim S, Krinsky N, Shklover J, et al. Chapter 24 - Scope of biosensors, commercial aspects, and miniaturized devices for point-of-care testing from lab to clinics applications. In: Elnour AAM, editor. Cancers (Basel) [Internet], vol. 13(1). 2022. p. 21. Available from: https://doi.org/10.1186/s13148-019-0736-8.
38. Yadav S, Saini A, Devi R, Lata S. Transducers in biosensors. In: Biomaterials-based sensors: recent advances and applications. Springer; 2023. p. 101–25.
39. Ranjan Srivastava V, Kumari R, Chandra P. Miniaturized surface engineered technologies for multiplex biosensing devices. Electroanalysis. 2023;35(8):e202200355.
40. Kumari S, Islam M, Gupta A. Based multiplex biosensors for inexpensive healthcare diagnostics: a comprehensive review. Biomed Microdevices. 2023;25(2):17.
41. Zheng Y, Song X, Fredj Z, Bian S, Sawan M. Challenges and perspectives of multi-virus biosensing techniques: a review. Anal Chim Acta. 2023;1244:340860.
42. Jarockyte G, Karabanovas V, Rotomskis R, Mobasheri A. Multiplexed nanobiosensors: current trends in early diagnostics. Sensors [Internet]. 2020;20(23). Available from: https://www.mdpi.com/1424-8220/20/23/6890.
43. Cai Z, Li Z, Ravaine S, He M, Song Y, Yin Y, et al. From colloidal particles to photonic crystals: advances in self-assembly and their emerging applications. Chem Soc Rev [Internet]. 2021;50(10):5898–951. Available from: https://doi.org/10.1039/D0CS00706D.
44. Pauliukaite R, Voitechovič E. Multisensor systems and arrays for medical applications employing naturally-occurring compounds and materials. Sensors [Internet]. 2020;20(12). Available from: https://www.mdpi.com/1424-8220/20/12/3551.
45. Aslam M, Rani A, Khan J, Pant BN, Pandey G. In: Bose S, Shukla AC, Baig MR, Banerjee S, editors. Applications of biotechnology in pharmaceutical product analysis BT - concepts in pharmaceutical biotechnology and drug development. Singapore: Springer Nature Singapore; 2024. p. 43–66. Available from: https://doi.org/10.1007/978-981-97-1148-2_4.
46. Chandra P. Affordable and sustainable biosensing technology. Nanotheranostics. 2025;9(1):63–6.
47. Plastic Europe. Scholar (12). 2020.
48. Warsi I, Khurshid Z, Shazam H, Umer MF, Imran E, Khan MO, et al. Saliva exhibits high sensitivity and specificity for the detection of SARS-COV-2. Diseases. 2021;9(2):38.
49. Kovács A, Palásti P, Veréb D, Bozsik B, Palkó A, Kincses ZT. The sensitivity and specificity of chest CT in the diagnosis of COVID-19. Eur Radiol. 2021;31:2819–24.
50. Vervoort N, Goossens K, Baeten M, Chen Q. Recent advances in analytical techniques for high throughput experimentation. Anal Sci Adv. 2021;2(3–4):109–27.
51. Mahjour B, Zhang R, Shen Y, McGrath A, Zhao R, Mohamed OG, et al. Rapid planning and analysis of high-throughput experiment arrays for reaction discovery. Nat Commun. 2023;14(1):3924.
52. Alwosheel A, Van Cranenburgh S, Chorus CG. Is your dataset big enough? Sample size requirements when using artificial neural networks for discrete choice analysis. J Choice Model. 2018;28:167–82.
53. Deans ZC, Butler R, Cheetham M, Dequeker EMC, Fairley JA, Fenizia F, et al. IQN path ASBL report from the first European cfDNA consensus meeting: expert opinion on the minimal requirements for clinical ctDNA testing. Virchows Arch. 2019;474:681–9.
54. Murray LP, Mace CR. Usability as a guiding principle for the design of paper-based, point-of-care devices–a review. Anal Chim Acta. 2020;1140:236–49.
55. Blanchard IE, Kozicky R, Dalgarno D, Simms J, Goulder S, Williamson TS, et al. Community paramedic point of care testing: validity and usability of two commercially available devices. BMC Emerg Med. 2019;19:1–10.
56. Shah B, Allen JLY, Chaudhury H, O'Shaughnessy J, Tyrrell CSB. The role of digital health in the future of integrated care. Clin Integr Care. 2022;15:100131.
57. Wang Q, Su M, Zhang M, Li R. Integrating digital technologies and public health to fight Covid-19 pandemic: key technologies, applications, challenges and outlook of digital healthcare. Int J Environ Res Public Health. 2021;18(11):6053.

58. Sanghera S, Coast J, Martin RM, Donovan JL, Mohiuddin S. Cost-effectiveness of prostate cancer screening: a systematic review of decision-analytical models. BMC Cancer. 2018;18:1–15.
59. Sathianathen NJ, Konety BR, Alarid-Escudero F, Lawrentschuk N, Bolton DM, Kuntz KM. Cost-effectiveness analysis of active surveillance strategies for men with low-risk prostate cancer. Eur Urol. 2019;75(6):910–7.
60. Zhang R, Belwal T, Li L, Lin X, Xu Y, Luo Z. Nanomaterial-based biosensors for sensing key foodborne pathogens: advances from recent decades. Compr Rev Food Sci Food Saf. 2020;19(4):1465–87.
61. Zhang L, Gu C, Wen J, Liu G, Liu H, Li L. Recent advances in nanomaterial-based biosensors for the detection of exosomes. Anal Bioanal Chem [Internet]. 2021;413(1):83–102. Available from: https://doi.org/10.1007/s00216-020-03000-0.
62. de Mirres ACM, de da Silva BEPM, Tessaro L, Galvan D, de Andrade JC, Aquino A, et al. Recent advances in nanomaterial-based biosensors for pesticide detection in foods. Biosensors [Internet]. 2022;12(8). Available from: https://www.mdpi.com/2079-6374/12/8/572.
63. Bidarra D, Constâncio V, Barros-Silva D, Ramalho-Carvalho J, Moreira-Barbosa C, Antunes L, et al. Circulating microRNAs as biomarkers for prostate cancer detection and metastasis development prediction. Front Oncol. 2019;9:900.
64. Salciccia S, Capriotti AL, Laganà A, Fais S, Logozzi M, De Berardinis E, et al. Biomarkers in prostate cancer diagnosis: from current knowledge to the role of metabolomics and exosomes. Int J Mol Sci. 2021;22(9):4367.
65. Chen E, Cario CL, Leong L, Lopez K, Márquez CP, Chu C, et al. Cell-free DNA concentration and fragment size as a biomarker for prostate cancer. Sci Rep [Internet]. 2021;11(1):5040. Available from: https://doi.org/10.1038/s41598-021-84507-z.
66. Galvão-Lima LJ, Morais AHF, Valentim RAM, Barreto EJSS. miRNAs as biomarkers for early cancer detection and their application in the development of new diagnostic tools. Biomed Eng Online [Internet]. 2021;20(1):21. Available from: https://doi.org/10.1186/s12938-021-00857-9.
67. Li Y, Shi X, Jia E, Qin S, Yu F. Extracellular vesicle biomarkers for prostate cancer diagnosis: a systematic review and meta-analysis. Urol Oncol Semin Orig Investig [Internet]. 2023;41(11):440–53. Available from: https://www.sciencedirect.com/science/article/pii/S1078143923002958.
68. Filella X, Fernandez-Galan E, Fernandez Bonifacio R, Foj L. Emerging biomarkers in the diagnosis of prostate cancer. Pharmgenom Pers Med. 2018:83–94.
69. Kwong GA, Ghosh S, Gamboa L, Patriotis C, Srivastava S, Bhatia SN. Synthetic biomarkers: a twenty-first century path to early cancer detection. Nat Rev Cancer. 2021;21(10):655–68.
70. Song C, Chen H, Chen L, Ru G, Guo J, Ding Q. The potential of microRNAs as human prostate cancer biomarkers: a meta-analysis of related studies. J Cell Biochem. 2018;119(3):2763–86.
71. Choksi AU, Khan AI, Lokeshwar SD, Segal D, Weiss RM, Martin DT. Functionalized nanoparticles targeting biomarkers for prostate cancer imaging and therapy. Am J Clin Exp Urol. 2022;10(3):142.
72. Aidoo-Brown J, Moschou D, Estrela P. Multiplexed prostate cancer companion diagnostic devices. Sensors [Internet]. 2021;21(15). Available from: https://www.mdpi.com/1424-8220/21/15/5023.
73. Jones A, Dhanapala L, Kankanamage RNT, Kumar CV, Rusling JF. Multiplexed immunosensors and immunoarrays. Anal Chem [Internet]. 2020;92(1):345–62. Available from: https://doi.org/10.1021/acs.analchem.9b05080.
74. Munge BS, Stracensky T, Gamez K, DiBiase D, Rusling JF. Multiplex immunosensor arrays for electrochemical detection of cancer biomarker proteins. Electroanalysis. 2016;28(11):2644–58.
75. O'Brien C, Khor CK, Ardalan S, Ignaszak A. Multiplex electrochemical sensing platforms for the detection of breast cancer biomarkers. Front Med Technol [Internet]. 2024;6. Available from: https://www.frontiersin.org/journals/medical-technology/articles/10.3389/fmedt.2024.1360510.

76. Kaur B, Kumar S, Kaushik BK. Recent advancements in optical biosensors for cancer detection. Biosens Bioelectron [Internet]. 2022;197:113805. Available from: https://www.sciencedirect.com/science/article/pii/S0956566321008423.
77. Chung YK, Reboud J, Lee KC, Lim HM, Lim PY, Wang KY, et al. An electrical biosensor for the detection of circulating tumor cells. Biosens Bioelectron [Internet]. 2011;26(5):2520–6. Available from: https://www.sciencedirect.com/science/article/pii/S0956566310007591.
78. Wang L, Sipe DM, Xu Y, Lin Q. A MEMS thermal biosensor for metabolic monitoring applications. J Microelectromech Syst. 2008;17(2):318–27.
79. Shahbazi F, Jabbari M, Esfahani MN, Keshmiri A. Microfluidic-integrated biosensors BT. In: Azizi A, editor. Applied complex flow: applications of complex flows and CFD. Singapore: Springer Nature Singapore; 2023. p. 21–42. Available from: https://doi.org/10.1007/978-981-19-7746-6_2.
80. Cho Y, Choi Y, Jang Y, Seong H. Nanomaterial-enhanced biosensing: mechanisms and emerging applications. Adv Healthc Mater [Internet]. 2025;14:2500189. Available from: https://advanced.onlinelibrary.wiley.com/doi/abs/10.1002/adhm.202500189.
81. Usman A. Nanoparticle enhanced optical biosensing technologies for prostate specific antigen biomarker detection. IEEE Rev Biomed Eng. 2020;15:122–37.
82. Li H, Wang X, Wu H, Wang W, Zheng A, Zhu J, et al. Simultaneous noninvasive ultrasensitive detection of prostate specific antigen and lncRNA PCA3 using multiplexed dual optical microfibers with strong plasmonic nanointerfaces. Biosens Bioelectron. 2024;264:116672.
83. Zamri AZM, Mustafa MK, Awang NA, Zalkepali NUHH, Mahmud NNHEN, Muhammad NAM. Fiber-laser based on D-shaped fiber biosensor for prostate cancer biomarker detection. Mater Today Proc [Internet]. 2024. Available from: https://www.sciencedirect.com/science/article/pii/S2214785324002591.
84. Ravindran N, Kumar S, Rajeshwari S, Mamathi CA, Thirunavookarasu SN, Sunil CK. Recent advances in Surface Plasmon Resonance (SPR) biosensors for food analysis: a review. Crit Rev Food Sci Nutr. 2023;63(8):1055–77.
85. Zhou J, Qi Q, Wang C, Qian Y, Liu G, Wang Y, et al. Surface plasmon resonance (SPR) biosensors for food allergen detection in food matrices. Biosens Bioelectron. 2019;142:111449.
86. Kushwaha AS, Kumar A, Kumar R, Srivastava SK. A study of surface plasmon resonance (SPR) based biosensor with improved sensitivity. Photonics Nanostructures-Fundam Appl. 2018;31:99–106.
87. Wang Q, Ren ZH, Zhao WM, Wang L, Yan X, Zhu AS, et al. Research advances on surface plasmon resonance biosensors. Nanoscale. 2022;14(3):564–91.
88. Girigoswami K, Akhtar N. Nanobiosensors and fluorescence based biosensors: an overview. Int J Nano Dimens. 2019;10(1):1–17.
89. Sharma A, Majdinasab M, Khan R, Li Z, Hayat A, Marty JL. Nanomaterials in fluorescence-based biosensors: defining key roles. Nano-structures Nano-objects. 2021;27:100774.
90. Li P, Long F, Chen W, Chen J, Chu PK, Wang H. Fundamentals and applications of surface-enhanced Raman spectroscopy–based biosensors. Curr Opin Biomed Eng [Internet]. 2020;13:51–9. Available from: https://www.sciencedirect.com/science/article/pii/S2468451119300273.
91. Pyrak E, Krajczewski J, Kowalik A, Kudelski A, Jaworska A. Surface enhanced Raman spectroscopy for DNA biosensors—how far are we? Molecules. 2019;24(24):4423.
92. Zhu D, Liu B, Wei G. Two-dimensional material-based colorimetric biosensors: a review. Biosensors [Internet]. 2021;11(8). Available from: https://www.mdpi.com/2079-6374/11/8/259.
93. Qian S, Cui Y, Cai Z, Li L. Applications of smartphone-based colorimetric biosensors. Biosens Bioelectron X. 2022;11:100173.
94. Yang T, Luo Z, Tian Y, Qian C, Duan Y. Design strategies of AuNPs-based nucleic acid colorimetric biosensors. TrAC Trends Anal Chem [Internet]. 2020;124:115795. Available from: https://www.sciencedirect.com/science/article/pii/S0165993619305989.
95. Yu L, Li N. Noble metal nanoparticles-based colorimetric biosensor for visual quantification: a mini review. Chem Int. 2019;7(4). Available from: https://www.mdpi.com/2227-9040/7/4/53.

96. Zhang F, Liu J. Label-free colorimetric biosensors based on aptamers and gold nanoparticles: a critical review. Anal Sens. 2021;1(1):30–43.
97. Wu J, Liu H, Chen W, Ma B, Ju H. Device integration of electrochemical biosensors. Nat Rev Bioeng. 2023;1(5):346–60.
98. Singh A, Sharma A, Ahmed A, Sundramoorthy AK, Furukawa H, Arya S, et al. Recent advances in electrochemical biosensors: applications, challenges, and future scope. Biosensors. 2021;11(9):336.
99. Cesewski E, Johnson BN. Electrochemical biosensors for pathogen detection. Biosens Bioelectron. 2020;159:112214.
100. Zhang L, Guo W, Lv C, Liu X, Yang M, Guo M, et al. Electrochemical biosensors represent promising detection tools in medical field. Adv Sens Energy Mater [Internet]. 2023;2(4):100081. Available from: https://www.sciencedirect.com/science/article/pii/S2773045X23000365.
101. Shabestani Monfared G, Ertl P, Rothbauer M. Microfluidic and lab-on-a-chip systems for cutaneous wound healing studies. Pharmaceutics [Internet]. 2021;13(6). Available from: https://www.mdpi.com/1999-4923/13/6/793.
102. Nikoleli GP, Siontorou CG, Nikolelis DP, Bratakou S, Karapetis S, Tzamtzis N. Chapter 13 - Biosensors based on microfluidic devices lab-on-a-chip and microfluidic technology. In: Nikolelis DP, Nikoleli GP, editors. Nanotechnology and biosensors [Internet], Advanced Nanomaterials. Elsevier; 2018. p. 375–94. Available from: https://www.sciencedirect.com/science/article/pii/B9780128138557000131.
103. Verma N, Pandya A. Chapter Twelve - Challenges and opportunities in micro/nanofluidic and lab-on-a-chip. In: Pandya A, Singh V, editors. Micro/Nanofluidics and lab-on-chip based emerging technologies for biomedical and translational research applications - Part A [Internet], Progress in Molecular Biology and Translational Science, vol. 186. Academic Press; 2022. p. 289–302. Available from: https://www.sciencedirect.com/science/article/pii/S1877117321001563.
104. Dekker S, Buesink W, Blom M, Alessio M, Verplanck N, Hihoud M, et al. Standardized and modular microfluidic platform for fast lab on chip system development. Sensors Actuators B Chem [Internet]. 2018;272:468–78. Available from: https://www.sciencedirect.com/science/article/pii/S0925400518306932.
105. Mozaffari S, Ghasemi H, Tchoukov P, Czarnecki J, Nazemifard N. Lab-on-a-Chip systems in asphaltene characterization: a review of recent advances. Energy Fuels [Internet]. 2021;35(11):9080–101. Available from: https://doi.org/10.1021/acs.energyfuels.1c00717.
106. Manimekala T, Sivasubramanian R, Dharmalingam G. Nanomaterial-based biosensors using field-effect transistors: a review. J Electron Mater [Internet]. 2022;51(5):1950–73. Available from: https://doi.org/10.1007/s11664-022-09492-z.
107. Chu SS, Nguyen HA, Zhang J, Tabassum S, Cao H. Towards multiplexed and multimodal biosensor platforms in real-time monitoring of metabolic disorders. Sensors [Internet]. 2022;22(14). Available from: https://www.mdpi.com/1424-8220/22/14/5200.
108. Liao Z, Wang J, Zhang P, Zhang Y, Miao Y, Gao S, et al. Recent advances in microfluidic chip integrated electronic biosensors for multiplexed detection. Biosens Bioelectron [Internet]. 2018;121:272–80. Available from: https://www.sciencedirect.com/science/article/pii/S0956566318306717.
109. Beduk T, Beduk D, Hasan MR, Guler Celik E, Kosel J, Narang J, et al. Smartphone-based multiplexed biosensing tools for health monitoring. Biosensors [Internet]. 2022;12(8). Available from: https://www.mdpi.com/2079-6374/12/8/583.
110. Ramirez JC, Grajales García D, Maldonado J, Fernández-Gavela A. Current trends in photonic biosensors: advances towards multiplexed integration. Chem Int. 2022;10(10). Available from: https://www.mdpi.com/2227-9040/10/10/398.
111. Cady NC, Tokranova N, Minor A, Nikvand N, Strle K, Lee WT, et al. Multiplexed detection and quantification of human antibody response to COVID-19 infection using a plasmon enhanced biosensor platform. Biosens Bioelectron [Internet]. 2021;171:112679. Available from: https://www.sciencedirect.com/science/article/pii/S0956566320306680.

112. Hu J, Liu F, Chen Y, Shangguan G, Ju H. Mass spectrometric biosensing: a powerful approach for multiplexed analysis of clinical biomolecules. ACS Sens. 2021;6(10):3517–35.
113. Canning AJ, Chen X, Li JQ, Jeck WR, Wang HN, Vo-Dinh T. miRNA probe integrated biosensor platform using bimetallic nanostars for amplification-free multiplexed detection of circulating colorectal cancer biomarkers in clinical samples. Biosens Bioelectron. 2023;220:114855.
114. Kaur S, Gupta N, Malhotra BD. Recent developments in wearable & non-wearable point-of-care biosensors for cortisol detection. Expert Rev Mol Diagn. 2023;23(3):217–30.
115. Haghayegh F, Norouziazad A, Haghani E, Feygin AA, Rahimi RH, Ghavamabadi HA, et al. Revolutionary point-of-care wearable diagnostics for early disease detection and biomarker discovery through intelligent technologies. Adv Sci. 2024;11(36):2400595.
116. Kaushik A, Mujawar MA. Point of care sensing devices: better care for everyone. Sensors. MDPI. 2018;18:4303.
117. Bhaiyya M, Panigrahi D, Rewatkar P, Haick H. Role of machine learning assisted biosensors in point-of-care-testing for clinical decisions. ACS Sens. 2024;9(9):4495–519.
118. Xu D, Huang X, Guo J, Ma X. Automatic smartphone-based microfluidic biosensor system at the point of care. Biosens Bioelectron. 2018;110:78–88.
119. Zhang M, Cui X, Li N. Smartphone-based mobile biosensors for the point-of-care testing of human metabolites. Mater Today Bio. 2022;14:100254.
120. Zhao W, Tian S, Huang L, Liu K, Dong L, Guo J. A smartphone-based biomedical sensory system. Analyst. 2020;145(8):2873–91.
121. Madrid RE, Ashur Ramallo F, Barraza DE, Chaile RE. Smartphone-based biosensor devices for healthcare: technologies, trends, and adoption by end-users. Bioengineering. 2022;9(3):101.
122. Tyagi AK, Richa KS. Smartphone-based sensors for biomedical applications. Artif Intell Blockchain Technol Digit Twin Smart Hosp. 2024:327–45.
123. Prabowo BA, Cabral PD, Freitas P, Fernandes E. The challenges of developing biosensors for clinical assessment: a review. Chemosensors. 2021;9(11):299.
124. Noreen S, Ishaq I, Saleem MH, Ali B, Muhammad Ali S, Iqbal J. Electrochemical biosensing in oncology: a review advancements and prospects for cancer diagnosis. Cancer Biol Ther. 2025;26(1):2475581.
125. Sen M, Seth S. Chapter 30 - Current challenges and future prospects of biosensors. In: Hasnain MS, Nayak AK, Aminabhavi TM, editors. Fundamentals of biosensors in healthcare [Internet]. Academic Press; 2025. p. 721–41. Available from: https://www.sciencedirect.com/science/article/pii/B9780443216589000085.
126. Kim ER, Joe C, Mitchell RJ, Gu MB. Biosensors for healthcare: current and future perspectives. Trends Biotechnol. 2023;41(3):374–95.
127. Goumas G, Vlachothanasi EN, Fradelos EC, Mouliou DS. Biosensors, artificial intelligence biosensors, false results and novel future perspectives. Diagnostics. 2025;15:1037.
128. Chatterjee N, Manna K, Mukherjee N, Das SK. Chapter 20 - Challenges and future prospects and commercial viability of biosensor-based devices for disease diagnosis. In: Khan R, Parihar A, Sanghi SK, editors. Biosensor based advanced cancer diagnostics [Internet]. Academic Press; 2022. p. 333–52. Available from: https://www.sciencedirect.com/science/article/pii/B9780128234242000132.
129. Yonet-Tanyeri N, Ahlmark BZ, Little SR. Advances in multiplexed paper-based analytical devices for cancer diagnosis: a review of technological developments. Adv Mater Technol [Internet]. 2021;6(8):2001138. Available from: https://doi.org/10.1002/admt.202001138.
130. Hao L, Zhao RT, Welch NL, Tan EKW, Zhong Q, Harzallah NS, et al. CRISPR-Cas-amplified urinary biomarkers for multiplexed and portable cancer diagnostics. Nat Nanotechnol [Internet]. 2023;18(7):798–807. Available from: https://doi.org/10.1038/s41565-023-01372-9.
131. Parums DV. Editorial: First regulatory approvals for CRISPR-Cas9 therapeutic gene editing for sickle cell disease and transfusion-dependent β-Thalassemia. Med Sci Monit. 2024;30:e944204.

132. Gray M, Meehan J, Ward C, Langdon SP, Kunkler IH, Murray A, et al. Implantable biosensors and their contribution to the future of precision medicine. Vet J [Internet]. 2018;239:21–9. Available from: https://www.sciencedirect.com/science/article/pii/S1090023318304180.
133. Singh A, Randive S, Breggia A, Ahmad B, Christman R, Amal S. Enhancing prostate cancer diagnosis with a novel artificial intelligence-based web application: synergizing deep learning models, multimodal data, and insights from usability study with pathologists. Cancers (Basel) [Internet]. 2023;15(23). Available from: https://www.mdpi.com/2072-6694/15/23/5659.
134. Shrivastava S, Trung TQ, Lee NE. Recent progress{,} challenges{,} and prospects of fully integrated mobile and wearable point-of-care testing systems for self-testing. Chem Soc Rev [Internet]. 2020;49(6):1812–66. Available from: https://doi.org/10.1039/C9CS00319C.
135. Hughes C, Sreenilayam SP, Afkham Y, Brabazon D. Emerging technology trends in point-of-care diagnostics. In: 2020 International Conference on Assistive and Rehabilitation Technologies (iCareTech); 2020. p. 109–14.
136. Ramesh M, Janani R, Deepa C, Rajeshkumar L. Nanotechnology-enabled biosensors: a review of fundamentals, design principles, materials, and applications. Biosensors [Internet]. 2023;13(1). Available from: https://www.mdpi.com/2079-6374/13/1/40.
137. Liao C, Wu Z, Lin C, Chen X, Zou Y, Zhao W, et al. Nurturing the marriages of urinary liquid biopsies and nano-diagnostics for precision urinalysis of prostate cancer. Smart Med. 2023;2(1):e20220020.
138. Saeidi Tabar F, Pourmadadi M, Yazdian F, Rashedi H, Rahdar A, Fathi-karkan S, et al. Ultrasensitive aptamer-based electrochemical nanobiosensor in diagnosis of prostate cancer using 2D:2D reduced graphene oxide/graphitic carbon nitride decorated with au nanoparticles. Eur J Med Chem Reports [Internet]. 2024;12:100192. Available from: https://www.sciencedirect.com/science/article/pii/S2772417424000645.
139. Sharifianjazi F, Jafari Rad A, Bakhtiari A, Niazvand F, Esmaeilkhanian A, Bazli L, et al. Biosensors and nanotechnology for cancer diagnosis (lung and bronchus, breast, prostate, and colon): a systematic review. Biomed Mater [Internet]. 2021;17(1):12002. Available from: https://doi.org/10.1088/1748-605X/ac41fd.
140. Chiou YE, Yu KJ, Pang SN, Yang YL, Pang ST, Weng WH. A highly sensitive urinary exosomal miRNAs biosensor applied to evaluation of prostate cancer progression. Bioengineering [Internet]. 2022;9(12). Available from: https://www.mdpi.com/2306-5354/9/12/803.
141. Roberts A, Gandhi S. A concise review on potential cancer biomarkers and advanced manufacturing of smart platform-based biosensors for early-stage cancer diagnostics. Biosens Bioelectron X [Internet]. 2022;11:100178. Available from: https://www.sciencedirect.com/science/article/pii/S2590137022000735.

Data Analysis from Biosensors by Artificial Intelligence and Machine Learning in the Detection of Prostate Cancer

10

Shriyansh Srivastava, Sakshi Patel, Subhashish Tripathy, and Mohd. Tariq

Abbreviations

AI	Artificial intelligence
cfDNA	Cell-free DNA
CNN	Convolutional neural network
CTC	Circulating tumor cell
DL	Deep learning
DRE	Digital rectal examination
FDA	Food and Drug Administration
fPSA	Free PSA
GDPR	General Data Protection Regulation
IoMT	Internet of Medical Things
k-NN	k-nearest neighbors
LASSO	Least absolute shrinkage and selection operator
LoC	Lab-on-a-chip

S. Srivastava
Department of Pharmacy, School of Medical and Allied Sciences, Galgotias University, Greater Noida, Uttar Pradesh, India

S. Patel
Department of Pharmaceutical Technology, Meerut Institute of Engineering & Technology, Meerut, Uttar Pradesh, India

S. Tripathy
BMS College of Pharmacy, Amethi, Tiloi, Uttar Pradesh, India

M. Tariq (✉)
Department of Academics, Sumandeep Vidyapeeth, Deemed to be University, Vadodara, Gujarat, India

Department of Biotechnology, Graphic Era (Deemed to be University), Dehradun, Uttarakhand, India

S. Srivastava et al. (eds.), *Biosensor Technologies for Prostate Cancer*, https://doi.org/10.1007/978-981-95-8644-8_10

miRNA	MicroRNA
ML	Machine learning
MRI	Magnetic resonance imaging
p2PSA	[−2]proPSA
PCA	Principal component analysis
PCA3	Prostate cancer antigen 3
PSA	Prostate-specific antigen
QCM	Quartz crystal microbalance
RF	Random forest
RFE	Recursive feature elimination
RNN	Recurrent neural network
SAW	Surface acoustic wave
SPR	Surface plasmon resonance
SVM	Support vector machine
TMPRSS2: ERG	Transmembrane protease, serine 2: ETS-related gene fusion
XAI	Explainable artificial intelligence

10.1 Introduction

Prostatic cancer follows breast cancer as the main health threat affecting men internationally, because it persists in growing in frequency, as elderly men now survive longer, and there is better cancer detection [1]. The GLOBOCAN 2024 report reveals that prostate cancer produces more than 1.6 million new cases each year, which places it at position two in cancer diagnoses and position five in cancer mortality among male patients (Table 10.1) [2]. Current advancements in screening and imaging have not solved the main scientific challenges because there are no dependable methods to identify early-stage aggressive or indolent prostate cancer without invasive procedures [3].

Standard prostate disease diagnostic tools, including prostate-specific antigen (PSA) testing and digital rectal examination (DRE), as well as biopsies, suffer from limitations, which include low test accuracy, high error rates, and possible incorrect diagnoses [5]. Patients suffer from high costs while experiencing unnecessary surgical procedures alongside psychological stress because of inadequate diagnostic procedures. A clinical urgency exists for improved diagnostics that are accurate, time-efficient, and user-friendly. Biosensors enable scientists to find solutions for current challenges while offering significant improvements in their techniques [6]. The detection devices with electrochemical or optical or nanomaterial transducing elements provide precise biomarker detection for prostate cancer through the analysis of PSA and

Table 10.1 Key epidemiological statistics for prostate cancer

Parameter	Statistic/value	References
Global incidence	Approximately 1.6 million new cases in 2024; projected to rise to 2.9 million by 2040	[4]
Leading cause of cancer death	The second leading cause of cancer-related death among men worldwide	[4]
Average age at diagnosis	Approximately 67 years	[4]
5-year survival rate	>98% (early stage), <30% (late stage)	[4]

prostate cancer antigen 3 (PCA3) together with microRNAs (miRNAs), exosomes, and circulating tumor DNA. Signal chips in modern biosensors have been reduced in size to create possibilities for medical testing at the patient's bedside, as well as for continuous patient observation [7]. New data challenges from biosensors lead to signal variability problems, as well as challenges in signal interpretation and signal-to-noise ratios [8]. Due to their importance, machine learning (ML) programs, along with artificial intelligence (AI) applications, prove indispensable for this task. Biosensor data becomes easier to analyze through ML methods, which discover patterns that are not readily apparent beyond regular analytic approaches [9]. Clinicians can use predictive analytics functionality to conduct ongoing progression surveillance through the integration of time-sensitive risk appraisal with ML/AI models. Advanced biosensors achieve performance enhancement when they incorporate support vector machines (SVMs), decision trees, and random forests (RFs), as well as convolutional neural networks (CNNs) and recurrent neural networks (RNNs) from deep learning (DL) frameworks. Explainable AI (XAI) frameworks serve as solutions to improve both the clinical trustworthiness of interpretable AI models and to handle their black box operations [10]. Healthcare providers must fulfill mandatory regulations from regulatory organizations about reporting medical choices through emerging technologies. The combination of biosensor technology with ML/AI transforms the way prostate cancer diagnosis operates in this setting. Such systems can detect prostate cancer early on and provide accurate diagnoses, tailoring treatment plans to individual needs, especially since early medical action has a direct impact on patient outcomes [11]. This chapter further explores the biosensors being used, along with data nature, together with AI implementation methods, which revolutionize contemporary prostate cancer detection and management practices. The integration of biosensor technologies with AI and ML enables a streamlined, real-time diagnostic process for prostate cancer from biological sampling to personalized decision support. A simplified overview of this workflow is illustrated in Fig. 10.1.

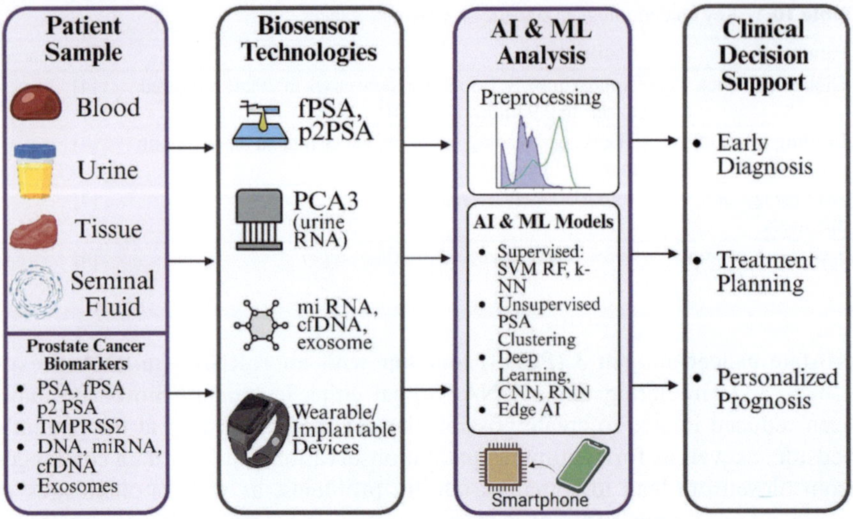

Fig. 10.1 Integrated workflow of biosensor-based prostate cancer diagnosis using AI and ML approaches

10.2 Biosensors for Prostate Cancer Detection

The application of biosensors for prostate cancer detection results in significant improvements to medical diagnostic systems, including early precise non-invasive methods [12]. Through biosensors, medical professionals gain permanent observation capabilities and unique patient health monitoring abilities that overcome traditional medical diagnostic systems. Biosensors of various types with their identified biomarkers are included in this section, along with design parameters and implementation challenges [13].

10.2.1 Classification of Biosensors for Prostate Cancer

Devices built as biosensors serve to identify biological molecules through signal conversion processes that produce electrical, optical, or mechanical signals for measurement [14]. The diagnosis of prostate cancer depends on biosensors to perform specific and sensitive tests of vital biomarkers present in biological fluids, which include blood, urine, and seminal plasma [15].

Designs of biosensors for prostate cancer detection are divided into two categories (Table 10.2), which describe their biological recognition elements along with transduction principles. The working principle of these biosensors relies on the classification system, which identifies their functionality while determining the diagnostic conditions they can address from early detection through monitoring of treatments [17].

Table 10.2 Comparison of biosensor types for prostate cancer

biosensor type	Detection principle	Biomarkers detected	Advantages	Limitations	References
Electrochemical	Current/ voltage	PSA, PCA3	High sensitivity, portable	Affected by environmental noise	[16]
Optical (SPR, fluorescence)	Light-based interaction	PCA3, miRNA, TMPRSS2: ERG	Label-free, real-time, multiplexing	Needs optical components	[16]
Mass-sensitive (QCM/SAW)	Frequency/ mass shift	Exosomes, PSA	Real-time interaction detection	Fragile, costly, sample-sensitive	[16]
Nano-biosensors	Nano-scale properties	miRNA, PSA, exosomes	Ultra-sensitive, LoC integration	Still in prototyping phase	[16]
Wearable/ implantable	Dynamic biomarkers in vivo	PSA, pH, metabolic markers	Continuous, remote monitoring	Power supply and biocompatibility	[16]

10.2.1.1 Electrochemical Biosensors

Electrochemical biosensors represent the most common diagnostic tool for cancer surveillance because they provide fast results at low costs with small physical dimensions and easy operation [18]. Biosensors detect target analytes through changes in electrical properties that lead to current changes detected with amperometric sensors and potential changes detected with potentiometric sensors, as well as impedance changes detected by impedimetric sensors. Prostate cancer diagnosis through biosensors commonly measures PSA levels because PSA stands as the most available, although controversial, biomarker that has limited accuracy [19]. The detection sensitivity alongside lower detection thresholds of these devices became possible by implementing gold nanoparticles (AuNPs) and graphene oxide with carbon nanotubes (CNTs) and conducting polymers. The detection of PSA reached femtomolar levels through the use of AuNPs in an electrode configuration, which generated better results than typical enzyme-linked immunosorbent assay (ELISA)-based testing. Single-stranded DNA or RNA aptamers serve as replacement elements for antibodies in aptamer-based electrochemical sensors to enhance stability with added benefits of reusability and improved functionalization [20]. Electrochemical sensors will integrate into compact mobile devices for real-time point-of-care (POC) diagnostics during the upcoming years particularly for underprivileged medical environments.

10.2.1.2 Optical Biosensors

The detection capabilities of optical biosensors include fluorescence and chemiluminescence, surface plasmon resonance (SPR), and interferometry, and they use light-based methods including colorimetry [21]. These biosensors offer high value because they detect substances in a real-time manner without destroying samples or requiring labels. Optical biosensors detect both PCA3 mRNA nucleic acids alongside exosomes, as well as the DNA mutations that include transmembrane protease, serine 2: ETS-related gene fusion (TMPRSS2: ERG) gene fusion, which occurs in about half of prostate cancer patients and indicates poor clinical outcomes [22]. The SPR-based biosensors deliver exceptional real-time kinetic analysis functions that make them suitable for their intended applications [21]. A sensor chip coated with gold allows scientists to detect biomarkers at high precision rates using prostate cancer-specific antibodies or aptamers immobilized on its surface in complex biological fluids such as urine and serum. Plasmonic nanorods made from gold serve as signal enhancement components when used to identify distinct miRNA biomarkers combined with epigenetic signatures at high levels of measurement accuracy [23]. Multi-analyte detection through multiplexing shows optical biosensors as an ideal solution for obtaining increased diagnostic confidence. The combination of biosensors and microfluidics systems and smartphone-based readers systems will fuel major advances in medical applications.

10.2.1.3 Mass-Sensitive Biosensors (e. g., QCM and SAW)

The detection using mass-sensitive biosensors relies on tracking modifications of mass and mechanical effects on sensors through platforms like quartz crystal microbalance (QCM) or surface acoustic wave (SAW). These platforms function by measuring frequency changes upon target molecule (PSA and exosome) binding to functionalized surfaces, which directly correlates with changes in surface mass [24]. Real-time interaction detection capabilities of the devices exist despite their sensitivity, while their adoption rate in clinical diagnostics remains slow because of sample preparation precision needs and high costs, combined with technical fragility issues. These devices provide important help for both research at universities and industries while studying biomolecular interactions, despite some practical implementation challenges [25]. Scientists today focus on developing smaller sensing instruments to integrate them into automated microfluidic platforms that suit medical diagnostics in the field [26]. Scientists are currently developing combination devices that unite mass detection methods with optical detection methods to create more powerful systems.

10.2.1.4 Nano-Biosensors and Lab-on-a-Chip Devices

The application of nanomaterial-based properties, such as large surface-to-volume area, quantum phenomena, and excellent conductance properties, improves biosensor performance. Different nano-biosensors utilize the properties of CNTs in addition to graphene, magnetic nanoparticles, quantum dots, dendrimers, and metal–organic frameworks [27]. Nano-biosensors have delivered high sensitivity capabilities for detecting PSA together with exosomal proteins and oncogenic miRNAs in prostate cancer cases. The graphene oxide-based field-effect transistor biosensor performs trace PSA and PCA3 detection by using exceptional sensitivity at attomolar concentration levels [28]. The lab-on-a-chip device unites three fields to run different diagnostic assays on small integrated systems through microfluidic technology and automatic systems. The device system needs small amounts of sample to function and generates results promptly. Accurate prostate cancer diagnosis depends on multiplex biomarker profiling; therefore, these devices prove perfect for this purpose because of the disease heterogeneity [29]. Total Laboratory of Chips platforms connect with AI/ML analytics systems, which support real-time health decisions directly at healthcare delivery points [30]. Several commercial startups, together with prototype devices, now exist to develop quick prostate cancer detection options for primary medical facilities [31].

10.2.1.5 Wearable and Implantable Biosensors

Future healthcare surveillance, along with continuous health monitoring, operates from the frontier of technology through wearable and implantable biosensors. Biosensors specifically perform dynamic biomarker monitoring through time to deliver understanding about tumor development, as well as disease relapse status and therapeutic effectiveness [32]. Biosensors available in wearable formats use skin patches, microneedle arrays, and smart tattoos, which perform biomarker analysis on fluids such as sweat and interstitial fluid, and through light transmission examination. Multiple biosensor prototypes apply fluorescence or electrochemical detection techniques to measure PSA and pH variations, which indicate tumor metabolism activities [33]. The placement of implantable biosensors occurs either beneath the skin surface or directly inside specific body organs. The devices enable continuous tumor-secreted protein and oxidative stress marker and extracellular pH monitoring, which supports precise therapy changes [34]. According to experimental research, scientists created an implantable microchip system to detect PSA levels while automatically delivering drugs beyond specific limits, thus enabling automated cancer treatment. This technology faces challenges related to regulatory approval and material safety standards, as well as power system limitations, but significant development of bioelectronic devices and wirelessly connected instruments and power self-sustaining sensors will enable its quick market growth [35].

10.2.2 Biomarkers Relevant to Prostate Cancer

The successful utilization of biosensors in prostate cancer diagnostics requires proper identification and implementation of dependable biomarkers that precisely indicate disease status and disease advancement [36]. Various biomarkers (Table 10.3) developed during the last two decades have increased diagnostic capabilities, thus outperforming traditional screening methods [37]. PSA stands as the primary serum biomarker that medical professionals utilize in their practice. PSA functions as a serine protease produced by prostate epithelial cells, yet increased PSA concentrations in blood frequently appear with prostate cancer but are not cancer-specific because benign prostatic hyperplasia, inflammation, and physical prostate contact can raise serum PSA levels [38]. The poor specificity of PSA testing has led researchers to evaluate related indicators, including free-to-total PSA ratio, along with PSA velocity, PSA density, and [−2] proPSA values. The advanced

Table 10.3 Key prostate cancer biomarkers and biosensor compatibility

Biomarker	Biological role	Sample source	Detection method	Clinical relevance	References
PSA	Serine protease, elevated in PCa	Blood	Electrochemical, ELISA	Primary screening biomarker	[42]
PCA3	Non-coding RNA, overexpressed in PCa	Urine	Optical, electrochemical	FDA-approved test, biopsy guide	[42]
TMPRSS2: ERG	Gene fusion, tumor progression	Urine	Optical, qPCR	Aggressive cancer indicator	[42]
miR-21, miR-141, miR-375	miRNAs, gene regulation	Blood, urine	Electrochemical, nano-biosensors	Subtyping, prognosis	[42]
Exosomes (with PCA3/ miRNA)	Tumor-derived vesicles	Blood, urine	SPR, microfluidic	Liquid biopsy, multiplex detection	[42]
cfDNA, CTCs	Tumor fragments/cells in circulation	Blood	Microfluidic, CRISPR	Mutation profiling, therapy guide	[42]

versions provide better risk assessment abilities, which help reduce both false diagnoses and unneeded biopsies when used alongside PSA measurements [39]. Non-coding RNA biomarkers represent an advanced solution that outperforms PSA specificity restrictions. The noncoding RNA PCA3 stands as a notable case of prostate cancer biomarkers because it shows intense overexpression within prostate cancer cell populations. PSA3 can identify itself in post-DRE urine specimens and delivers significantly superior detection performance compared to single PSA testing [40]. The PROGENSA PCA3 test with Food and Drug Administration (FDA) approval helps medical professionals determine additional prostate biopsy needs when patients show no signs of cancer, yet doctors remain concerned. Research has identified TMPRSS2: ERG gene fusion as a critical molecular target because it exists in almost 50% of prostate cancers, particularly affecting Western patients. The abnormal gene expression, which drives tumor progression, results from TMPRSS2 gene fusion with the oncogenic transcription factor ERG and the androgen-responsive TMPRSS2 gene [41]. The diagnostic performance of prostate cancer screening using urine samples becomes more precise through the combined analysis of the TMPRSS2: ERG mRNA marker with PCA3.

Scientific research now recognizes miRNAs as effective gene expression controllers that have the potential to function as non-invasive biomarkers. Research has established that prostate cancer development, as well as progression and metastatic spread, can be tracked through malfunctions in the expression patterns of miR-21 and the miR-141 and miR-375 miRNAs [43]. Multiple biological fluids, such as blood, urine, and seminal plasma, contain these molecules, providing strong options for liquid biopsy diagnostic methods. The easy integration of these molecules into modern biosensing systems is facilitated by their stability during circulation and their small structural size because they function with electrochemical and fluorescence-based biosensors, which perform single-nucleotide analyses [44]. Biosensors developed at an advanced level detect multiple miRNAs to create precise molecular profiles for characterizing prostate cancer subtypes and phenotypes. Exosomes, as nanoscale extracellular vesicles secreted by all cell types, have gained attention because they contain tumor-derived biomolecules such as proteins together with DNA and RNA. The isolation of exosomes from both urine and blood samples reveals that these vesicles contain significant biomarkers such as PCA3, TMPRSS2: ERG, together with specific miRNAs [45]. Due to their protected lipid bilayer membrane, exosomes represent reliable entities for diagnostic procedures that avoid invasive procedures. Researchers are developing numerous biosensor platforms with the capability to separate and analyze exosomes that incorporate optical detection capabilities, electrochemical methods, or membrane affinity detection systems. Such systems enable immediate molecular analysis with tiny sample amounts that advance personal medical strategies for treating prostate cancer [46]. The combination of circulating tumor cells (CTCs) together with cell-free DNA (cfDNA) stands as powerful biomarkers, which demonstrate strong potential to identify prostate cancer. CTCs indicate their link to metastasis through the metastasis of tumor cells into the bloodstream, while cfDNA shows the DNA fragments from deteriorating tumor cells that feature mutations such as changes in the androgen receptor variant (e.g., AR-V7) [47]. Manufacturing of microfluidic devices and the use of CRISPR-detection systems enable liquid biopsy platforms using biosensors to enhance their detection ability for both CTCs and cfDNA. Clinical research presents increased interest in three emerging biomarkers made up of sarcosine and kallikrein-related peptidases (KLK2/3), with gene methylation markers (such as GSTP1) among them [48]. The development of prostate cancer disease follows two key long non-coding RNAs named PCAT-1 and Scheme LAP1. The combination of biomarkers with automated biosensing systems and advanced ML data analysis brings revolutionary potential to prostate cancer diagnosis by enabling proactive precision-medicine strategies [49].

10.2.3 Sensor Design, Signal Processing, and Sensitivity

Different design aspects, together with operational specifications, determine how biosensors perform their functions in real-world diagnostic applications [50]. During development, the individual components of biosensors influence measurement quality by deciding how effectively they detect biomarkers linked to prostate cancer.

10.2.3.1 Surface Functionalization

Designing efficient sensors demands proper surface functionalization as the most important operational step. The surface of the sensor requires modification with special recognition elements to achieve proper biomolecule binding while reducing nonspecific attachments. Surface attachment of biological recognition elements, including antibodies and aptamers, also incorporates DNA/RNA probes, which are installed onto the sensor surface [51]. The target biomarkers react with recognition elements from the sensor, which generates detectable signals. Medical practitioners commonly employ antibodies binding specifically to PSA as well as PCA3 in prostate cancer diagnostic procedures [52]. Improper functionalization of sensor surfaces restricts both the specificity rate and sensitivity because it enhances biomolecule binding and blocks nonspecific binding contaminants. The optimization of biomarker interaction must be performed at suitable levels to achieve successful detection of target biomarkers while lowering diagnosis errors [53].

10.2.3.2 Nanomaterial Integration

Sensor technology experienced its most important advancement with the integration of nanomaterials into biosensors. Nanoparticles, including graphene alongside AuNPs and CNTs, bring three essential advantages to sensors: their large surface-to-volume ratio and their enhanced electrical capability, together with their ability to improve electron transfer in devices [54]. Sensor performance experiences significant enhancement due to the addition of these materials, which improves both signal-to-noise performance and biomolecule binding throughout the sensor process [55]. The biomolecular binding strength of sensors improves because AuNPs deliver additional surface space, which increases interaction opportunities between target molecules, and sensors become more sensitive [56]. The sensor achieves enhanced response time and accuracy using graphene, as this material exhibits high electrical conductivity and electron mobility. The sensor functions better when these materials are added to its design, which lowers the detection limitations so doctors can identify prostate cancer biomarkers at earlier stages, regardless of concentration levels [57].

10.2.3.3 Miniaturization and Portability

Biosensors become more practical when miniaturization techniques are used for applications involving POC [58]. When multiple operational features join within small compact devices, they become simpler to implement for clinical or remote applications. Microfabrication techniques that use microfluidics enabled scientists to design extremely portable and miniature biosensors [59]. Through recent advancements, researchers have achieved multiplexing by detecting different biomarkers in one single sample without using big and costly laboratory machines. Prostate cancer screening technology combines portable biosensors capable of delivering quick results to patients through POC testing, which substitutes the requirement of using invasive diagnostic methods [60]. Veterans in remote areas along with underserved regions, can benefit from the openness of these devices since diagnostic laboratory facilities are scarce in their region.

10.2.3.4 Signal Processing

Biosensor data interpretation must be precise because it determines the dependability of the diagnostic result. Biosensor outputs through electrical signals and emissions or physical data need strong processing methods to reveal useful information from their raw data [61]. Background noise elimination through baseline correction and weak signal amplification, and various signal processing techniques, allows users to recognize authentic signals from the surrounding noise [62]. Biosensor-generated complex data needs the application of advanced analytical methods, including AI and ML, to establish patterns in multidimensional datasets [63]. AI-based algorithms enhance medical diagnostics by enabling the review of extensive datasets for pattern identification and outcome prediction. Biosensors achieve precise and usable outcomes thanks to these techniques, especially when biomarkers exist at minimal concentration levels [64].

10.2.4 Challenges in Biosensor Data Handling and Interpretation

Multiple challenges prevent the full implementation of biosensor technologies due to significant hurdles regarding data analysis, medical applications, and interpretation issues. The requirements of standardization, together with biological complexity and complex analytics needs, hinder the implementation of biosensor platforms [65].

10.2.4.1 Data Variability and Noise

All biological samples exhibit high levels of complexity due to their often-extensive variations. Sensor readings come with noise brought on by biological heterogeneity and interacting factors, including sample composition and environmental conditions, which generate variations that potentially harm the accuracy of results [66]. During patient sample analysis, biosensor readings can become inaccurate because proteins, lipids, and numerous metabolites present in the samples will mask or distort sensor data signals, thereby delivering incorrect positive or negative results [67]. Research biomarker measurements become complex because the use of these products introduces unpredictable changes. Multiple issues can be solved through the development of standardized procedures for sample collection, data processing, and sensor calibration. Biosensor platforms become more reliable when integrated with both internal controls and reference biomarkers to detect and fix performance variations, thus improving their result consistency [68].

10.2.4.2 Standardization Issues

The general medical market rejects biosensor clinical implementation because different platforms employ inconsistent procedural standards. Each biosensor application features unique productive procedures, calibration methods, and interpretation techniques that differ notably from scientific investigations to commercial applications [69]. This variability between research studies and clinical use makes study result comparison challenging because it affects replication success. The process of obtaining wider regulatory approval needs standard protocols for biosensor operations [70]. Studies guarantee that sensors work consistently across all clinical settings. Additionally, it requires standard development protocols for sensors and data interpretation standards and calibration requirements for sensors.

10.2.4.3 Complex Biological Interactions

The sensor surface of biosensors shows non-specific binding behavior as additional biomolecules besides target molecules will attach themselves [71]. Two effects that result from this condition lead to incorrect sensor detection and decrease sensor sensitivity. The analysis of biological samples becomes difficult because of matrix effects, which occur when diverse biological elements interfere with data measurement equipment [72]. The high complexity of urine and blood samples makes these biological materials expose sensor devices to many molecular interactions and reduces the readability of target biomarker signals [73]. Sensor specificity can be improved through the development of enhanced surface functionalization techniques that use aptamers or antibody fragments, since these elements demonstrate strong specific biomarker binding properties. Compatibility intense diagnostic information emerges from detection systems utilizing multiple sensors while tracking several biomarkers, thus reducing the effects of biological complexity in samples [74].

10.2.4.4 Need for Advanced Analytics

Data produced by biosensing methods becomes challenging to analyze through conventional methods because it generates extensive amounts that require sophisticated analytics for interpretation [75]. The statistical analysis methods lack the necessary capacity to process combined datasets of several detected biomarkers and intricate signal patterns over time. Due to its vast quantity, ML algorithms and sophisticated AI systems must be used to extract relevant information from the data [76]. This toolset examines enormous datasets to identify valuable patterns that researchers use for producing specific outcome predictions based on the acquired biomarkers [77]. Standard AI algorithms use PSA measurement as well as imaging results alongside genetic markers to determine whether prostate cancer is benign or malignant. Through their analysis tools, these systems enhance both medical diagnostic accuracy and create personalized treatment plans and foresee treatment results [78].

10.2.4.5 Clinical Translation and Validation

The effective clinical implementation of biosensors faces tremendous challenges because of an ongoing problem between laboratory discoveries and the needs of clinical use [79]. Many promising biosensor technologies demonstrate research and preclinical performance yet need extensive validation work, together with regulatory certification and clinical value demonstration, before becoming clinical products [80]. Biomedical devices need thorough clinical testing for evaluating their precision as well as dependability, in addition to safety parameters, during actual healthcare operations. The diagnostic tools need to fulfill standards determined by the FDA and European Medicines Agency (EMA) before becoming officially available for clinical work [81]. Both accurate and affordable accessibility to wide healthcare settings must be demonstrated through successful cost-effectiveness studies as part of clinical validation measures [82].

10.3 Data Characteristics and Preprocessing

The so-called smart diagnostics era benefits from biosensors that are redefining both prostate cancer detection and its monitoring methods. Biosensors function in the medical field now as diagnostic allies that analyze volatility data streams to reveal tiny biological patterns that human vision cannot detect [83]. These powerful monitoring systems generate information that researchers may find disorganized and inconsistent, along with being filled with noise. Those tiny devices need appropriate data treatment methods to reveal their full potential. Different types of biosensors, including electrochemical, optical, microfluidic, and image-based, generate specific data expressions. Real-time PSA detectors generate voltage outputs through short millisecond periods [84]. An optical biosensor should produce multidimensional fluorescence spectral information when detecting PCA3 or TMPRSS2: ERG targets present in urine. The latest platforms merge several detection modes (Fig. 10.2) to create complicated combined datasets. A data science practitioner would view this system as simultaneously beneficial and dangerous [85]. The raw data outputs exist as Comma-Separated Values (CSV), Hierarchical Data Format version 5 (HDF5), and Tagged Image File Format (TIFF) files, but managing their content proves even more complex, as it contains signal drift combined with baseline changes and environmental disturbances, along with biological variations. The readings in urine testing will be altered when patients become dehydrated or when testing room temperatures deviate from standard conditions [86]. Trying to detect vital cancer biomarkers leads to the discovery of false results because of electromagnetic interference spikes. Preprocessing functions as the essential solution for resolving this challenge.

10.3.1 Taming the Chaos: Cleaning and Structuring the Data

Machines require cleaned signal data before they can analyze biosensor information. The cleaning process includes digital dust removal to preserve essential disease patterns,

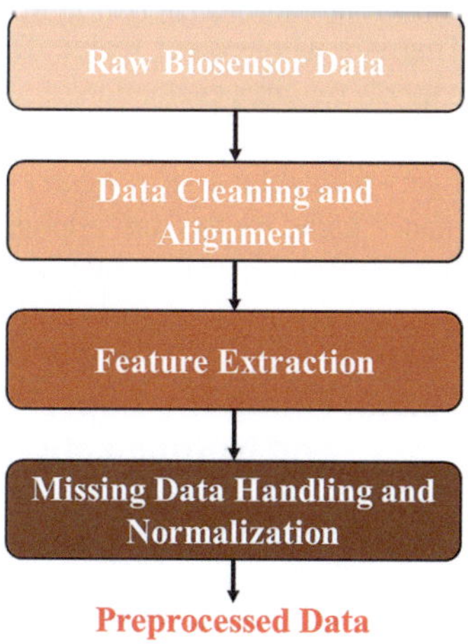

Fig. 10.2 Data preprocessing pipeline for biosensor data

as well as the removal of irrelevant signal noise [87]. The decomposition process of noise from signals becomes easier through wavelet transforms, which work through multiple levels. Through Savitzky-Golay filtering techniques, significant peaks remain intact when the algorithm smooths sudden signal variations. An exponential smoothing method, combined with polynomial fitting, enables the recovery of the original signal that remains unaffected by background drifts. The cleaning process for biosensor data does not eliminate every surprise from the original signals. Training algorithms become damaged when outliers appear, which are created by electrical blips or sample contamination [88]. The data assessment process becomes smoother through the application of Isolation Forest and Density-Based Spatial Clustering of Applications with Noise (DBSCAN) algorithms, which remove unorthodox data entries. There exists another essential concern that impacts the data collection process. Multiple biosensors need their data collection periods to match precisely for parallel operations. System alignment through dynamic time warping lets signals of differing timestamps integrate perfectly until their peak and valley patterns match, regardless of temporal mismatch. The system encounters issues when sensor versions exhibit calibration differences due to changes in environmental conditions between days [89]. All these need normalizations. Biological data processing techniques in modern research assure that researchers evaluate genuine biological signals rather than instrument-generated measurement fluctuations.

10.3.2 Extracting the Gold: Turning Signals Into Features

Now the data becomes ready to provide insights following the taming procedures. A biosensor signals the transition into machine-readable features during the stage of feature extraction, before machines apply predictions. Different signal features, including basic statistical properties and complex frequency transforms of data, exist between each data point that share specific information. Physical signals that measure enzyme kinetics require analysis of their rising times and falling slopes, and peak areas to capture the biochemical interaction between the analyzing molecules and sensor properties [90]. Measurable signal energies point at wavelet coefficient frequencies, which expose underlying cancer indications in spectral data. And in image-based sensors? That is a whole other realm. The discrimination between benign and malignant cell patterns requires evaluation of features that include texture patterns, shape characteristics, sharp edge definition, and deep features acquired through CNN extraction [91]. Every parameter does not carry an equivalent value. Model and computational performance gains result from applying Least Absolute Shrinkage and Selection Operator (LASSO) along with mutual information to select relevant features within the data [92].

10.3.3 Filling the Gaps: Handling Missing Data and Normalization

The performance of biosensor systems operating in real-world conditions never meets absolute perfection levels. Missing data points mostly result from power incidents, obstructed fluid streams, or random system failures [93]. The method to address missing data points depends on the situation and includes statistical filling by mean or median and k-nearest neighbor (k-NN)-based similarity techniques, along with predictive MICE approaches for missing value completion [94]. Time-series data interpolation through splines and predictive models employing Kalman filters produces very accurate recreations of absent information sections [95]. The goal? This data system needs to generate uninterrupted trustworthy results that precisely represent biological facts [96]. Annihilation of all disparities stands as the last step. The model performance remains unaltered when variables possess different measurement units through Z-score normalization. Uniform value compression is the main objective of min-max scaling. Identical interpretation results are achieved across different hardware setups due to histogram equalization and color deconvolution techniques for image data.

10.3.4 Wrapping Up: From Chaos to Clinical Clarity

Biosensor-generated data is naturally difficult to control, and this situation does not imply that it has no value. A well-built pipeline consisting of cleaning, denoising, alignment, enrichment, and normalization of data transforms disorder into structured information [97]. The foundation steps of cancer diagnostics will gain new importance, while we aim to develop real-time AI diagnostics for cancer. Clean data does not define the sole purpose of preprocessing [98]. The process of respecting biological principles entails both understanding technological capabilities and creating conditions that enable algorithms to produce accurate life-saving results.

10.4 ML for Biosensor Data Analysis

The true power of biosensor data emerges when the data processing work finishes, since algorithmic intervention from ML programs (Table 10.4) enables humans to see biological signals beyond human perceptual limits [99]. The signals processed by ML produce diagnostic knowledge which enables predictions about disease existence, together with disease development and reaction to treatments [100]. Achieving valuable results from biosensor outputs requires a proper selection of algorithms alongside complete clarity about their working principles. The following discussion outlines different ML methods that process biosensor data, starting with supervised classifiers and continuing to unsupervised pattern seekers, ensemble powerhouses, and success metrics [101].

10.4.1 Supervised Learning Algorithms: SVM, RF, K-NN, and More

Biosensor diagnostics use supervised learning as its analytical base when datasets contain proper labels. The SVM algorithm creates exact boundary definitions that help distinguish cancerous signals from non-cancerous ones in complex data domains

Table 10.4 AI and ML techniques for biosensor data

Model type	Examples	Best suited for	Advantages	References
Supervised ML	SVM, RF, k-NN	PSA classification, subtype prediction	High accuracy with labeling data	[109]
Unsupervised ML	K-means, DBSCAN, PCA	Biomarker pattern discovery, feature grouping	No labels required, pattern discovery	[110]
Dl	CNNs, RNNs, DNNs	Image/signal analysis, time-series data	Learns complex patterns automatically	[111]
Ensemble models	RF, boosting, stacking	Handling biological variation, improving recall	Improved robustness and accuracy	[107]

[102]. The voting mechanism of RF utilizes multiple decision trees to extract robust and noise-resistant outputs, while k-NN bases its decision-making on policies for new examples using known classifications. The lightweight and interpretable models, including logistic regression together with Naïve Bayes, remain excellent choices for limited resources in specific environments [103]. Such methods succeed with organized datasets that align perfectly with clinical biosensor information systems that prioritize precise diagnostic outcomes. Supervised learning models achieve clinical clarity along with predictive accuracy when used with care by medical staff.

10.4.2 Unsupervised Learning for Pattern Discovery and Biomarker Exploration

Unsupervised learning approaches the problem when there is a lack of available dataset labels. K-means clustering and DBSCAN produce groups of biosensor data that can discover unknown disease variants as well as biomarker signatures in naturally occurring ways. High-dimensional data becomes more visualizable and detectable of anomalies through two techniques, namely, principal component analysis (PCA) and autoencoders [104]. Through DL technology, t-Distributed Stochastic Neighbor Embedding (t-SNE) provides users with visual data relationships that show delicate connections between points. The approach delivers substantial value to biosensor analysis during early stages of biomarker scouting or exploration of unknown diagnostic fields.

10.4.3 Feature Selection and Dimensionality Reduction: RFE, LASSO, PCA, and More

The raw data obtained from biosensors contains numerous elements, where some elements will be useful, but others prove useless. Selection methods alongside reduction techniques assist in clearing the data noise. Recursive feature elimination (RFE) and

LASSO manage both feature prediction and feature reduction through an optimal variable selection process [105]. Features selected based on statistical relevance by mutual information and Analysis of Variance (ANOVA) measures, along with PCA/LDA techniques, minimize dimensions without losing meaning from the original data structure. The payoff? A leaner, faster, and more interpretable model exists, which maintains its high accuracy level across diverse sets of patients alongside multiple sensor conditions [106].

10.4.4 Ensemble Learning Techniques: Bagging, Boosting, and Stacking

The problem of insufficient single-model performance leads ensemble techniques to take charge. RFs implement bagging by creating several predictive models, combining their averaged results to prevent overfitting. Among boosting methods, XGBoost enhances prediction accuracy sequentially by addressing past mistakes to achieve powerful performance in complex data [107]. Stacking creates meta-learning by combining multiple models to produce judgments from diverse perspectives. Ensemble learning enables reliable biosensor diagnostics that actively address biological variations and mitigate sensor drift problems [108].

10.4.5 Model Evaluation Metrics: Accuracy, Precision, Recall, Receiver Operating Characteristic - Area Under the Curve (ROC-AUC), and Confusion Matrix

No ML model is complete without rigorous evaluation. *Accuracy* gives a general idea of performance, but in imbalanced datasets (like early cancer detection), metrics such as *Precision* and *Recall* are more telling, indicating how well true positives are identified versus false alarms [112]. The *F1 Score* balances both, while *ROC-AUC* quantifies the model's ability to distinguish between classes. A detailed *Confusion Matrix* reveals strengths and blind spots in predictions. For clinical deployment, these metrics are not just numbers but they also represent trust, safety, and informed decisions for patients [113].

10.4.6 ML as the Diagnostic Brain of Biosensor Systems

ML serves as the main procedure that converts biosensor data into actionable medical knowledge [114]. ML systems empower biosensors by enabling them to execute diagnoses and make predictions, which in turn support clinical decision-making processes. The evolution of biosensors relies on ML, as it enables the processing of biological information through individual data points [115].

10.5 AI and DL Techniques

Traditional ML becomes nonsuited due to the high-scale biosensor data points containing time-series signals alongside microscopic images. AI with DL represents the new model generation, which generates systems through the replication of human brain learning mechanisms, perception abilities, and memory pathways [116]. This section evaluates modern, top-of-the-line techniques that utilize both deep neural systems and XAI to enhance biosensor diagnostics capabilities.

10.5.1 Deep Neural Networks and Their Application

Deep neural network (DNNs) operate as vital components of modern-day AI, making it possible to analyze challenging biosensor data properly. The human brain tissue arrangement gets replicated in sophisticated neural networks that use various linked nodes to evolve higher-level data characteristics from basic inputs [117]. The implementation of direct DNNs operates on biosensor information to extract features from electrical signals, as well as optical intensity data and multi-parameter results before performing analysis without human involvement. The neural networks handle high-dimensional inputs and noise effectively because their design structure supports superior performance in these operational environments. Training of DNN systems enables them to learn the ability to identify prostate cancer status from combined biosensor measurement datasets [118]. The diagnostic models provide reliable solutions for multiple sensor systems, supporting high accuracy while processing a variety of sensing data types. Clinical information integration is possible through age combination with PSA level and genetic marker variables, allowing individualized medical assessment.

10.5.2 CNNs for Signal/Image-Based Biosensor Data

CNNs represent specialized DNNs that revolutionized computer vision before they started transforming biosensor data processing, particularly when the data has image or structured signal map formats [119]. CNNs possess the ability to discover spatial relationships in data, thereby allowing them to detect key patterns within biosensor-generated outputs, which include 2D fluorescence microscopy images, electrochemical signal heatmaps, and also reshapable spectral curves [119]. CNN models determine prostate cancer diagnostic indicators through their analysis of biosensor microscope cellular images, as well as their analysis of biomarker distribution patterns on microfluidic platforms. Their multi-layered structure helps detectors analyze basic elements such as edges and curves and complex tissue forms, which prove essential for determining between benign and malignant tissue samples [120]. The diagnostic process becomes faster, and human errors decrease as CNNs both improve visual analysis automation and refine their understanding through self-learning from the processed data.

10.5.3 Recurrent Networks for Time-Series Biosensor Data

Biomarker level variations that are time-dependent require RNNs and their improved version, long short-term memory (LSTM) networks, for effective performance [121]. RNNs contain an integrated memory operation that sustains contextual data between several time steps to assist sequential input processing. Diagnostics and monitoring devices based on biosensors automatically perform amplitude detection and abnormal event identification and produce future trend predictions using their analysis of historical measurement data [122]. The LSTM model predicts prostate cancer relapse by analyzing biosensor-derived data on inflammatory markers and hormonal levels. Static information collections alone cannot detect continuous modifications and sudden spikes, but the networks execute this function better than human analysts. RNNs function as diagnostic prediction tools because their dynamic input system gives healthcare solutions future-oriented capabilities that extend past routine responses [123].

10.5.4 Transfer Learning and Federated Learning in Healthcare

Ample medical data collection becomes difficult for institutions as expert XXXlabeling work requires payment, and patients demand confidentiality for their medical information. On a large scale, both transfer learning and federated learning prove themselves as appropriate solutions [124]. Pre-educated models that have trained on extensive repositories can use transfer learning processes to adapt their operations to smaller datasets from specific domains. This method shortens biosensor data training durations so that the system becomes more effective in cancer type work and rare biomarker identification [125]. The training operations within feder ated learning allow source institutions to retain full authority over their data through local processing without data exchange. After performing training operations at research facilities and medical institutions as separate locations, the acquired model parameters from these sites merge into a universal aggregated model. Effective patient data security and institutional data protection occur through this method, which enables collaborative work without compromising health records privacy. Complex AI solutions become possible through the integration of transfer learning with federated learning for hospital deployments across institutions that have limited data and privacy risks [126].

10.5.5 XAI and Interpretability in Medical AI

Medical staff must trust AI systems more than ever since these systems are starting to become deeply integrated into clinical operations. XAI offers a solution to this issue by producing accessible explanations about the internal functions of complex models for both clinicians and researchers [127]. The high-risk cancer diagnostic setting requires more than a black-box approach due to its potential to modify life-course treatments. Using XAI techniques enables users to track the diagnostic process of a model through the identification of crucial features in addition to signal regions or image segments that shaped its predictive outcome. Heatmaps generated through XAI show physicians which image sections led to positive or negative results in CNN analyses of biosensor-produced images [128]. The attention mechanisms enable time-series models to identify crucial durations of time which helped predict disease outbreaks. The generated biological insights through XAI both authenticate the AI model's computational process and provide novel vital signs about disease classifications and human genetics. The implementation of XAI successfully connects automated decisions with human understanding, which leads to the ethical deployment of AI in medical diagnostic systems.

10.6 Integration of Multi-Modal Data Sources

Standard healthcare practices in precision medicine require multiple data sources to comprehend the complete picture of a disease. Simple diagnosis of prostate cancer requires integrating diverse data sources such as biosensors and clinical reports with genomic information, imaging results, and more [129]. The process of linking multiple data types, named multi-modal data integration, provides stronger diagnostic abilities that permit personalized care and lead healthcare toward all-encompassing approaches [130]. The current state of ML and AI makes it possible to unite separate datasets into whole and smart analytical models that mimic the approach doctors use to integrate all medical information for diagnostic purposes.

10.6.1 Combining Biosensor Data with Clinical and Genomic Data

Biosensors deliver critical physiological information about hormones and enzymes and electrical signals, yet their clinical value becomes exponential when medical data from tests and genomic data from gene sequences and DNA changes are added to the analysis [131]. The combination of PSA detection through biosensor technology with genomic risk variants assessment and patient medical records allows doctors to predict both cancer diagnosis and metastasis risk levels. By employing this approach, ML models gain the ability to view disease biological signatures within the complete framework of patient medical profiling alongside genetic risk profiles [132]. The method converts basic detection into an understanding based on multiple components, which improves forecasting and therapeutic response and disease tracking capabilities. Integrated research frameworks facilitate researchers to reveal genotype-phenotype correlations that remained hidden when data remained separate.

10.6.2 Data Fusion Strategies: Early, Intermediate, and Late Fusion

The process of uniting multiple data types requires significant effort. The three categories of biosensor signals alongside clinical text documents and genomic sequences maintain individual structural elements with distinct scales and noise characteristics throughout the system. The process requires data fusion strategies to work effectively [133]. Early fusion performs a singular input space consolidation of unprocessed research data prior to ML model processing. However, the normalization process should be performed with attention during execution because it serves best for time or space synchronized datasets [134]. The intermediate fusion technique in DL creates separate sub-networks for each data kind (clinical data and sensor readings) before combining their learned representations at a central processing point. The method lets each data source maintain individual interpretation understanding until it creates a joint predictive output. The late fusion method constructs independent models for different modalities after which their results can be merged using voting methods, averaged, or with a new prediction system [135]. The method enables analysis when data collection runs asynchronously while handling values that may be missing. Early fusion presents advantages for detecting low-level relationships at the same time intermediate fusion offers balanced complexity combined with synergy between the streams, while late fusion maintains independent processing modules. The combination of several approaches is typically employed during biosensor system implementation to merge information (Fig. 10.3) between wearable tech data and electronic health records and genomic analysis results [136].

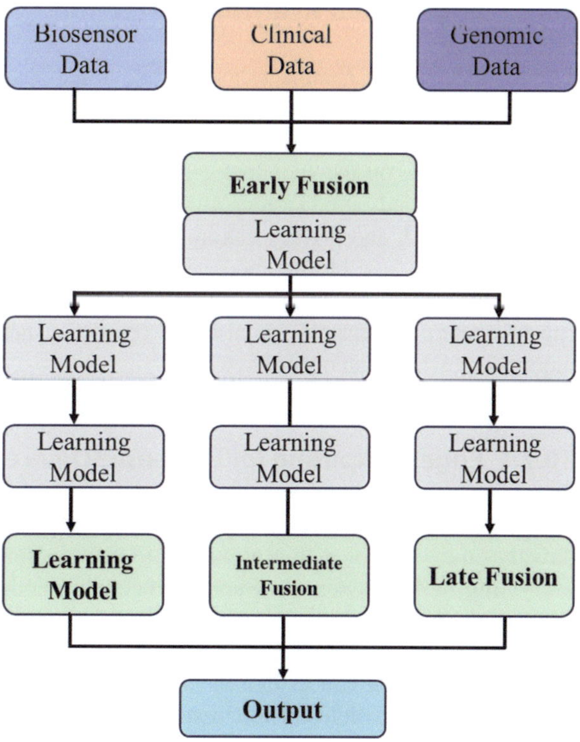

Fig. 10.3 Fusion strategies in multi-modal learning

10.6.3 Case Studies Using Multi-Modal ML Models

The healthcare field adopts multi-modal ML technology to transform how healthcare professionals work in their daily practice [137]. Medical researchers have combined biosensor-detected proteomic patterns with magnetic resonance imaging (MRI) imaging data and patient genomics through models that predict prostate cancer tumor grades exceptionally well [138]. The research combined a DL model containing separate branches for different data types, where biosensor signals entered a CNN network parallel to a dense network handling clinical parameters and then sending genomic features through an attention module before producing a combined diagnostic performance. The result? The predictive model bettered standard single-modality systems because it achieved superior performance in both sensitivity detection and specificity identification [139]. Clinical recovery plans for patients after surgery benefit from the combination of wearable biosensor readings with patient feedback and drug resistance markers, which guide their treatment process. Such models used in clinical trials enable the identification of early signs of relapse by identifying subtle biosensor variations that appear before clinical symptoms develop. The fuser technology creates analytical power beyond accuracy improvement because it enables novel capabilities for dynamic risk assessment and real-time therapeutic performance feedback while providing extended monitoring capabilities [140].

10.7 Edge AI and Real-Time Detection

The advancement of healthcare toward individual-based care depends on the integration of Edge AI (Fig. 10.4) technology with biosensor platforms, which provides a progressive method to diagnose and monitor prostate cancer efficiently [141]. Edge AI provides on-the-spot device-based complex biosensor data analysis instead of using only cloud-based systems for processing. Device-to-data processing speeds have accelerated, and privacy has improved while system reliability has strengthened, making it suitable for medical diagnostic and wearable usages [142]. The combination of biosensors and microprocessors enabled by AI technology develops capabilities to transform hospital-based reactive cancer tests into personal health monitoring, which can occur anywhere.

10.7.1 Edge Computing for Biosensor Devices

Edge computing describes the process that performs biosensor data collection directly on devices or within proximity to information sources instead of sending everything to distant servers. Such a processing method becomes essential when addressing medically sensitive latency data, including PSA levels and biomarker spikes that signal tumor advancement or disease recurrence [143]. A diagnostic kit holding the prostate cancer biosensor grants real-time biochemical analysis capabilities on-site and delivers test results instantly, ignoring the need for Internet

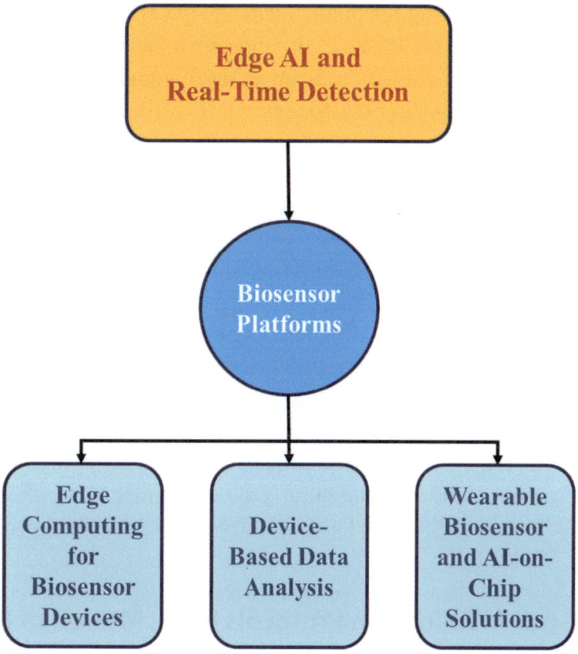

Fig. 10.4 Edge AI-enabled biosensor system for real-time prostate cancer monitoring

access. These architectures implement AI models that have been optimized to run with minimal power consumption on embedded devices that include Raspberry Pi, as well as NVIDIA Jetson Nano and microcontrollers with Tensor Processing Unit / Neural Processing Unit (TPU/NPUs) [144]. The device-based location of data storage provides improved patient data safety by isolating complete information from external networks.

10.7.2 Wearable Biosensors and AI-on-Chip Solutions

Wearable biosensors, when combined with AI-on-chip technologies, deliver the most revolutionary developments at present [145]. Microscopic devices, insertable into smartwatches, patches, or clothing, function to detect prostate cancer biomarkers such as PSA, PCA3, or miRNA in interstitial fluids, blood, and sweat samples. Medical biosensors now combine with Edge TPU AI chips from Google, along with Intel Movidius processors and specific application-specific integrated circuits that complete tasks, including pattern detection, signal processing, and anomaly identification, while staying inside the device [146]. The cooperative operation of software with hardware systems enables uninterrupted health tracking capabilities, eliminating the need for bulky medical testing devices. Modern medical devices continue to advance in intelligence and power efficiency, which allows their deployment in remote healthcare services for patients who need constant monitoring without needing hospital-based care [147]. Research indicates that advanced cancer surveillance systems will use biosensors with AI and communication components in one compact element to form an intelligent disease surveillance system always running and acquiring knowledge while available for all [148].

10.8 Validation, Clinical Trials, and Regulatory Aspects

The swift development of AI-driven biosensors requires rigorous testing and standard trial integration, and must strictly fulfill ethical and regulatory prerequisites for clinical application [149]. Medical organizations require clear verification of safety, along with effectiveness and reproducibility, before implementing a model, despite its accuracy. Stringent clinical evaluations must exist for prostate cancer diagnosis because the consequences of wrong diagnosis and improper treatment or detection remain high [150]. This section examines the steps for deploying AI biosensor models through rigorous validation research protocols, integrating them into trial procedures, and achieving global regulatory approval for operational use in clinical conditions.

10.8.1 Validation Protocols for AI Models in Healthcare

The initial step to gain trust in AI-driven biosensor tools is validation. Healthcare AI systems require clinical verification with patients of diverse types who utilize AI across multiple settings, unlike standard consumer models. Model validation implements a sequential three-part procedure [151]. The single dataset includes three validation strategies for baseline assessment: training/testing splits, cross-validation, and bootstrapping. Insights about model generalizability are obtained when performing external validation by analyzing an independent dataset that originates from different institutions and geographic regions. The model receives new unseen clinical data points in real time through a live laboratory or clinical environment during prospective validation. Performance metrics, including sensitivity and specificity, as well as ROC-AUC measures and precision-recall scores, and F1 score, require calculation before they can be checked against established clinical benchmarks [152]. During validation, the use of explainability tools, including SHAP and LIME, becomes essential to disclose model-driven choices, thus aiding clinician trust and model enhancement. The validation process for biosensors requires co-validation between biosensor hardware and software components to confirm their shared performance under different environmental and biological conditions.

10.8.2 Clinical Trial Integration of AI-Biosensor Systems

Structured clinical trials are a requirement for obtaining medical approval of AI-powered diagnostic devices. These tests evaluate both safety and effectiveness, investigating usability elements and how patients respond to the system and its workflow compatibility [153]. Multiple issues arise when testing AI-biosensor systems, as these devices combine hardware-based biosensors with software-based AI models and human-machine interaction elements [154]. Clinical trials include five sequential phases for integration, which are as follows: During Phase 0/I and Pilot Trials, researchers assess how well devices work by collecting effective data while producing dependable output results; FDA requires that Early-Phase Clinical Trials conduct system evaluations by comparing diagnostic output with established diagnostic methods which include PSA testing, biopsy, and MRI; the Phase III Pivotal Trials evaluate if the AI-biosensor system creates better patient results while improving clinical decisions; and Post-Market Surveillance (Phase IV) tracks long-term performance and side effects in broader populations. The testing process must be registered on ClinicalTrials.gov and subject to approval by an ethical review board. Performance monitoring remains essential for adaptive AI models since their operational behavior transforms with exposure to new information. The new clinical trial frameworks Developmental and Exploratory Clinical Investigation of DEcision support systems driven by Artificial Intelligence (DECIDE-AI) and Standard Protocol Items: Recommendations for Interventional Trials–Artificial Intelligence (SPIRIT-AI) provide guidance on how to integrate AI components into established clinical research protocols [155].

10.8.3 Ethical and Regulatory Considerations (FDA, GDPR, etc.)

Implementing AI in healthcare practice requires more than technical solutions, as it entails both ethical and legal obligations. Different regulatory bodies, together with privacy frameworks, control the entire lifecycle of AI-biosensor system development, testing, and deployment [156]. The U.S. FDA operates its Digital Health Centre of Excellence to oversee AI/ML-based Software as a Medical Device (SaMD) under its regulatory authority throughout the United States. AI-enabled biosensors need to fulfill several sets of requirements, which include safety and efficacy standards, before review from the U.S. FDA [157]. Testing and assessment at the premarket stage serve to ensure both the safety and effectiveness of operations. Good Machine Learning Practices require adaptive algorithms to have change control procedures in place. Additionally, real-world performance monitoring is necessary. Strict guidelines are enforced in the European Union under the General Data Protection Regulation (GDPR) and the Medical Device Regulation regarding device classification and CE marking, transparency in AI decision-making, and consent and data protection for personal health data. The ethical domain consists of algorithmic bias, together with data sovereignty, informed consent, and right to explanation, which becomes crucial when dealing with life-altering decisions during oncology applications [158]. Models require developers to take multiple population groups into model training to prevent health-related inequalities and need frequent audits to maintain fairness and equity. Both ISO 13485 (medical device quality management) and ISO/IEC 27001 (data security) have become mandatory industry standards that biosensor-AI platforms must obtain before entering clinical and commercial use [159].

10.9 Challenges, Limitations, and Future Directions

The advancement of prostate cancer diagnostic methods through AI and biosensor integration remains quick-paced, even though numerous obstacles and new developments lead its direction [160]. The following part explains major obstacles while reviewing innovative technological solutions, alongside examining new platforms and discussing the necessary ethical and regulatory criteria required for moving this solution into routine medical practice [161].

10.9.1 Technical Challenges in Real-World Implementation

The implementation of AI-biosensor systems has several technical and practical barriers that limit their effectiveness. The main obstacle to overcome is model generalization because many AI systems operate using dataset samples, which omit demographic and clinical diversity, leading to system flaws and reduced applicability across patient demographics [162]. Tools used for medical diagnosis on one patient group often deliver suboptimal performance when tested on different patient groups, thus leading to increased healthcare discrepancies [163]. The durability and dependability of biosensors pose challenges for their operational use. Medical devices used for distant or wearable monitoring must handle changing environmental factors that include temperature extremes and humidity levels, together with patient bodily motions [164]. The operation of sensors becomes degraded due to three primary factors: sensor drift, power loss, and sample contamination [165]. To build trustworthy and extended usable systems, these technologies require self-calibrating capabilities with automated redundancy elements and power-saving hardware components [166]. The primary challenge lies in integrating biosensors into established clinical workflow procedures. Existing hospital Electronic Health Record (EHR) systems from the past reflect legacy systems, which fail to support immediate biosensor data transmission and AI prediction capabilities [167]. Full health system integration demands compatible technical standards together with easy-to-use interfaces that work with clinical workflows, so medical staff do not face process complexity [168].

10.9.2 Innovations Reshaping the Future of Cancer Diagnostics

New technological advances enable new possibilities to emerge in prostate cancer diagnosis. The creation of digital twins represents a major advance by creating virtual patient copies that predict illness conduct and reaction to therapies by analyzing real-time biosensor information with genomic sequences and medical documentation. Such dynamic predictive models support healthcare providers in creating individualized care routes [169]. Researchers find that quantum computing demonstrates potential value for processing the large nonlinear biosensor datasets that exist [170]. Quantum AI processing expands biosensor data analysis speed by its exponential capacity compared to standard computers, which makes difficult biomarker relationships accessible to AI algorithms. AI technologies have introduced a new method for predicting therapeutic outcomes. The monitoring of PSA, miRNA, and metabolic profiles using biosensors enables clinicians to track patient drug responses with the aid of AI for analysis [171]. The upcoming generation of these platforms will become therapeutic feedback systems that adjust medication doses in real time in accordance with biosensor feedback.

10.9.3 Integrating with Future Health Platforms and Virtual Care

The biosensor-based AI system operates within technological networks, which encompass metaverse systems and virtual health management platforms. Healthcare users experience constructive features because innovative tools present diagnostic information through 3D models and let patients meet with doctors digitally and function with self-monitoring AI treatments [172]. Through this technology, both remote patients and rural residents, as well as patients with mobility difficulties, receive superior advantages. With AI-on-chip systems embedded in biosensors, people can obtain passive cancer detection capabilities through wearable sensors without patient intervention [173]. The combination of microelectronics devices and smartwatches with adhesive patches or clothing allows biological signal information to pass through neural networks linked directly with real-time federated learning modules [174]. The deployment of ongoing context-sensitive healthcare systems will enable hospitals to switch from regular scheduled visits to sustained, accurate tracking outside medical facilities for early treatment under lower hospital loads and increased patient-community partnership [175].

10.9.4 Ethical, Regulatory, and Data Governance Considerations

Field deployment of biosensor-AI systems requires attendance to numerous complex ethical and regulatory requirements. Healthcare devices, along with remote diagnostic solutions, face ongoing challenges in securing privacy and maintaining security for constantly recorded sensitive patient data [176]. The GDPR (EU), together with HIPAA (USA), establishes specific compliance requirements that demand permission-based data handling, along with encryption protocols, and secure access management. Technical systems designed for future security need to implement edge computing techniques to prevent dangers related to data transmission and central storage systems [177]. SaMD digital devices need standardized protocols from the FDA, EMA, and national health authorities during their development, especially when applied to adaptive AI systems where updates occur throughout their operational period [178]. The validation of biosensor-AI platforms requires extensive assessment through clinical trials at different locations, along with real-time field testing and continual post-release monitoring of their operational security, precision, and prejudice. The ethical development process requires developers to resolve matters concerning algorithm visibility together with patient rights and AI system explanation capabilities. SHAP and Grad-CAM should become integrated into clinical decision support systems that enable clinicians and patients to understand how AI systems develop their recommendations [179]. To match the progress in technology, the ethical frameworks need development, as the advancement of innovation must never exceed responsible governance.

10.10 Conclusion

This chapter presents an in-depth exploration of a study on the diagnostic and tracking advancements of prostate cancer through biosensor integration with AI and ML systems. The research evaluated four fundamental biosensors, including electrochemical and optical sensors, as well as nano sensors and wearable units, to demonstrate their information processing capabilities for making diagnostic decisions. This chapter explains biosensor data analysis procedures, starting from data cleaning and proceeding through DL model deployment, which enables the processing of biological signals using multi-modal fusion methods under edge computing for real-time operations. The combination of AI and ML technology enables biological sensor-based diagnostics to provide both higher accuracy and faster operation speed, as well as adjustable design frameworks. The system monitors prostate cancer biomarkers in real-time alongside predictive analytics features, which help patients receive new medical solutions that lead to earlier diagnosis. This section demonstrates that AI transforms medical tests from threshold-based examinations to pattern-recognition systems, enabling the deployment of portable healthcare instruments to medical facilities and remote locations. The development of an extended AI-biosensor system requires both laboratory testing and adherence to ethical standards to demonstrate its value for clinical use before approval. Manufacturers must dedicate focus to compliance requirements, fairness measures, privacy standards, and clinician trust programs when developing healthcare systems. The digital twin technology, operated by AI, will be utilized in conjunction with quantum computing to develop customized active cancer prevention services through virtual care solutions. Future healthcare applications rely on biosensor-AI systems for precise oncology applications, thanks to their ongoing development.

10.11 Summary

This chapter examines how the early detection and monitoring of prostate cancer are being revolutionized by the combination of biosensors with AI and ML technologies. It begins by discussing the drawbacks of conventional diagnostic techniques, such as PSA testing, and emphasizes how contemporary biosensors, including electrochemical, optical, nano, and wearable technologies, enable the non-invasive, real-time monitoring of key biomarkers such as PSA, PCA3, and TMPRSS2: ERG. The chapter describes the preprocessing, filtering, and analysis of biosensor-generated data using a variety of AI/ML models, such as DL (CNNs and RNNs), supervised learning (SVM and RF), and unsupervised learning (PCA and K-means). It also highlights how crucial edge computing is for on-device diagnostics, which makes healthcare more accessible and individualized. In addition, the chapter examines XAI, regulatory standards, multimodal data integration, and potential future developments, such as digital twins and quantum computing. All things considered, it provides a comprehensive overview of AI-driven biosensor systems as powerful tools for enhancing prostate cancer precision diagnosis.

Glossary

AI The use of computer systems to mimic human intelligence.

Biosensor A device that detects biological signals and converts them into measurable output.

Biomarker Biological molecule used as an indicator of disease or a health state.

Digital Twin A virtual model of a patient used to simulate and monitor real-world outcomes.

DL A class of ML using neural networks with multiple layers for feature learning.

Edge Computing Data processing performed locally at the device level, not in the cloud.

ML Subset of AI that uses data to train models for prediction or classification.

Personalized Diagnostics Diagnostic systems tailored to an individual's biological data.

Signal Processing Manipulation and analysis of sensor data to extract meaningful features.

XAI AI systems that offer transparent, interpretable decision-making processes.

References

1. Teng Y, Li W, Gunasekaran S. Biosensors based on single or multiple biomarkers for diagnosis of prostate cancer. Biosens Bioelectron X. 2023;15:100418. https://www.sciencedirect.com/science/article/pii/S2590137023001152
2. Chan KM, Gleadle JM, O'Callaghan M, Vasilev K, MacGregor M. Prostate cancer detection: a systematic review of urinary biosensors. Prostate Cancer Prostatic Dis. 2022;25(1):39–46. https://doi.org/10.1038/s41391-021-00480-8.
3. Kim H, Park S, Jeong IG, Song SH, Jeong Y, Kim CS, et al. Noninvasive precision screening of prostate cancer by urinary multimarker sensor and artificial intelligence analysis. ACS Nano. 2020;15(3):4054–65.
4. Schafer EJ, Laversanne M, Sung H, Soerjomataram I, Briganti A, Dahut W, et al. Recent patterns and trends in global prostate cancer incidence and mortality: an update. Eur Urol. 2025;87(3):302–13.

5. Rodrigues VC, Soares JC, Soares AC, Braz DC, Melendez ME, Ribas LC, et al. Electrochemical and optical detection and machine learning applied to images of genosensors for diagnosis of prostate cancer with the biomarker PCA3. Talanta. 2021;222:121444. https://www.sciencedirect.com/science/article/pii/S0039914020307359
6. Kokabi M, Tahir MN, Singh D, Javanmard M. Advancing healthcare: synergizing biosensors and machine learning for early cancer diagnosis. Biosensors. 2023;13(9). https://www.mdpi.com/2079-6374/13/9/884
7. Wasilewski T, Kamysz W, Gębicki J. AI-assisted detection of biomarkers by sensors and biosensors for early diagnosis and monitoring. Biosensors. 2024;14(7).
8. Ahmed Taha B, Kadhim AC, Addie AJ, Haider AJ, Azzahrani AS, Raizada P, et al. Advancing cancer diagnostics through multifaceted optical biosensors supported by nanomaterials and artificial intelligence: a panoramic outlook. Microchem J. 2024;205:111307. https://www.sciencedirect.com/science/article/pii/S0026265X2401419X
9. Wu Y, Wang Y, Huang Z, Liu Q. Recent advances in analysis technology for detection of prostate cancer biomarkers. Microchem J. 2023;190:108740. https://www.sciencedirect.com/science/article/pii/S0026265X23003582
10. Choi JY, Park S, Shim JS, Park HJ, Kuh SU, Jeong Y, et al. Explainable artificial intelligence-driven prostate cancer screening using exosomal multi-marker based dual-gate FET biosensor. Biosens Bioelectron. 2025;267:116773.
11. Alnaimi A, Al-Hamry A, Makableh Y, Adiraju A, Kanoun O. Gold nanoparticles-MWCNT based Aptasensor for early diagnosis of prostate cancer. Biosensors 2022;12(12). https://www.mdpi.com/2079-6374/12/12/1130
12. Terjung A, Kummer S, Friedrich M. Simultaneous 24 h-infusion of high-dose 5-fluorouracil and sodium-folinate as alternative to capecitabine in advanced breast cancer. Anticancer Res. 2014;34(12):7233–8.
13. Singh S, Gill AAS, Nlooto M, Karpoormath R. Prostate cancer biomarkers detection using nanoparticles based electrochemical biosensors. Biosens Bioelectron. 2019;137:213–21. https://www.sciencedirect.com/science/article/pii/S0956566319302441
14. Takita S, Nabok A, Mussa M, Kitchen M, Lishchuk A, Smith D. Ultrasensitive prostate cancer marker PCA3 detection with impedimetric biosensor based on specific label-free aptamers. Biosens Bioelectron X. 2024;18:100462. https://www.sciencedirect.com/science/article/pii/S2590137024000268
15. Najeeb MA, Ahmad Z, Shakoor RA, Mohamed AMA, Kahraman R. A novel classification of prostate specific antigen (PSA) biosensors based on transducing elements. Talanta. 2017;168:52–61.
16. Akbari Nakhjavani S, Tokyay BK, Soylemez C, Sarabi MR, Yetisen AK, Tasoglu S. Biosensors for prostate cancer detection. Trends Biotechnol. 2023;41(10):1248–67. https://doi.org/10.1016/j.tibtech.2023.04.001.
17. Xu L, Wen Y, Pandit S, Mokkapati VRSS, Mijakovic I, Li Y, et al. Graphene-based biosensors for the detection of prostate cancer protein biomarkers: a review. BMC Chem. 2019;13(1):112. https://doi.org/10.1186/s13065-019-0611-x.
18. Wu J, Liu H, Chen W, Ma B, Ju H. Device integration of electrochemical biosensors. Nat Rev Bioeng. 2023;1(5):346–60.
19. Sumitha MS, Xavier TS. Recent advances in electrochemical biosensors—a brief review. Hybrid Adv. 2023;2:100023.
20. Singh A, Sharma A, Ahmed A, Sundramoorthy AK, Furukawa H, Arya S, et al. Recent advances in electrochemical biosensors: applications, challenges, and future scope. Biosensors. 2021;11(9):336.
21. Kaur B, Kumar S, Kaushik BK. Recent advancements in optical biosensors for cancer detection. Biosens Bioelectron. 2022;197:113805. https://www.sciencedirect.com/science/article/pii/S0956566321008423
22. Khansili N, Rattu G, Krishna PM. Label-free optical biosensors for food and biological sensor applications. Sensors Actuators B Chem. 2018;265:35–49.

23. Lei Z, Guo B. 2D material-based optical biosensor: status and prospect. Adv Sci. 2022;9(4):2102924.
24. Ozgür E, Saylan Y, Akgönüllü S, Denizli A. Mass-sensitive based biosensors. In: Biosensors. CRC Press; 2022. p. 89–104.
25. Mujahid A, Afzal A, Dickert FL. An overview of high frequency acoustic sensors—QCMs, SAWs and FBARs—chemical and biochemical applications. Sensors. 2019;19(20).
26. Huang X, Chen Q, Pan W, Yao Y. Advances in the mass sensitivity distribution of quartz crystal microbalances: A Review. Sensors. 2022;22(14).
27. Khan NI, Song E. Lab-on-a-chip systems for aptamer-based biosensing. Micromachines. 2020;11(2):220.
28. Nikoleli GP, Siontorou CG, Nikolelis DP, Bratakou S, Karapetis S, Tzamtzis N. Chapter 13 - Biosensors Based on Microfluidic Devices Lab-on-a-Chip and Microfluidic Technology. In: Nikolelis DP, Nikoleli GP, editors. Nanotechnology and Biosensors. Elsevier; 2018. p. 375–94. (Advanced Nanomaterials). https://www.sciencedirect.com/science/article/pii/B9780128138557000131.
29. Sengupta J, Adhikari A, Hussain CM. Graphene-based analytical lab-on-chip devices for detection of viruses: a review. Carbon Trends. 2021;4:100072.
30. Arfin T. 9—Emerging trends in lab-on-a-chip for biosensing applications. In: Hussain CM, Shukla SK, Joshi GM, editors. Functionalized Nanomaterials Based Devices for Environmental Applications. Elsevier; 2021. p. 199–218. (Micro and Nano Technologies).
31. Dkhar DS, Kumari R, Malode SJ, Shetti NP, Chandra P. Integrated lab-on-a-chip devices: fabrication methodologies, transduction system for sensing purposes. J Pharm Biomed Anal. 2023;223:115120.
32. Zhang P, Zhu B, Du P, Travas-Sejdic J. Electrochemical and electrical biosensors for wearable and implantable electronics based on conducting polymers and carbon-based materials. Chem Rev. 2024;124(3):722–67.
33. Rodrigues D, Barbosa AI, Rebelo R, Kwon IK, Reis RL, Correlo VM. Skin-integrated wearable systems and implantable biosensors: a comprehensive review. Biosensors. 2020;10(7).
34. Li P, Lee GH, Kim SY, Kwon SY, Kim HR, Park S. From diagnosis to treatment: recent advances in patient-friendly biosensors and implantable devices. ACS Nano. 2021;15(2):1960–2004. https://doi.org/10.1021/acsnano.0c06688.
35. Gao W, Yu C. Wearable and implantable devices for healthcare. Vol. 10, Advanced Healthcare Materials. Wiley Online Library; 2021. p. 2101548.
36. Eyrich NW, Morgan TM, Tosoian JJ. Biomarkers for detection of clinically significant prostate cancer: contemporary clinical data and future directions. Transl Androl Urol. 2021;10(7):3091–103.
37. Filella X, Fernandez-Galan E, Fernandez Bonifacio R, Foj L. Emerging biomarkers in the diagnosis of prostate cancer. Pharmgenomics Pers Med. 2018;Volume 11:83–94.
38. Nevo A, Navaratnam A, Andrews P. Prostate cancer and the role of biomarkers. Abdom Radiol. 2020;45:2120–32.
39. Song C, Chen H, Chen L, Ru G, Guo J, Ding Q. The potential of microRNAs as human prostate cancer biomarkers: a meta-analysis of related studies. J Cell Biochem. 2018;119(3):2763–86.
40. Lamy PJ, Allory Y, Gauchez AS, Asselain B, Beuzeboc P, de Cremoux P, et al. Prognostic biomarkers used for localised prostate cancer management: a systematic review. Eur Urol Focus. 2018;4(6):790–803. https://www.sciencedirect.com/science/article/pii/S2405456917300652
41. Kohaar I, Petrovics G, Srivastava S. A rich array of prostate cancer molecular biomarkers: opportunities and challenges. Int J Mol Sci. 2019;20(8):1813.
42. Romero Otero J, Garcia Gomez B, Campos Juanatey F, Touijer KA. Prostate cancer biomarkers: an update. Urol Oncol Semin Orig Investig. 2014;32(3):252–60. https://www.sciencedirect.com/science/article/pii/S1078143913003979
43. Scott E, Munkley J. Glycans as biomarkers in prostate cancer. Int J Mol Sci 2019;20(6). https://www.mdpi.com/1422-0067/20/6/1389

44. Chistiakov DA, Myasoedova VA, Grechko A V, Melnichenko AA, Orekhov AN. New biomarkers for diagnosis and prognosis of localized prostate cancer. In: Seminars in cancer biology. Elsevier; 2018. p. 9–16.
45. Kdadra M, Höckner S, Leung H, Kremer W, Schiffer E. Metabolomics biomarkers of prostate cancer: a systematic review. Diagnostics. 2019;9(1):21.
46. Gómez-Cebrián N, Rojas-Benedicto A, Albors-Vaquer A, López-Guerrero JA, Pineda-Lucena A, Puchades-Carrasco L. Metabolomics contributions to the discovery of prostate cancer biomarkers. Meta. 2019;9(3).
47. Cucchiara V, Cooperberg MR, Dall'Era M, Lin DW, Montorsi F, Schalken JA, et al. Genomic markers in prostate cancer decision making. Eur Urol. 2018;73(4):572–82.
48. Salciccia S, Capriotti AL, Laganà A, Fais S, Logozzi M, De Berardinis E, et al. Biomarkers in prostate cancer diagnosis: from current knowledge to the role of metabolomics and exosomes. Int J Mol Sci. 2021;22(9):4367.
49. Fredsøe J, Rasmussen AKI, Thomsen AR, Mouritzen P, Høyer S, Borre M, et al. Diagnostic and prognostic MicroRNA biomarkers for prostate cancer in cell-free urine. Eur Urol Focus. 2018;4(6):825–33. https://www.sciencedirect.com/science/article/pii/S2405456917300664
50. Toth R, Schiffmann H, Hube-Magg C, Büscheck F, Höflmayer D, Weidemann S, et al. Random forest-based modelling to detect biomarkers for prostate cancer progression. Clin Epigenetics. 2019;11(1):148. https://doi.org/10.1186/s13148-019-0736-8.
51. Yang R, Zhang W, Tiwari N, Yan H, Li T, Cheng H. Multimodal sensors with decoupled sensing mechanisms. Adv Sci. 2022;9(26):2202470.
52. Posada-Quintero HF, Chon KH. Innovations in electrodermal activity data collection and signal processing: a systematic review. Sensors. 2020;20(2):479.
53. Ji B, Zhou Q, Hu B, Zhong J, Zhou J, Zhou B. Bio-inspired hybrid dielectric for capacitive and triboelectric tactile sensors with high sensitivity and ultrawide linearity range. Adv Mater. 2021;33(27):2100859.
54. He J, Xiao P, Lu W, Shi J, Zhang L, Liang Y, et al. A universal high accuracy wearable pulse monitoring system via high sensitivity and large linearity graphene pressure sensor. Nano Energy. 2019;59:422–33.
55. Ashrafizadeh M, Aghamiri S, Tan SC, Zarrabi A, Sharifi E, Rabiee N, et al. Nanotechnological approaches in prostate cancer therapy: integration of engineering and biology. Nano Today. 2022;45:101532. https://www.sciencedirect.com/science/article/pii/S1748013222001591
56. Barani M, Sabir F, Rahdar A, Arshad R, Kyzas GZ. Nanotreatment and nanodiagnosis of prostate cancer: recent updates. Nano. 2020;10(9):1696.
57. Hao B, Wei L, Cheng Y, Ma Z, Wang J. Advanced nanomaterial for prostate cancer theranostics. Front Bioeng Biotechnol. 2022;10:1046234.
58. Wongkaew N. Nanofiber-integrated miniaturized systems: an intelligent platform for cancer diagnosis. Anal Bioanal Chem. 2019;411(19):4251–64.
59. Ranjan P, Singhal A, Sadique MA, Yadav S, Parihar A, Khan R. Chapter 24 - scope of biosensors, commercial aspects, and miniaturized devices for point-of-care testing from lab to clinics applications. In: Khan R, Parihar A, Sanghi SK, editors. Biosensor based advanced cancer diagnostics [internet]. Academic Press; 2022. p. 395–410. https://www.sciencedirect.com/science/article/pii/B9780128234242000041.
60. Aidoo-Brown J, Moschou D, Estrela P. Multiplexed prostate cancer companion diagnostic devices. Sensors 2021;21(15). https://www.mdpi.com/1424-8220/21/15/5023
61. Wang L, Ji Y, Wang L, zheng S, Chen Y, Xu X, et al. Ratio fluorescence/colorimetric dual mode aptasensor and smartphones-assisted miniaturized device for early diagnosis of prostate cancer. Chem Eng J. 2024;485:150152. https://www.sciencedirect.com/science/article/pii/S1385894724016383
62. Schatten H. Brief overview of prostate cancer statistics, grading, diagnosis and treatment strategies. In: Schatten H, editor. Cell {\&} Molecular Biology of Prostate Cancer: Updates, Insights and New Frontiers. Cham: Springer International Publishing; 2018. p. 1–14. doi:https://doi.org/10.1007/978-3-319-95693-0_1.

63. Akinnuwesi BA, Olayanju KA, Aribisala BS, Fashoto SG, Mbunge E, Okpeku M, et al. Application of support vector machine algorithm for early differential diagnosis of prostate cancer. Data Sci Manag. 2023;6(1):1–12.
64. Tzeng S, Tsai C, Chao T, Chou Y, Yang Y, Tsai M, et al. O-glycosylation-mediated signaling circuit drives metastatic castration-resistant prostate cancer. FASEB J. 2018;32(12):6869–82.
65. Moradi A, Srinivasan S, Clements J, Batra J. Beyond the biomarker role: prostate-specific antigen (PSA) in the prostate cancer microenvironment. Cancer Metastasis Rev. 2019;38:333–46.
66. Carobene A, Guerra E, Locatelli M, Cucchiara V, Briganti A, Aarsand AK, et al. Biological variation estimates for prostate specific antigen from the European biological variation study; consequences for diagnosis and monitoring of prostate cancer. Clin Chim Acta. 2018;486:185–91.
67. Gresser E, Schachtner B, Stüber AT, Solyanik O, Schreier A, Huber T, et al. Performance variability of radiomics machine learning models for the detection of clinically significant prostate cancer in heterogeneous MRI datasets. Quant Imaging Med Surg. 2022;12(11):4990–5003.
68. Malagi AV, Netaji A, Kumar V, Baidya Kayal E, Khare K, Das CJ, et al. IVIM–DKI for differentiation between prostate cancer and benign prostatic hyperplasia: comparison of 1.5 T vs. 3 T MRI. Magn Reson Mater Physics, Biol Med 2022;35(4):609–620.
69. Larson PEZ, Chen H, Gordon JW, Korn N, Maidens J, Arcak M, et al. Investigation of analysis methods for hyperpolarized 13C-pyruvate metabolic MRI in prostate cancer patients. NMR Biomed. 2018;31(11):e3997.
70. Xiang J, Wang X, Wang X, Zhang J, Yang S, Yang W, et al. Automatic diagnosis and grading of prostate cancer with weakly supervised learning on whole slide images. Comput Biol Med. 2023;152:106340.
71. Gu S, Hou P, Liu K, Niu X, Wei B, Mao F, et al. NOL8, the binding protein for beta-catenin, promoted the growth and migration of prostate cancer cells. Chem Biol Interact. 2018;294:40 7.
72. El-Gammal OA, Mohamed FS, Rezk GN, El-Bindary AA. Structural characterization and biological activity of a new metal complexes based of Schiff base. J Mol Liq. 2021;330:115522.
73. Anaya-Eugenio GD, Rebollar-Ramos D, del Carmen González M, Raja H, Mata R, Carcache de Blanco EJ. Apoptotic activity of xanthoquinodin JBIR-99, from Parengyodontium album MEXU 30054, in PC-3 human prostate cancer cells. Chem Biol Interact 2019;311:108798.
74. Jiang X, Guo S, Wang S, Zhang Y, Chen H, Wang Y, et al. EIF4A3-induced circARHGAP29 promotes aerobic glycolysis in docetaxel-resistant prostate cancer through IGF2BP2/c-Myc/LDHA signaling. Cancer Res. 2022;82(5):831–45.
75. Ku SY, Gleave ME, Beltran H. Towards precision oncology in advanced prostate cancer. Nat Rev Urol. 2019;16(11):645–54.
76. Kelly SP, Anderson WF, Rosenberg PS, Cook MB. Past, current, and future incidence rates and burden of metastatic prostate cancer in the United States. Eur Urol Focus. 2018;4(1):121–7.
77. Nevedomskaya E, Baumgart SJ, Haendler B. Recent advances in prostate cancer treatment and drug discovery. Int J Mol Sci. 2018;19(5). https://www.mdpi.com/1422-0067/19/5/1359
78. Rebuzzi SE, Rescigno P, Catalano F, Mollica V, Vogl UM, Marandino L, et al. Immune checkpoint inhibitors in advanced prostate cancer: current data and future perspectives. Cancers (Basel). 2022;14(5).
79. He H, Liu L, Morin EE, Liu M, Schwendeman A. Survey of clinical translation of cancer Nanomedicines lessons learned from successes and failures. Acc Chem Res. 2019;52(9):2445–61. https://doi.org/10.1021/acs.accounts.9b00228.
80. Hwang YC, Cho SY, Ku JH, Jeong SJ, Oh SJ. Translation and linguistic validation of Korean version of the expanded prostate cancer index composite for clinical practice for patients with prostate cancer. Int Neurourol J. 2021 Dec;25(4):296–309.
81. Yekula A, Muralidharan K, Kang KM, Wang L, Balaj L, Carter BS. From laboratory to clinic: translation of extracellular vesicle based cancer biomarkers. Methods. 2020;177:58–66.

82. Koo KM, Mainwaring PN, Tomlins SA, Trau M. Merging new-age biomarkers and nanodiagnostics for precision prostate cancer management. Nat Rev Urol. 2019;16(5):302–17.
83. Ali AM, Mohammed AA. Improving classification accuracy for prostate cancer using noise removal filter and deep learning technique. Multimed Tools Appl. 2022;81(6):8653–69.
84. Momenzadeh N, Hafezalseheh H, Nayebpour MR, Fathian M, Noorossana R. A hybrid machine learning approach for predicting survival of patients with prostate cancer: a SEER-based population study. Informatics Med Unlocked. 2021;27:100763.
85. Kuo RJ, Su PY, Zulvia FE, Lin CC. Integrating cluster analysis with granular computing for imbalanced data classification problem—a case study on prostate cancer prognosis. Comput Ind Eng. 2018;125:319–32.
86. Liberda D, Pięta E, Pogoda K, Piergies N, Roman M, Koziol P, et al. The impact of preprocessing methods for a successful prostate cell lines discrimination using partial least squares regression and discriminant analysis based on Fourier transform infrared imaging. Cells. 2021;10(4).
87. Casotti MC, Meira DD, Zetum ASS, Campanharo CV, da Silva DRC, Giacinti GM, et al. Integrating frontiers: a holistic, quantum and evolutionary approach to conquering cancer through systems biology and multidisciplinary synergy. Front Oncol 2024;14:1419599.
88. Paul D. Cancer as a form of life: musings of the cancer and evolution symposium. Prog Biophys Mol Biol. 2021;165:120–39.
89. Erenpreisa J, Giuliani A, Yoshikawa K, Falk M, Hildenbrand G, Salmina K, et al. Spatial-temporal genome regulation in stress-response and cell-fate change. Int J Mol Sci. 2023;24(3)
90. Eskra JN, Rabizadeh D, Pavlovich CP, Catalona WJ, Luo J. Approaches to urinary detection of prostate cancer. Prostate Cancer Prostatic Dis. 2019;22(3):362–81. https://doi.org/10.1038/s41391-019-0127-4.
91. García G, Colomer A, Naranjo V. First-stage prostate cancer identification on histopathological images: hand-driven versus automatic learning. Entropy. 2019;21(4).
92. Bax C, Taverna G, Eusebio L, Sironi S, Grizzi F, Guazzoni G, et al. Innovative diagnostic methods for early prostate cancer detection through urine analysis: a review. Cancers (Basel). 2018;10(4). https://www.mdpi.com/2072-6694/10/4/123
93. Jeong CW, Washington SL, Herlemann A, Gomez SL, Carroll PR, Cooperberg MR. The new surveillance, epidemiology, and end results prostate with watchful waiting database: opportunities and limitations. Eur Urol. 2020;78(3):335–44.
94. Koshkin VS, Patel VG, Ali A, Bilen MA, Ravindranathan D, Park JJ, et al. PROMISE: a real-world clinical-genomic database to address knowledge gaps in prostate cancer. Prostate Cancer Prostatic Dis. 2022;25(3):388–96.
95. Ahuja G, Kaur I, Lamba PS, Virmani D, Jain A, Chakraborty S, et al. Prostate cancer prognosis using machine learning: a critical review of survival analysis methods. Pathol - Res Pract. 2024;264:155687.
96. Le Boutillier C, Urch C, King A, Barry C, Mansfield L, Archer S. 'Still living with it even though it's gone': using interpretive phenomenological analysis to explore shared experiences of living with and beyond breast, prostate, and colorectal cancer. Eur J Oncol Nurs. 2022;56:102067.
97. Salem AF, Wang S, Billet S, Chen JF, Udompholkul P, Gambini L, et al. Reduction of Circulating Cancer Cells and Metastases in Breast-Cancer Models by a Potent EphA2-Agonistic Peptide–Drug Conjugate. J Med Chem. 2018;61(5):2052–61.
98. Dadhich R, Kapoor S. Lipidomic and membrane mechanical signatures in triple-negative breast cancer: scope for membrane-based Theranostics. Mol Cell Biochem. 2022;477(11):2507–28.
99. Banerjee A, Maity S, Mastrangelo CH. Nanostructures for biosensing, with a brief overview on cancer detection, IoT, and the role of machine learning in smart biosensors. Sensors. 2021;21(4). https://www.mdpi.com/1424-8220/21/4/1253
100. Lee S, Jue M, Lee K, Paulson B, Oh J, Cho M, et al. Early-stage diagnosis of bladder cancer using surface-enhanced Raman spectroscopy combined with machine learning algorithms in a rat model. Biosens Bioelectron. 2024;246:115915.

101. Liyanage T, Alharbi B, Quan L, Esquela-Kerscher A, Slaughter G. Plasmonic-based biosensor for the early diagnosis of prostate cancer. ACS Omega. 2022;7(2):2411–2418. https://doi.org/10.1021/acsomega.1c06479.
102. Wu N, Zhang XY, Xia J, Li X, Yang T, Wang JH. Ratiometric 3D DNA machine combined with machine learning algorithm for ultrasensitive and high-precision screening of early urinary diseases. ACS Nano. 2021;15(12):19522–34.
103. Dubey P, Kumar S. Advancing prostate cancer detection: a comparative analysis of PCLDA-SVM and PCLDA-KNN classifiers for enhanced diagnostic accuracy. Sci Rep. 2023;13(1):13745.
104. Naji MA, El FS, Bouhlal M, Benlahmar ELH, Abdelouhahid RA, Debauche O. Breast cancer prediction and diagnosis through a new approach based on majority voting ensemble classifier. Procedia Comput Sci. 2021;191:481–6.
105. Mylona E, Zaridis DI, Kalantzopoulos CN, Tachos NS, Regge D, Papanikolaou N, et al. Optimizing radiomics for prostate cancer diagnosis: feature selection strategies, machine learning classifiers, and MRI sequences. Insights Imaging. 2024;15(1):265.
106. Sahran S, Albashish D, Abdullah A, Shukor NA, Hayati Md Pauzi S. Absolute cosine-based SVM-RFE feature selection method for prostate histopathological grading. Artif Intell Med 2018;87:78–90.
107. Emegano DI, Mustapha MT, Ozsahin DU, Ozsahin I. Machine learning prediction of overall survival in prostate adenocarcinoma using ensemble techniques. Comput Biol Med. 2025;189:110008.
108. Mostafaei S, Abdollahi H, Kazempour Dehkordi S, Shiri I, Razzaghdoust A, Zoljalali Moghaddam SH, et al. CT imaging markers to improve radiation toxicity prediction in prostate cancer radiotherapy by stacking regression algorithm. Radiol Med. 2020;125(1):87–97.
109. Onumaku Mbcs V. A comparative and predictive analysis of prostate cancer diagnosis and treatment using decision tree, neural network, support vector machine, random Forest and K-nearest neighbor KNN classification algorithms OGUOMA IKECHUKWU STANLEY 1, UKA KANAYO KIZITO 2, VICTORY CHIBUIKE ONUMAKU 3, ONUNJOKU CHARLES ENYINNAYA 4, NNEDINMA CHRISTIANA NJOKU 5, CHUKWU ALPHONSUS CHEKWUBE. 2024;
110. Morakis D, Adamopoulos A. Hybrid machine learning algorithms to evaluate prostate cancer. Algorithms. 2024;17(6).
111. Cao-Van K, Minh TC, Minh LG, Quyen TTB, Tan HM. Soft-voting ensemble model: an efficient learning approach for predictive prostate cancer risk. Vietnam J Comput Sci. 2024;11(04):531–52. https://doi.org/10.1142/S2196888824500155.
112. Emegano DI, Mustapha MT, Ozsahin I, Ozsahin DU, Uzun B. Advancing prostate cancer diagnostics: a ConvNeXt approach to multi-class classification in underrepresented populations. Bioengineering. 2025;12(4).
113. Yang E, Shankar K, Kumar S, Seo C, Moon I. Equilibrium optimization algorithm with deep learning enabled prostate cancer detection on MRI images. Biomedicine. 2023;11(12).
114. Solovieva S, Karnaukh M, Panchuk V, Andreev E, Kartsova L, Bessonova E, et al. Potentiometric multisensor system as a possible simple tool for non-invasive prostate cancer diagnostics through urine analysis. Sensors Actuators B Chem. 2019;289:42–7. https://www.sciencedirect.com/science/article/pii/S0925400519304290
115. Beeram R, Vepa KR, Soma VR. Recent trends in SERS-based Plasmonic sensors for disease diagnostics, biomolecules detection, and machine learning techniques. Biosensors. 2023;13(3).
116. Tătaru OS, Vartolomei MD, Rassweiler JJ, Virgil O, Lucarelli G, Porpiglia F, et al. Artificial intelligence and machine learning in prostate cancer patient management—current trends and future perspectives. Diagnostics 2021;11(2). https://www.mdpi.com/2075-4418/11/2/354
117. Mehralivand S, Yang D, Harmon SA, Xu D, Xu Z, Roth H, et al. Deep learning-based artificial intelligence for prostate cancer detection at biparametric MRI. Abdom Radiol. 2022;47(4):1425–34.

118. Hassan MR, Islam MF, Uddin MZ, Ghoshal G, Hassan MM, Huda S, et al. Prostate cancer classification from ultrasound and MRI images using deep learning based explainable artificial intelligence. Futur Gener Comput Syst. 2022;127:462–72.
119. Duran-Lopez L, Dominguez-Morales JP, Gutierrez-Galan D, Rios-Navarro A, Jimenez-Fernandez A, Vicente-Diaz S, et al. Wide & Deep neural network model for patch aggregation in CNN-based prostate cancer detection systems. Comput Biol Med. 2021;136:104743.
120. Abdelhalim I, Badawy MA, Abou El-Ghar M, Ghazal M, Contractor S, van Bogaert E, et al. Multi-branch CNNFormer: a novel framework for predicting prostate cancer response to hormonal therapy. Biomed Eng Online. 2024;23(1):131.
121. Sushentsev N, Rundo L, Abrego L, Li Z, Nazarenko T, Warren AY, et al. Time series radiomics for the prediction of prostate cancer progression in patients on active surveillance. Eur Radiol. 2023;33(6):3792–800.
122. Srinivasan US, Pavithra V, Sutha K, Ramachandiran S, Indumathi N. An innovative analysis of time series-based detection models for improved cancer detection in modern healthcare environments. Eng Proc. 2023;59(1).
123. Kovacs KD, Beres B, Kanyo N, Szabó B, Peter B, Bősze S, et al. Single-cell classification based on label-free high-resolution optical data of cell adhesion kinetics. Sci Rep. 2024;14(1):11231.
124. Albalawi E, T.R. M, Thakur A, Kumar VV, Gupta M, Khan SB, et al. Integrated approach of federated learning with transfer learning for classification and diagnosis of brain tumor. BMC Med Imaging. 2024;24(1):110.
125. S S, Dharani Devi G, V R, Jeyalakshmi J. Privacy-preserving breast cancer classification: a federated transfer learning approach. J imaging informatics Med. 2024;37(4):1488–504.
126. Rajagopal A, Redekop E, Kemisetti A, Kulkarni R, Raman S, Sarma K, et al. Federated learning with research prototypes: application to multi-center MRI-based detection of prostate cancer with diverse histopathology. Acad Radiol. 2023;30(4):644–57.
127. Ramírez-Mena A, Andrés-León E, Alvarez-Cubero MJ, Anguita-Ruiz A, Martinez-Gonzalez LJ, Alcala-Fdez J. Explainable artificial intelligence to predict and identify prostate cancer tissue by gene expression. Comput Methods Prog Biomed. 2023;240:107719.
128. Bertsimas D, Margonis GA. Explainable vs. interpretable artificial intelligence frameworks in oncology. Vol. 12, Translational cancer research China; 2023. p. 217–220.
129. Esteva A, Feng J, van der Wal D, Huang SC, Simko JP, DeVries S, et al. Prostate cancer therapy personalization via multi-modal deep learning on randomized phase III clinical trials. npj Digit Med. 2022;5(1):71.
130. Boehm KM, Khosravi P, Vanguri R, Gao J, Shah SP. Harnessing multimodal data integration to advance precision oncology. Nat Rev Cancer. 2022;22(2):114–26.
131. Yu Y, Chen D, Zhu Y. Multi-modal predictive modeling in prostate cancer radiotherapy: a radiomics and dosiomics approach. J Radiat Res Appl Sci. 2025;18(2):101518.
132. Ayyad SM, Abdel-Hamid NB, Ali HA, Labib LM. Multimodality imaging in prostate cancer diagnosis using artificial intelligence: basic concepts and current state-of-the-art. Multimed Tools Appl. 2025;84:42649.
133. Sedghi A, Mehrtash A, Jamzad A, Amalou A, Wells WM, Kapur T, et al. Improving detection of prostate cancer foci via information fusion of MRI and temporal enhanced ultrasound. Int J Comput Assist Radiol Surg. 2020;15(7):1215–23.
134. Ren S, Li J, Dorado J, Sierra A, González-Díaz H, Duardo A, et al. From molecular mechanisms of prostate cancer to translational applications: based on multi-omics fusion analysis and intelligent medicine. Heal Inf Sci Syst. 2023;12(1):6. https://doi.org/10.1007/s13755-023-00264-5.
135. Zhu M, Liang Z, Feng T, Mai Z, Jin S, Wu L, et al. Up-to-date imaging and diagnostic techniques for prostate cancer: a literature review. Diagnostics. 2023;13(13).
136. Li Y, El Habib Daho M, Conze PH, Zeghlache R, Le Boité H, Tadayoni R, et al. A review of deep learning-based information fusion techniques for multimodal medical image classification. Comput Biol Med. 2024;177:108635.

137. Morote J, Miró B, Hernando P, Paesano N, Picola N, Muñoz-Rodriguez J, et al. Developing a Predictive Model for Significant Prostate Cancer Detection in Prostatic Biopsies from Seven Clinical Variables: Is Machine Learning Superior to Logistic Regression? Cancers (Basel). 2025;17(7).
138. Kline A, Wang H, Li Y, Dennis S, Hutch M, Xu Z, et al. Multimodal machine learning in precision health: a scoping review. npj Digit Med. 2022;5(1):171.
139. Arya N, Saha S, Mathur A, Saha S. Improving the robustness and stability of a machine learning model for breast cancer prognosis through the use of multi-modal classifiers. Sci Rep. 2023;13(1):4079.
140. Singh A, Randive S, Breggia A, Ahmad B, Christman R, Amal S. Enhancing prostate cancer diagnosis with a novel artificial intelligence-based web application: synergizing deep learning models, multimodal data, and insights from usability study with pathologists. Cancers (Basel). 2023;15(23). https://www.mdpi.com/2072-6694/15/23/5659
141. Talyshinskii A, Hameed BMZ, Ravinder PP, Naik N, Randhawa P, Shah M, et al. Catalyzing precision medicine: artificial intelligence advancements in prostate cancer diagnosis and management. Cancers (Basel). 2024;16(10). https://www.mdpi.com/2072-6694/16/10/1809
142. Horasan A, Güneş A. Advancing prostate cancer diagnosis: a deep learning approach for enhanced detection in MRI images. Diagnostics. 2024;14(17).
143. Perera RH, de Leon A, Wang X, Wang Y, Ramamurthy G, Peiris P, et al. Real time ultrasound molecular imaging of prostate cancer with PSMA-targeted nanobubbles. Nanomed Nanotechnol Biol Med 2020;28:102213.
144. Li H, Lee CH, Chia D, Lin Z, Huang W, Tan CH. Machine learning in prostate MRI for prostate cancer: current status and future opportunities. Diagnostics. 2022;12(2). https://www.mdpi.com/2075-4418/12/2/289
145. Bahramian H, Gholinejad J, Yazdanpanah GA. Folded flexure MOEMS for the detection of PSA and hepatitis DNA as biosensor for prostate cancer and viruses. Sci Rep. 2024;14(1):22881.
146. Sohrabi H, Bolandi N, Hemmati A, Eyvazi S, Ghasemzadeh S, Baradaran B, et al. State-of-the-art cancer biomarker detection by portable (bio) sensing technology: a critical review. Microchem J. 2022;177:107248. https://www.sciencedirect.com/science/article/pii/S0026265X22000765
147. Dehghani P, Karthikeyan V, Tajabadi A, Assi DS, Catchpole A, Wadsworth J, et al. Rapid near-patient Impedimetric sensing platform for prostate cancer diagnosis. ACS Omega. 2024;9(12):14580–91. https://doi.org/10.1021/acsomega.4c00843.
148. Xu T, Song Y, Gao W, Wu T, Xu LP, Zhang X, et al. Superwettable electrochemical biosensor toward detection of cancer biomarkers. ACS Sens. 2018;3(1):72–8.
149. Mota JM, Armstrong AJ, Larson SM, Fox JJ, Morris MJ. Measuring the unmeasurable: automated bone scan index as a quantitative endpoint in prostate cancer clinical trials. Prostate Cancer Prostatic Dis. 2019;22(4):522–30.
150. Jamaspishvili T, Berman DM, Ross AE, Scher HI, De Marzo AM, Squire JA, et al. Clinical implications of PTEN loss in prostate cancer. Nat Rev Urol. 2018;15(4):222–34. https://doi.org/10.1038/nrurol.2018.9.
151. Nagpal K, Foote D, Liu Y, Chen PHC, Wulczyn E, Tan F, et al. Development and validation of a deep learning algorithm for improving Gleason scoring of prostate cancer. NPJ Digit Med. 2019;2(1):48.
152. Pantel K, Hille C, Scher HI. Circulating tumor cells in prostate cancer: from discovery to clinical utility. Clin Chem. 2019;65(1):87–99.
153. Goumas G, Vlachothanasi EN, Fradelos EC, Mouliou DS. Biosensors, Artificial intelligence biosensors, false results and novel future Perspectives. Diagnostics. 2025;15.
154. Parameswari R, Babujanarthanam R, Yogesh T, Janani Iswarya S, Ganesamoorthy R. Electroanalysis and sensors for biomedical and clinical applications. In: Kasinathan K, Ladchumananandasivam R, Mohamed SB, editors. New Technologies for Energy Transition Based on sustainable development goals: factors contributing to global warming. Singapore: Springer Nature Singapore; 2024. p. 67–94.

155. Golden GJ, Opiekun M, Martin-Taylor T, Kimball BA. Training the domestic ferret to discriminate odors associated with wildlife disease. PLoS One. 2021;16(11):e0259415.
156. Bouderhem R. Privacy and regulatory issues in wearable health technology. Eng Proc. 2023;58(1):87.
157. Gerke S, Minssen T, Cohen G. Ethical and legal challenges of artificial intelligence-driven healthcare. In: Artificial intelligence in healthcare. Elsevier; 2020. p. 295–336.
158. Massella M, Dri DA, Gramaglia D. Regulatory considerations on the use of machine learning based tools in clinical trials. Health Technol (Berl). 2022;12(6):1085–96.
159. Donovan SM, Abrahams M, Anthony JC, Bergia R, Blander G, Brisbois TD, et al. Perspective: challenges for personalized nutrition in the current United States regulatory framework and future opportunities. Adv Nutr. 2025;16(3):100382.
160. Swami U, McFarland TR, Nussenzveig R, Agarwal N. Advanced prostate cancer: treatment advances and future directions. Trends in Cancer. 2020;6(8):702–15. https://doi.org/10.1016/j.trecan.2020.04.010.
161. Varaprasad GL, Gupta VK, Prasad K, Kim E, Tej MB, Mohanty P, et al. Recent advances and future perspectives in the therapeutics of prostate cancer. Exp Hematol Oncol. 2023;12(1):80. https://doi.org/10.1186/s40164-023-00444-9.
162. Stabile A, Giganti F, Rosenkrantz AB, Taneja SS, Villeirs G, Gill IS, et al. Multiparametric MRI for prostate cancer diagnosis: current status and future directions. Nat Rev Urol. 2020;17(1):41–61. https://doi.org/10.1038/s41585-019-0212-4.
163. Crawford ED, Heidenreich A, Lawrentschuk N, Tombal B, Pompeo ACL, Mendoza-Valdes A, et al. Androgen-targeted therapy in men with prostate cancer: evolving practice and future considerations. Prostate Cancer Prostatic Dis. 2019;22(1):24–38. https://doi.org/10.1038/s41391-018-0079-0.
164. Sebastian AM, Peter D. Artificial intelligence in cancer research: trends, challenges and future directions. Life. 2022;12(12):1991.
165. Sekhoacha M, Riet K, Motloung P, Gumenku L, Adegoke A, Mashele S. Prostate cancer review: genetics, diagnosis. Treatment Options, and Alternative Approaches Molecules. 2022:27(17). https://www.mdpi.com/1420-3049/27/17/5730
166. Kim TJ, Koo KC. Current status and future perspectives of checkpoint inhibitor immunotherapy for prostate cancer: a comprehensive review. Int J Mol Sci. 2020;21(15):5484.
167. Tufail AB, Ma YK, Kaabar MKA, Martínez F, Junejo AR, Ullah I, et al. Deep learning in cancer diagnosis and prognosis prediction: a minireview on challenges, recent trends, and future directions. Comput Math Methods Med. 2021;2021(1):9025470.
168. Dagar G, Gupta A, Masoodi T, Nisar S, Merhi M, Hashem S, et al. Harnessing the potential of CAR-T cell therapy: progress, challenges, and future directions in hematological and solid tumor treatments. J Transl Med. 2023;21(1):449.
169. Bhoir S, De Benedetti A. Beyond the horizon: rethinking prostate cancer treatment through innovation and alternative strategies. Cancers (Basel). 2025;17(1). https://www.mdpi.com/2072-6694/17/1/75
170. Feretzakis G, Juliebø-Jones P, Tsaturyan A, Sener TE, Verykios VS, Karapiperis D, et al. Emerging trends in AI and Radiomics for bladder, kidney, and prostate cancer: a critical review. Cancers (Basel). 2024;16(4). https://www.mdpi.com/2072-6694/16/4/810
171. Dhoundiyal S, Srivastava S, Kumar S, Singh G, Ashique S, Pal R, et al. Radiopharmaceuticals: navigating the frontier of precision medicine and therapeutic innovation. Eur J Med Res. 2024;29(1):26.
172. Homewood DC, Mcdonald J, Valaydon Z, Ogluszko C, Sukocheva OA, Tse E, et al. eHealth platforms facilitate prostate cancer shared care: a systematic review. Healthcare. 2024;12(17).
173. Young K, Xiong T, Pfisterer KJ, Ng D, Jiao T, Lohani R, et al. A qualitative study on healthcare professional and patient perspectives on nurse-led virtual prostate cancer survivorship care. Commun Med. 2023;3(1):159.
174. Pham Q, Hearn J, Gao B, Brown I, Hamilton RJ, Berlin A, et al. Virtual care models for cancer survivorship. npj Digit Med. 2020;3(1):113.

175. Clarke AL, Roscoe J, Appleton R, Parashar D, Muthuswamy R, Khan O, et al. Promoting integrated care in prostate cancer through online prostate cancer-specific holistic needs assessment: a feasibility study in primary care. Support Care Cancer. 2020;28(4):1817–27.
176. Omar MI, Roobol MJ, Ribal MJ, Abbott T, Agapow PM, Araujo S, et al. Introducing PIONEER: a project to harness big data in prostate cancer research. Nat Rev Urol. 2020;17(6):351–62.
177. Sanchini V, Marelli L, Monturano M, Bonizzi G, Peruzzotti G, Orecchia R, et al. A comprehensive ethics and data governance framework for data-intensive health research: lessons from an Italian cancer research institute. Account Res. 2025;32(1):59–76.
178. Cacciamani GE, Chen A, Gill IS, Hung AJ. Artificial intelligence and urology: ethical considerations for urologists and patients. Nat Rev Urol. 2024;21(1):50–9.
179. Kucera R, Pecen L, Topolcan O, Dahal AR, Costigliola V, Giordano FA, et al. Prostate cancer management: long-term beliefs, epidemic developments in the early twenty-first century and 3PM dimensional solutions. EPMA J. 2020;11(3):399–418. https://doi.org/10.1007/s13167-020-00214-1.

Current Challenges in Prostate Cancer Biosensing

11

Brijesh Shukla, Rahul Kumar, Dhruv Vasishtha, and Farzad Taghizadeh-Hesary

Abbreviations

AI	artificial intelligence
BPH	benign prostatic hyperplasia
CDSS	clinical decision support system
ctDNA	circulating tumor DNA
DRE	digital rectal examination
EMA	European Medicines Agency
FDA	U.S. Food and Drug Administration
FHIR	Fast Healthcare Interoperability Resources
GDPR	General Data Protection Regulation
HER	electronic health record
HIPAA	Health Insurance Portability and Accountability Act
HL7	Health Level Seven (data exchange standard)
LMICs	low- and middle-income countries

B. Shukla
Seiko College of Pharmacy, Lucknow, Uttar Pradesh, India

R. Kumar
Faculty of Pharmacy, Vidya University, Meerut, Uttar Pradesh, India

D. Vasishtha
Department of Pharmacy, School of Medical and Allied Sciences, Galgotias University, Greater Noida, Uttar Pradesh, India

F. Taghizadeh-Hesary (✉)
Breast Cancer Research Center, Iran University of Medical Sciences, Tehran, Iran

ENT and Head and Neck Research Center and Department, The Five Senses Health Institute, School of Medicine, Iran University of Medical Sciences, Tehran, Iran
e-mail: taghizadeh_hesary.f@iums.ac.ir

S. Srivastava et al. (eds.), *Biosensor Technologies for Prostate Cancer*,
https://doi.org/10.1007/978-981-95-8644-8_11

MIP	molecularly imprinted polymer
miRNA	microRNA
ML	machine learning
PSA	prostate-specific antigen
SOPs	standard operating procedures
SPR	surface plasmon resonance
VOC	volatile organic compound
XAI	explainable artificial intelligence

11.1 Introduction

Prostate cancer rates continue to rank as a leading male cancer worldwide because of population aging and rising socio-economic conditions in developing regions [1]. The detection methods of digital rectal examination, prostate-specific antigen (PSA) testing, and biopsy maintain their status as fundamental diagnostic tools, yet encounter various sensitiveness and specific performance-related shortcomings along with invasive characteristics. Biosensors demonstrate great potential in developing methods that deliver sensitive prostate cancer biomarker detection through non-invasive techniques at different stages of cancer progression [2]. The wide range of biosensor development platforms during the previous decade, which included electrochemical, optical, piezoelectric, and microfluidic systems, has not overcome translational barriers for their use in medical environments [3].

The application of prostate cancer biosensors faces three major challenges: poor technical performance in signal detection and biological problems produced by tissue differences and a shortage of biomarkers, along with insufficient validation procedures [4]. The 2023 Biosensors and Bioelectronics paper reported that cancer detection biosensors progress to clinical trials at only 8% of the time due to major barriers between laboratory development and healthcare delivery [5]. The combination of multi-capability biosensors with artificial intelligence (AI) technology results in enhanced difficulties when interpreting data results and complying with regulatory requirements. Prostate cancer molecular detection tools, which measure circulating tumor DNA (ctDNA), exosomes, and microRNAs, must be developed by biosensor platforms because the disease manifests as multiple distinct genetic entities instead of one distinct clinical type [6]. Implementation of prostate cancer biosensors requires both technological advancement and innovative team development methods that integrate knowledge from oncology with molecular biology, data science, and health systems research disciplines [7]. The chapter analyzes all current issues (Table 11.1) that stop biosensors from becoming mainstream devices for prostate cancer diagnostics [8]. Biosensing needs to overcome technical, biological, clinical, and economic, as well as ethical obstacles to reach maximum effectiveness in detecting prostate cancer early on, while supporting personalized treatment approaches.

These multifaceted barriers are graphically illustrated in Fig. 11.1, which summarizes the core domains hindering the clinical translation of prostate cancer biosensors.

Table 11.1 Summary of major challenges in prostate cancer biosensing

Challenge domain	Key issues	Impact	References
Technological	Sensitivity/specificity limits, miniaturization, signal noise	Poor clinical translation, device instability	[3]
Biological	Heterogeneity, biomarker variability, low early-stage marker availability	Low diagnostic accuracy, overtreatment	[5]
Clinical/ translational	Regulatory delays, reproducibility, insufficient validation	Market entry difficulty, lack of trust	[5]
Economic	High costs, poor access in LMICs, manufacturing complexity	Limited affordability and adoption	[9]
Data integration	Multiplex signal complexity, AI misinterpretation	Risk of diagnostic errors, lack of clinical integration	[10]

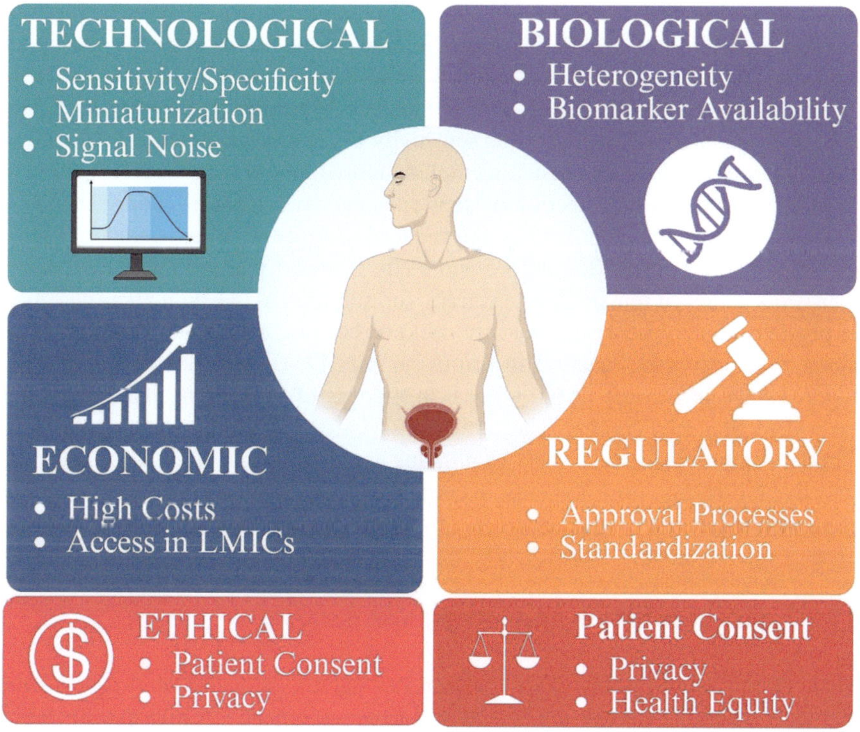

Fig. 11.1 Multifactorial challenges in the clinical translation of prostate cancer biosensors

11.2 Technological Limitations in Biosensor Development

Biosensors designed to detect prostate cancer show a strong prospect for change because they deliver quick results with high precision rates within healthcare locations [11]. Current technological barriers prevent the move from laboratory design specifications to developing clinically effective biosensor devices. There exist significant limitations in prostate cancer diagnostics that need proper resolution to prevent stagnation in early detection progress, as well as personalized patient care methods [12].

11.2.1 Sensitivity and Specificity Constraints

A biosensor's fundamental operational assessment relies on three key factors, which include the limit of detection (LOD), sensitivity, and specificity. The picomolar to femtomolar detection levels of state-of-the-art biosensors for PSA and other biomarkers remain questionable due to the imprecise diagnostic power of these biomarkers [13]. Although widely used, PSA shows limited value in diagnosis because its levels rise frequently during benign prostatic hyperplasia and prostatitis, and even after ejaculation. The detection sensitivity of biosensors increases when using nanomaterials, such as graphene, in combination with gold nanoparticles (AuNPs) or MXenes [14]. These detection devices encounter two main problems: inconsistent performance between batches and reduced stability when used under physiological situations. The 2022 ACS Nano study revealed that graphene field-effect transistors achieved remarkable sensitivity for microRNA-141 biomarker detection of prostate cancer, yet their durability declined because of sample oxidation combined with unspecific reaction in serum samples [15]. False positives alongside negatives act as barriers to the clinical usefulness of biosensors, particularly for early detection applications. The critical task is to improve biosensor selectivity without compromising sensitivity by utilizing aptamers or monoclonal antibodies as selective bio-recognition elements, in conjunction with stability and reproducibility elements [16].

11.2.2 Miniaturization and Integration Issues

Medical and point-of-care (POC) biosensors require miniaturization to become clinically viable. The reduction of device dimensions typically results in diminished signal quality, while fluid management becomes challenging, and the manufacturing protocols get more intricate [17]. Although lab-on-a-chip devices show potential, they struggle with controlling microfluidics, as well as difficulties in handling samples prior to testing, and problems in gaining popularity. The main challenge in miniaturizing a system stems from the need to sustain reliable signal transmission across microscale dimensions [18]. The control of devices at small sizes reduces volumetric forces to surface forces, which can produce unexpected electrochemical problems while increasing background noise requirements and demanding refined signal boosting approaches. Scale-up processes for biomarker enrichment, together with sample pre-processing steps into automated units, pose significant technological barriers for compact systems [19].

11.2.3 Signal Interference and Noise Challenges

Whole blood, urine, and serum samples can cause problematic signal disturbances that limit accurate measurements in diagnostic systems. Chemical effects introduced through changes in solution pH, along with variations in native enzyme and protein amounts, severely disrupt the readings produced by the sensor [20]. Electrochemical biosensors face two major drawbacks during operation, which include non-specific adsorption and electrode fouling that result in reduced reproducibility and reliability over extended use. Surface passivation and nanostructured anti-fouling coatings, as well as blocking agents exemplified by bovine serum albumin, represent approaches used to mitigate this issue. These modifications tend to slow down target binding reaction rates while diminishing the overall sensitivity of the sensor [21]. Surface plasmon resonance (SPR)-based optical biosensors encounter operational problems due to baseline irregularities, which necessitate accurate continuous monitoring of angular or wavelength shifts, thereby making their deployment challenging in uncontrolled environments outside laboratories [22]. Biosensors with multiple detection channels face communication issues between channels, resulting in confusing or wrong result outputs. Successful solutions to this problem (Table 11.2) require advancements in architectural sensors, along with fluidic separation protocols and modern signal processing mechanisms [23].

Table 11.2 Comparative overview of current vs. next-generation biosensors for prostate cancer

Feature	Current biosensors	Next-generation biosensors (proposed)	References
Biomarker targeting	Primarily PSA	Multiplexed: PSA, PCA3, TMPRSS2-ERG, miRNAs, ctDNA	[24]
Sensitivity range	Nanomolar to micromolar	Femtomolar to picomolar with enhanced nanomaterials	[25]
Specificity	Moderate, often false positives/negatives	High, via aptamer/antibody hybrid bio-recognition	[26]
Sample type	Serum or biopsy	Non-invasive: urine, plasma, exosomes	[27]
Integration capability	Standalone devices	Lab-on-a-chip with AI/ML data processing	[28]
Stability and reusability	Low, especially in physiological conditions	Improved via anti-fouling coatings and signal amplification	[29]
Clinical validation status	Rarely beyond lab testing	Designed with regulatory and clinical trial pathways in mind	[30]

11.3 Biomarker Limitations and Biological Complexity

Prostate cancer biosensors strictly depend on accurate reliable biomarkers that match biological measurements during their detection process [31]. The biological protocols, including proteins and nucleic acids together with metabolites and extracellular vesicles, face fundamental restrictions that block both diagnostic accuracy and medical applications of sensing platforms [32].

11.3.1 Variability and Heterogeneity in Biomarkers

Several molecular subtypes of prostate cancer exist because this cancer displays various genetic and epigenetic changes throughout its diverse entity [33]. Multiple molecular heterogeneities within tumors, as well as between patients, directly alter biomarker expressions. As a widely used biomarker, PSA provides limited discrimination between aggressive tumor types and non-aggressive cases due to its lack of molecular markers of harm. Overtreatment, along with excessive biopsies, occurs because of this limitation, which increases both healthcare expenses and patient morbidity [34]. The detection biomarkers PCA3, along with TMPRSS2-ERG fusion gene and microRNAs, including miR-21 and miR-141, and exosomal cargo, demonstrate better specificity, yet they express differently according to tumor grade, patient ethnicity, inflammation status, and circadian rhythms [35]. A study in the European Urology Oncology journal demonstrated that microRNA expression profiles change drastically by more than 40% based on the choice of collection methods, storage environments, and patient dietary conditions at the time of collection. The diagnosis of prostate cancer at all stages proves impossible through the use of solitary biomarkers [36]. Advanced multiplexed biosensing platforms should be developed to simultaneously run multiple complementary biomarkers because such challenges increase the difficulty of designing sensors while complicating data integration and clinical interpretation.

11.3.2 Challenges in Multiplex Detection

Multiplexed biosensors demonstrate great potential because they can analyze diverse sets of biological molecules (proteins, RNAs, and metabolites) through single measurement assays. Multiple analysis detection presents technical and biological difficulties, which become significant factors during measurement [37]. A technological requirement exists for each detected analyte to have its own dedicated recognition element, while the signal transduction pathway requires precise adjustment to prevent interference with detection [38]. These biomarkers possess dissimilar concentration ranges that vary extensively from one another. PSA exists at nanogram per milliliter concentrations, and some microRNAs appear only at femtomolar levels. This disparity necessitates ultra-sensitive and dynamic biosensing mechanisms. Current biological evidence shows that researchers agree minimally about which biomarker combinations provide optimal predictive ability [39]. The clinical value of PSA, PCA3, and TMPRSS2-ERG together has proved promising but still needs to be fully validated for clinical use. Interpreting multiple analytical variables in tests becomes complex because each needs context-specific evaluation along with disease-related metadata, including patient age, racial background, and family medical history [40].

11.3.3 Limited Availability of Early-Stage Biomarkers

There exists an urgent diagnostic problem with prostate cancer because of insufficient reliable biomarkers during early detection [41]. Current diagnostic markers, such as PSA, exhibit significant changes only during late stages of tumorigenesis and when tumors reach considerable sizes. Current biosensing systems perform inadequately when applied to pre-symptomatic detection, which would lead to actual outcome improvements [42]. Researchers now investigate malignant potential through two early indicator measures, which include ctDNA together with DNA methylation signatures in Glutathione S-Transferase Pi 1 (GSTP1) or adenomatous polyposis coli (APC) genes [43]. The detection of ctDNA requires extremely sensitive platforms because this biomarker exists in sparse amounts as tumors begin to develop and must be differentiated from the normal cfDNA background signal [44]. The analysis of urinary biomarkers represents a promising non-invasive testing method, though it produces inconsistent results because of hydration levels and kidney functions, as well as handling variations [45]. Biosensors cannot deliver reliable early diagnosis until there exists a simultaneous effort to discover new biomarkers along with their validation through clinical standardization.

11.4 Clinical and Translational Barriers

The potential of biosensors for prostate cancer assessment through technological advancements and scientific advancements does not readily translate into widespread clinical use [46]. Clinically useful biosensors require the successful completion of complex regulatory tasks alongside logistical and standardization requirements, which link laboratory innovations to clinical applications at the bedside [47]. Advanced biosensors need the resolution of translational challenges to fulfill their clinical potential beyond laboratory settings.

11.4.1 Regulatory Hurdles for Clinical Adoption

Medical diagnostic biosensors need to complete demanding regulatory examinations before acquiring permission because they must demonstrate effectiveness for patient protection, along with reliable data generation [48]. Medical diagnostic biosensors must undergo controlled preclinical testing to meet regulatory standards for reproducibility data and biocompatibility results. This process also requires submission of clinical trial reports to the U.S. Food and Drug Administration and the European Medicines Agency to obtain diagnostic approval [49]. The regulatory approval of biosensors becomes strained due to their use of innovative diagnostic systems to measure new and complex biomarkers, such as exosomes, microRNAs, and ctDNA [50]. The ability to approve these biomarkers as regulatory elements is hindered by unclear clinical thresholds and a lack of agreement on their pathological significance. Oncological biosensor technologies remain ineligible for market authorization, as the Global Biosensing Alliance reports that in 2023, fewer than 5% of under-development devices achieved regulatory approval due to the absence of harmonized evaluation protocols and clinical data [51]. The existing regulatory frameworks must change due to the emerging difficulties posed by AI-assisted biosensors, as well as wearable diagnostic devices, which regulatory systems have not sufficiently developed. Startups alongside academic research institutions and development expenses are delayed due to an ambiguous regulatory structure, which also prevents clinical translation work [52].

11.4.2 Reproducibility and Standardization Issues

Executing biosensors successfully faces a substantial challenge when striving for identical measurement results between separate laboratories. Biosensors that demonstrate outstanding results in laboratory conditions often produce unsatisfactory outcomes throughout various patient groups and actual operational environments [53]. Biosensor inconsistency appears because laboratories do not use standardized protocols for fabrication and calibration, and for handling samples and interpreting data during testing. The performance of electrochemical and optical biosensors depends heavily on environmental conditions, including temperature and sample medium composition, along with medium water content. Standard operating procedures, when rigorously enforced, enable consistent results, yet the absence of these procedures makes it hard to duplicate findings inside the same laboratory environment [54]. Evaluation benchmarks represent a fundamental problem that cannot be ignored in the field. The biosensor industry has not established standard controls and guidelines that are comparable to those used in molecular diagnostics, such as Reverse Transcription Polymerase Chain Reaction (RT-PCR), through guides like Minimum Information for Publication of Quantitative Real-Time PCR Experiments (MIQE) for Quantitative Polymerase Chain Reaction (qPCR) [55]. Different laboratories struggle to implement standard performance reporting due to widespread variations in their detection methods (e.g., LOD, specificity, and signal-to-noise ratio). The Biosensor Technologies and Standards for Diagnostics by 2030 (BIOSENS2030) initiative with EU funding supports the development of testing requirements and clinical benchmarking data for biosensors as part of a new interdisciplinary collaboration model [56]. The current initiatives to develop these standards remain immature, while they need worldwide collaborative efforts.

11.4.3 Challenges in Clinical Validation and Trials

Testing and validation of diagnostic biosensors demand the highest number of resources within the product development process and span over an extended period of time [57]. Biosensor validation requires ongoing assessments of various patient groups and specimen types, together with clinical applications for official diagnostic confirmation. The lack of appropriate biobank samples for early-stage prostate cancer represents a major challenge because it reduces our ability to properly measure biosensor performance throughout disease evolution [58]. Medical trials often yield non-generalizable results because of disparities that occur within the design framework, especially when including sample preparation procedures, patient selection protocols, and observed outcomes. Sensitive detection platforms that work with minimally abundant biomarkers need to operate effectively in different biological substances, such as whole blood, plasma, and urine. The matrices produce complicated patterns that early validation protocols fail to include. An SPR-based biosensor designed for urinary PCA3 detection achieved 92% sensitivity in laboratory assessments, yet its clinical trial results in multiple sites declined to 65% sensitivity because of urine management inconsistencies and hydration effects in patients [59]. Financial limitations impact the situation as well [60]. Biosensor testing receives less financial support than drug testing, especially when performing preliminary validation studies. Tight budget constraints at both academic institutions and startup companies that work on biosensor development prevent them from performing the necessary large-scale clinical studies needed for regulatory approval. Figure 11.2 outlines the sequential decision-making

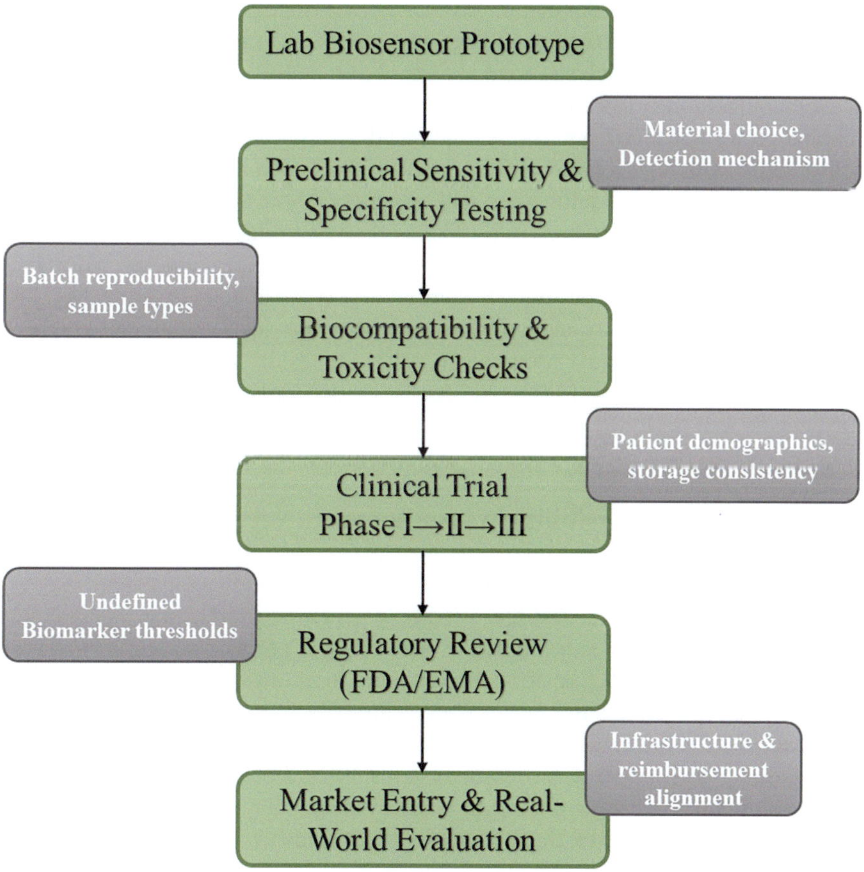

Fig. 11.2 Decision pipeline for biosensor clinical translation

pipeline required for the clinical translation of prostate cancer biosensors, from initial validation to regulatory approval and clinical integration [61].

11.5 Cost and Accessibility Issues

The development and implementation of prostate cancer diagnostic biosensors frequently lead to major expenses and difficulties with scalability [62]. The actual clinical utility and affordability of these diagnostic devices for POC applications prove challenging for researchers, specifically in low- and middle-income countries (LMICs) and underserved geographic regions [63].

11.5.1 High Development and Manufacturing Costs

The biosensor development lifecycle from conceptual design to clinical deployment requires considerable investment in materials, fabrication infrastructure, and validation studies [64]. The production of advanced biosensors, which combine nanomaterials such as AuNPs, carbon nanotubes, and graphene, or integrated microfluidics with AI-based signal analysis, requires expensive budgetary resources for large-scale manufacturing. The advances in screen printing, 3D printing, and roll-to-roll fabrication methods have not lowered the manufacturing expenses for reproducible sensor chips with high sensitivity. The precision needed to integrate biological recognition elements (e.g., antibodies and aptamers) onto nanostructured surfaces affects the production quality [65]. The high cost of biosensor manufacturing becomes more complex because biological elements deteriorate quickly, while sensors demand refrigerated transport systems throughout their delivery route [66]. The total commercialization expenses of biosensors become significantly higher due to the necessity of intellectual property licensing alongside quality control requirements and compliance with ISO and regulatory standards such as ISO 13485 for medical devices [67].

11.5.2 Economic Feasibility in Low-Resource Settings

The long-term biosensor development objective focuses on making cancer diagnosis more affordable and accessible, yet implementation shortages create a major barrier for resource-limited healthcare systems [68]. A portable real-time biosensor has the potential to create transformative changes in settings with limited pathology lab and imaging facilities in LMICs. Preserving biosensor use remains impossible due to the lack of proper infrastructure, qualified personnel, and budgetary support in developing nations. Moist biosensor systems utilize technological advancements from smartphones to handheld potentiometers and optical readers, as well as microfluidic controllers; however, these devices are not readily accessible in global rural and underserved areas [69]. Many biosensors deployed today use Western patient samples for testing purposes, while Western populations differ from global ethnic and regional disease patterns. Quality diagnostic testing becomes problematic because it compromises both accuracy and clinical usefulness in multiple populations. The reimbursement systems for healthcare services are often driven by the development of new diagnostic technologies [70]. The lack of specific reimbursement rules for new biosensor diagnostics within public healthcare programs complicates their clinical adoption even when innovative tools are ready for use. Future research requiring interdisciplinary efforts should prioritize three essential elements: design focused on minimizing costs alongside the development of both open-source electronic devices and local material procurement procedures and platform development at community-based settings [71]. The subsidy of biosensor adoption, together with infrastructure development for decentralized cancer diagnostics, must receive support from public–private partnerships and global health initiative programs such as the World Health Organization's Digital Health Strategy [72].

11.6 Data Integration and Interpretation Challenges

The advancement of prostate cancer biosensing platforms into complex diagnostic systems that detect multiple parameters in real time has led to the generation of complex high-dimensional datasets [73]. The diagnostic potential of these datasets increases substantially because they contain properties such as molecular concentrations together with electrochemical signals, spectral patterns, and patient metadata and temporal trends [74]. The process of integrating, clinically interpreting, and translating multi-stream data presents significant challenges.

11.6.1 Complex Data From Multiplexed and Multi-Modal Sensors

Current biosensors achieve better diagnosis through their simultaneous analysis of several biomarkers or their combination of electrochemical, along with optical and acoustic physical signatures [75]. Such multi-modal and multiplexed platforms produce highly complex, non-linear, multidimensional data that exceeds the output of conventional laboratory testing methods. When using a nano-plasmonic biosensor that detects PSA, Prostate Cancer Antigen 3 (PCA3), and Transmembrane Protease, Serine 2–ETS-Related Gene fusion (TMPRSS2-ERG) fusion genes simultaneously, it generates distinct optical signatures for each target substance. The signatures that a system produces at various concentrations will be impacted simultaneously by the environment and the complexity of the sample, and the state of the sensor calibration system [76]. Simultaneous detection of multiple targets in multiplexed platforms creates signal interferences among analytes, which results in erroneous interpretation of results. Technical capabilities alone do not resolve this problem because the analysis of optical data represents the primary issue [77]. Technical experts must develop advanced mathematical methods in conjunction with complex

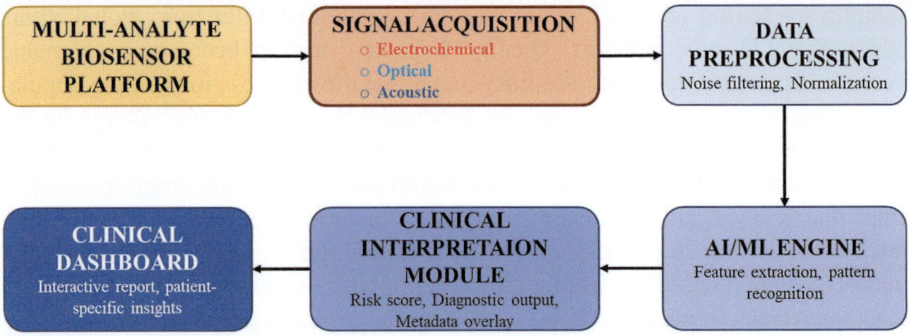

Fig. 11.3 Integrated AI-based multiplex biosensor workflow

signal-processing procedures to extract crucial clinical data from these biomarker signals. Healthcare practitioners risk exploiting clinical outcomes through incorrect signal interpretation or erroneous classification when they fail to handle platform complexity adequately because this leads to problems with overfitting and data misinterpretation, which harms both patient safety and clinical trust [78].

11.6.2 Role of AI and Machine Learning

Both AI and machine learning (ML) technologies are implemented in biosensing platforms to solve interpretative issues that exist in biosensing [79]. Deep learning pipelines and other algorithms, including support vector machines (SVMs), neural networks, and convolutional architectures, facilitate the detection of correlations in biosensor data that exceed human detection capabilities. The stepwise architecture of AI-assisted biosensor interpretation is illustrated in Fig. 11.3, demonstrating how multiplex biomarker inputs are processed through ML models to support clinical decision-making [80]. Research indicates that AI-based biosensors achieve better prostate cancer diagnosis by combining biosensor signals with patient characteristics, including age, PSA density, and Gleason score [81]. Engineering researchers presented an AI interpretation framework for electrochemical biosensors targeting PSA and miR-141 in the IEEE Transactions on Biomedical Engineering, which achieved 96% blade-test performance.

Integrating AI creates new technical barriers, which consist of the following components: data privacy and security. Mobile devices used with clinical biosensors must comply with both the Health Insurance Portability and Accountability Act (HIPAA) and the General Data Protection Regulation (GDPR) data privacy regulations and security requirements. Health organizations must maintain data security measures for both data transmission and storage, as well as the secure handling of patient-sensitive medical information [82]. *Model generalizability*: The particular population characteristics or controlled laboratory conditions used for AI model training produce poor diagnostic results when deployed in diverse clinical settings of real medical practice [83]. The issue poses a specific challenge to prostate cancer diagnosis because biomarker attributes, together with disease evolution, change according to ethnic background, individual health factors, and age groups. *Explainability and clinical trust*: Healthcare professionals cannot easily trust black-box AI models because they lack explainability during important medical decisions that impact patient health [84]. Explainable AI (XAI) frameworks that offer explainability and traceability in biosensor-assisted diagnosis receive increasing demand from the market.

11.6.3 Interfacing with Clinical Decision Systems

Clinical decision support systems (CDSSs) require the inclusion of biosensor output data to realize practical implementation. The integration faces problems because biosensors fail to work with current electronic health records systems due to both record differences and divergent data formatting, as well as conflicting medical threshold definitions [85]. Biosensor data becomes effective for clinical workflow enhancement through standardized presentation in combination with interpretability and actionability, while using Electronic Health Records (EHR)-compatible dashboards and mobile applications with real-time alert capabilities and visualization options [86]. Standard data protocols, such as Health Level Seven (HL7) or Fast Healthcare Interoperability Resources (FHIR), require agreement to work alongside engineers and healthcare personnel who collaborate on system development. Clinical staff require biosensors that enable extended data observation, as this capability enables doctors to track disease progression alongside treatment effects and make informed treatment adjustments. Table 11.3 summarizes key barriers to biosensor-CDSS integration and corresponding solutions to support real-time clinical workflows [87]. Analyzing time-series data includes multiple analytical challenges because it requires developers to manage non-continuous data points, combined with temporal offset changes and live system calibration adjustments [88]

Table 11.3 Challenges and proposed strategies for clinical integration of biosensor data

Challenge	Proposed strategy	References
Data format incompatibility	Use HL7/FHIR for EHR integration	[89]
Lack of real-time interoperability	Develop Active Pharmaceutical Ingredient (API)-based communication modules	[89]
Time-series data complexity	Employ adaptive time-series AI models with calibration drift correction	[89]
Visualization gaps	Implement clinician dashboards with actionable alerts	[89]

11.6.4 Clinical Validation of Data Interpretation Models

The last step before medical utilization involves verifying that algorithm-produced outcomes precisely represent the patient's medical status to achieve beneficial clinical outcomes [90]. Multiple centers test biosensors on different patients through trials, which must confirm their results against diagnostic tests, including histopathology, alongside imaging and molecular testing methods [67]. A major challenge exists because medical evaluation metrics remain unavailable. The clinical usefulness of biosensor-based decision models remains difficult to evaluate through standard accuracy, sensitivity, and specificity measurements [91]. Biosensor data evaluation benefits from new performance indicators, including net reclassification improvement, decision curve analysis, and clinical impact curves, for assessing diagnostic workflow opportunities. Developing biosensors poses dual challenges because developers should construct both sensor devices alongside complete frameworks that connect analytical control systems to computational systems and to clinical and regulatory networks that enhance direct patient healthcare benefits [91].

11.7 Ethical and Privacy Considerations in Biosensor Deployment

Recent advancements in biosensor manufacturing for prostate cancer detection create widespread ethical, legal, and social complications [92]. The deployment of devices that link to clinical health data needs thorough investigation regarding their impact on bioethics, alongside data control and the process of consenting patients and health equity standards [93].

11.7.1 Patient Autonomy and Informed Consent

Wearable and home-use biosensors give diagnostic control to decentralized patient settings and doctors' offices instead of laboratory facilities. These adjustments empower patients in healthcare, but they also impact how subsequent consent processes operate [94]. The process of obtaining consent depends on clinicians to guide their patients along the consent pathway during routine medical diagnostics. Biosensor systems used in POC or at-home testing provide their consent forms digitally through interface click-through agreements [95]. Patients face increased risks of not comprehending the extent of collected data, along with diagnostic limitations and the consequences of test false positives and false negatives. Numerous experts advocate for layered consent models that provide users with multimedia education about data flow, algorithm interpretations, and clinical pathways, as this approach can enable the ethical deployment of AI [96]. Patients must have the ability to change or cancel consent rights as their medical situation transforms, together with their preferences [97].

11.7.2 Privacy, Data Protection, and Surveillance Risks

The transmission of health-sensitive information, including biomarkers, disease status reports, and genetic details, happens through wireless technologies and cloud platforms. Data privacy, together with cybersecurity, suffers from major weaknesses when sensitive health information is communicated using wireless or cloud-based systems [98]. The well-rated npj Digital Medicine study from 2024 established that over 30% of health apps using biosensors presented insufficient end-to-end encryption alongside data sharing with third-party vendors without proper user consent in almost half of the cases [99]. Robust data governance frameworks should be established because they guarantee compliance with both the GDPR within the EU and HIPAA in the United States. For proper ethical application of biosensor data, sovereignty needs to be recognized because it represents the fundamental right of people and nation-states to regulate data they produce within their respective territories [100]. Certain population groups view biosensor-based diagnostics as a form of digital colonial expansion when data extraction fails to deliver benefits or involves insufficient local capacity development or group collaboration. Health monitoring and surveillance are two closely related, yet ethically ambiguous, activities. The use of biosensors in insurance and workplace or correctional environment settings creates the potential for coercive situations because individuals may need to employ diagnostic tools to maintain their employment, receive benefits, or parole from the system. These approaches might result in increased discrimination against the population and diminish the public trust in digital health solutions.

11.7.3 Algorithmic Bias and Health Disparities

The implementation of AI algorithms with ML in biosensor evaluation raises concerns about the potential problem of algorithmic bias, which can lead to misidentification or reduced performance for individuals belonging to minority communities [101]. A combination of problems arises from bias in the training datasets or structural flaws in the model architecture, which inadvertently benefit some biomarkers or clinical data points [102]. The analysis of a 2023 commercial prostate cancer AI tool using biosensors revealed that it predicted lower cancer risk for African American patients by 23% because its training dataset did not include enough minority participants [103]. The existence of bias compromises medical precision, exacerbating existing health inequalities. Multiple solutions are needed to address this problem [104]: inclusive training datasets that represent diverse ethnic, geographic, and socio-economic populations; bias-detection audits throughout the algorithm development lifecycle; and engagement with community advisory boards to co-develop culturally sensitive deployment strategies. The development of biosensor-based AI systems requires researchers and developers to implement the Fairness, Accountability, and Transparency (FAT) guidelines to prevent the reinforcement or intensification of social inequality [105].

11.7.4 Equity in Access and Use

Testing biosensors with ML techniques can introduce systematic errors, as the predictive systems often show reduced accuracy or misdiagnose individuals who do not belong to the primary population groups. AI models can develop limitations from bias issues because both training databases have inadequate diversity selection and intrinsic biases within their structural design choices [106]. A 2023 audit discovered that a commercial prostate cancer AI tool underdiagnosed risk in African Americans by 23% since its training dataset had inadequate minority representation. Clinically accurate results become incomplete because of such biases, which simultaneously promote existing healthcare gaps [107]. Multiple solutions are needed to address this problem: inclusive training datasets that represent diverse ethnic, geographic, and socio-economic populations; bias-detection audits throughout the algorithm development lifecycle; and engagement with community advisory boards to co-develop culturally sensitive deployment strategies. The development of biosensor-based AI systems requires researchers and developers to implement the FAT guidelines to prevent the reinforcement or intensification of social inequality [108].

11.7.5 Ethical Frameworks and Global Governance

To prevent technical barriers within biosensors' managerial applications, a cross-sectoral ethical framework needs immediate development for their proper innovation process. The WHO Global Strategy on Digital Health (2020–2025) and IEEE's Ethically Aligned Design provide general guidelines; however, scientists are currently developing more specialized guidelines for biosensing technologies used in oncology [109]. Such ethical governance systems require adaptability to conduct ongoing updates that match changing technologies, as well as cultural values and social expectations. The development of ethical biosensing technologies in oncology requires active participation from scientists, clinicians, ethicists, patients, regulators, technologists, and insurers [110]. Biosensors aimed at prostate cancer diagnosis will succeed when they fulfill ethical standards and align with both societal values and public trust elements. As outlined in Table 11.4, addressing biosensor ethics requires the integration of technical safeguards and inclusive design practices [111].

Table 11.4 Ethical challenges vs. technical safeguards in biosensor deployment

Ethical challenge	Technical or policy safeguard	References
Informed consent	Layered consent via multimedia and real-time opt-out	[112]
Data privacy and sovereignty	End-to-end encryption; local data storage options	[112]
Algorithmic bias	Bias audits, diverse datasets, XAI	[112]
Environmental sustainability	Modular design, biodegradable components	[112]

Real-time ethics monitoring systems should be studied to strengthen governance, as they can track unintended effects, misuse, and clinical outcome disparities for biosensor-based diagnostics, just as pharmacovigilance tracks drug safety [113]. A new structure known as algorithmic stewardship should be formalized through interdisciplinary teams that inspect, update, and protect the responsible development of AI models that interpret biosensor data. Biosensor systems with predictive features that forecast medical trajectories necessitate ethical decision-making regarding the presentation of data to patients when therapy options are scarce [114]. The ethical framework needs to analyze the psychological impact of continuous self-assessment because it can generate health anxiety and behavior changes in patients who receive regular diagnostic alerts [115]. The assessment of ethical conduct regarding automatic behavior change prompts from biosensor systems must determine whether these nudges have a persuasive impact without being coercive, thereby preserving user autonomy and advancing health literacy. Future biosensor ethics must address sustainability standards through research on the ecological challenges posed by waste from disposable components, as well as battery-powered devices and microelectronic components [116]. The developers should include circular design principles in their work with biodegradable materials combined with modular components that reduce waste while maintaining diagnostic precision. Equity requires consideration as a fundamental principle for accessing new innovations as well as diagnostics [117]. The development of biosensors for underprivileged groups and uncommon aggressive prostate cancer types should be a focused area for funding by academic institutions, together with biotech companies and funding bodies. Such an approach in research and peer-review procedures ensures inclusion and social awareness in biosensor research.

11.8 Future Perspectives and Innovation Pathways

11.8.1 Convergence of Multimodal Biosensing and Intelligent Diagnostics

The evolution of diagnostic technology will lead to biosensor development for prostate cancer that includes multi-biomarker detection in addition to multiple omics datasets analysis [118]. The next generation of biosensors integrates different types of biomarkers, including PSA, hK2 protein biomarkers, PCA3 mRNA and TMPRSS2-ERG fusion genes, and exosomal RNA and ctDNA mutations and oncometabolites under one diagnostic platform [119]. The combination of different analytical techniques leads to better tumor aggressiveness detection accuracy, as well as increased sensitivity at the early stages of diagnosis [120]. The detection process for scarce heterogenic markers will improve using Clustered Regularly Interspaced Short Palindromic Repeats diagnostics alongside aptamer arrays, along with molecularly imprinted polymers and antibody-mimetic scaffolds. Several novel biosensor prototypes are currently under development, as detailed in Table 11.5, offering expanded multiplexing and predictive capability

Table 11.5 Next-generation biosensor technologies in development

Technology	Target biomarkers	Analytical method	Sensing mechanism	Clinical stage	Key advantages	References
Sweat-based VOC sensor	Metabolic VOCs (e.g., hexanal)	Gas chromatography with sensor arrays	Chemo-resistive + nanoporous sensors	Pre-clinical	Non-invasive, wearable integration	[123]
Microfluidic ctDNA chip	ctDNA (AR mutations, TMPRSS2-ERG)	Digital PCR	Electrochemical readout	Early validation	Ultra-sensitive, sample-efficient	[124]
AI-coupled electrochemical array	PSA, hK2, miR-141, exosomal RNA	Multiplex ELISA + AI classifier	Graphene-based transduction	Clinical prototyping	Multiplexed, predictive analytics	[125]
Digital Twin-integrated patch	PSA + IL-6 + cortisol (stress)	Bio-affinity + digital modeling	Wearable, Bluetooth-enabled	Conceptual	Continuous monitoring, dynamic feedback	[126]

[121]. ML systems based on ensemble models and deep learning play crucial roles in interpreting biosensor information, which enables physicians to perform contextualized diagnoses using both individual health records and broader population health statistics, as well as known medical conditions. The transition leads to "diagnostics-as-a-service," which allows online processing of biosensor data into practical healthcare decisions through predictive analysis and individualized risk assessments [122].

11.8.2 Wearable, Implantable, and Decentralized Monitoring Platforms

Biosensors now enable continuous decentralized monitoring of biological indicators through devices that are either embedded or worn on the body [127]. Active researchers work on wearable devices that can identify prostate cancer-related biomarkers present in both sweat and interstitial fluid, as well as breath. Two possible options for non-invasive tumor activity monitoring involve the assessment of sweat volatile organic compounds (VOCs) together with electrochemical markers. The implantable nanosensors represent a promising surveillance system for biochemical recurrence monitoring after treatment by offering real-time in vivo measurement abilities of cytokines, as well as enzymes and PSA variants [128]. Smart fabrics, microneedle patches, and ingestible sensors will continually track diagnostic data and wirelessly transmit it to healthcare professionals, hence allowing early treatment action. This will shape future healthcare platforms. The new innovations support continuous treatment observation by delivering enhanced access to medical services in sparsely populated areas [129]. Technological integration of biosensors into mobile health (mHealth) and telehealth platforms allows AI-based triage systems to operate while generating dynamic risk reports and providing immediate virtual consultation services that distribute cancer care outside tertiary facilities [130].

11.8.3 Digital Twins, Sustainability, and Ethical-Driven Innovation

Biosensor science will adopt predictive simulation tools, especially digital twins, which are virtual patient models created from prolonged biosensor data in the future [131]. Simulated disease paths, intervention outcomes, and therapeutic responses become feasible with these models, which allow medical practitioners to verify treatment approaches virtually before clinical use. The privacy of patients remains protected through the use of federated learning, as this method enables the training of biosensor AI models across separate datasets. The upcoming generation of biosensors will implement both ethical criteria in their design alongside sustainable environmental practices [132]. The planned deployment of mass biosensors will become more sustainable through the use of auditable polymers with materials designed for recycling, along with low-power electronic components. Updateable modular system designs will enable migration of sensor components when biomarkers require modification [133]. The development of ethical biosensors needs worldwide components working together to harmonize sensor development with fair resource distribution and both medical benefits and governmental transparency. Multiple organizational partnerships between academic institutions, corporate sectors, regulatory offices, and patient advocacy networks must maintain biosensor technology development with proper governance and universal access in advanced healthcare systems and basic health care facilities.

11.9 Conclusions

Global male mortality statistics demonstrate that prostate cancer remains one of the primary cancer-related causes of death, thereby requiring immediate, efficient, early-stage diagnostic solutions. The current challenges in prostate cancer biosensing encompass multiple scientific, technological, clinical, and ethical barriers, as well as translational barriers, which must be addressed for biosensors to reach their full potential. The examination started by discussing prostate cancer's biologically complicated nature and diverse characteristics, which serve as a barrier to finding consistent, reliable biomarkers. The deficiencies of PSA as a single biomarker, along with its inability to differentiate between aggressive and harmless cancers, make it crucial to develop disease-stage and risk-factor-specific multi-omics biomarker panels. The discussion regarding technology highlighted the challenges faced by existing biosensors in detecting both rare and unstable biomarkers in complex biological samples during real-time measurements. The clinical application of nanomaterials and advanced transducers faces obstacles due to operational stability issues, as well as challenges in reducing biofouling and ensuring reliability and consistency. The pathways described in this chapter predict an exciting development of biosensing instrumentation, which will upgrade devices from single tests to combined tests and interface with intelligent, connected devices. Clinical applications of biosensors remain limited due to regulatory uncertainties, the absence of clinical validation, and insufficient standards for sensor development, as well as testing methodologies and readout interpretation methods. Biosensor platforms face significant adoption barriers in LMIC regions due to their high prices, especially when incorporating nanofabrication and AI integration technologies, which restrict their availability to patients in these areas. This section explains that although AI systems integrated with cloud platforms improve medical precision and individualized care, they also challenge healthcare providers with data confidentiality issues, discriminatory automated programs, and system compatibility matters, as well as compliance with rules and regulations. The realization of intelligent diagnostics depends on strong ethical and technical systems that protect patient trust from failures resulting from unsystematic implementation. Most of the chapter examined the ethical, legal, and social consequences that arise when deploying prostate cancer biosensors. The successful deployment of prostate cancer biosensors requires active management of five primary topics: continued monitoring, consent protocols, algorithmic solutions and their impact, sustainable practices, and fair accessibility. These challenges should be resolved through design-oriented ethics principles in unification with adaptable regulatory structures and functional stakeholder collaboration. Public standards for biosensors must be standardized worldwide because this will stop regulatory evasion and build systematic protection systems in every medical sector. The solution to current prostate cancer biosensing obstacles requires an approach that combines scientific progress with ethical foresight, while bringing together experts from diverse fields and focusing on designs that cater to all users, and delivering services tailored to patient needs. Moving forward, biosensors will establish themselves as critical instruments to combat prostate cancer through their ability to create uninterrupted intelligent treatment monitoring systems, which result in enhanced patient outcomes across the board.

11.10 Summary

This chapter examines how the early detection and monitoring of prostate cancer are being revolutionized by the combination of biosensors with AI and ML technologies. It starts by discussing the drawbacks of conventional diagnostic techniques like PSA testing and emphasizes how contemporary biosensors, electrochemical, optical, nano, and wearable, allow for the non-invasive, real-time monitoring of important biomarkers such as PSA, PCA3, and TMPRSS2: ERG. The chapter describes the preprocessing, filtering, and analysis of biosensor-generated data using a variety of AI/ML models, such as deep learning (convolutional neural networks and recurrent neural networks), supervised learning (SVM and random forest), and unsupervised learning (PCA and K-means). It also highlights how crucial edge computing is for on-device diagnostics, which makes healthcare more accessible and individualized. In addition, the chapter examines XAI, regulatory standards, multi-modal data integration, and potential future developments such as digital twins and quantum computing. All things considered, it offers a thorough vision of AI-driven biosensor systems as potent instruments for improving prostate cancer precision diagnosis.

Glossary

Biosensor A device that uses biological molecules to detect chemical or biological targets, producing a measurable signal.

Biomarker A biological molecule found in blood, urine, or tissues that indicates a normal or abnormal process or condition.

PSA A protein produced by prostate cells, commonly used in prostate cancer screening.
Microfluidics The manipulation of small amounts of fluids in microscale channels for testing and diagnostics.
Nanomaterials Materials engineered at the nanometer scale, often used in biosensors to improve sensitivity and specificity.
ctDNA DNA fragments from tumor cells found in the bloodstream, used as a cancer biomarker.
Exosomes Nano-sized extracellular vesicles secreted by cells, containing biomolecules useful for diagnostics.
AI/ML Computational technologies used for pattern recognition and predictive analytics in complex datasets.
Digital Twin A virtual model of a patient created using real-time sensor data, enabling personalized simulation and care planning.
Signal-to-noise ratio A measure comparing the level of a desired signal to the level of background noise, affecting biosensor accuracy.
Biorecognition element A molecule like an antibody or aptamer that specifically binds the biomarker of interest in a biosensor.

References

1. Bertok T, Bertokova A, Hroncekova S, Chocholova E, Svecova N, Lorencova L, et al. Novel prostate cancer biomarkers: aetiology, clinical performance and sensing applications. Chem Int. 2021;9(8). Available from: https://www.mdpi.com/2227-9040/9/8/205.
2. Khan R, Arshad F, Hassan IU, Naikoo GA, Pedram MZ, Zedegan MS, et al. Advances in nanomaterial-based immunosensors for prostate cancer screening. Biomed Pharmacother [Internet]. 2022;155:113649. Available from: https://www.sciencedirect.com/science/article/pii/S0753332222010381.
3. Deshmukh R, Singh V, Harwansh RK, Agrawal R, Garg A, Singh S, et al. Emerging trends of nanomedicines in the management of prostate cancer: perspectives and potential applications. Pharmaceutics [Internet]. 2024;16(3). Available from: https://www.mdpi.com/1999-4923/16/3/297.
4. Sánchez-Salcedo R, Miranda-Castro R, de-los-Santos-Álvarez N, Lobo-Castañón MJ. Dual electrochemical genosensor for early diagnosis of prostate cancer through lncRNAs detection. Biosens Bioelectron [Internet]. 2021;192:113520. Available from: https://www.sciencedirect.com/science/article/pii/S0956566321005571.
5. Dehghani P, Salehirozveh M, Tajabadi A, Yeung CC, Lam M, Leung HY, et al. Next-gen point-of-care tool for ultra-sensitive detection of urinary spermine for prostate cancer diagnosis. ACS Sens [Internet]. 2025;10(4):2640–51. Available from: https://doi.org/10.1021/acssensors.4c03250.
6. Berenguer CV, Pereira F, Pereira JAM, Câmara JS. Volatilomics: an emerging and promising avenue for the detection of potential prostate cancer biomarkers. Cancers (Basel). 2022;14(16).
7. Yao J, Wang Y, Dai Y, Liu CC. Bioconjugated, single-use biosensor for the detection of biomarkers of prostate cancer. ACS Omega [Internet]. 2018;3(6):6411–8. Available from: https://doi.org/10.1021/acsomega.8b00634.
8. Ji S, Lee M, Kim D. Detection of early stage prostate cancer by using a simple carbon nanotube@paper biosensor. Biosens Bioelectron. 2018;102:345–50.

9. Luhar S, Ghosh R, Chatterjee PB, Srivastava DN. An impedometric sensor based on boronic acid @ plastic chip electrode for sensitive detection of prostate cancer biomarker spermine. Biosens Bioelectron X [Internet]. 2022;12:100219. Available from: https://www.sciencedirect.com/science/article/pii/S2590137022001121.
10. Nair RR, Debnath S, Das S, Wakchaure P, Ganguly B, Chatterjee PB. A highly selective turn-on biosensor for measuring spermine/spermidine in human urine and blood. ACS Appl Bio Mater [Internet]. 2019;2(6):2374–87. Available from: https://doi.org/10.1021/acsabm.9b00084.
11. Dejous C, Krishnan UM. Sensors for diagnosis of prostate cancer: looking beyond the prostate specific antigen. Biosens Bioelectron. 2021;173:112790.
12. Kshirsagar P, Seshacharyulu P, Muniyan S, Rachagani S, Smith LM, Thompson C, et al. DNA-gold nanoprobe-based integrated biosensing technology for non-invasive liquid biopsy of serum miRNA: a new frontier in prostate cancer diagnosis. Nanomed Nanotechnol Biol Med [Internet]. 2022;43:102566. Available from: https://www.sciencedirect.com/science/article/pii/S1549963422000521.
13. Khan T, Altamimi MA, Hussain A, Ramzan M, Ashique S, Alhuzani MR, et al. Understanding of PSA biology, factors affecting PSA detection, challenges, various biomarkers, methods, and future perspective of prostate cancer detection and diagnosis. Adv Cancer Biol - Metastasis [Internet]. 2022;5:100059. Available from: https://www.sciencedirect.com/science/article/pii/S2667394022000338.
14. Prabowo BA, Cabral PD, Freitas P, Fernandes E. The challenges of developing biosensors for clinical assessment: a review. Chemosensors. 2021;9(11):299.
15. Mayoral-Peña K, González Peña OI, Orrantia Clark AM, Flores-Vallejo R d C, Oza G, Sharma A, et al. Biorecognition engineering technologies for cancer diagnosis: a systematic literature review of non-conventional and plausible sensor development methods. Cancers (Basel) [Internet]. 2022;14(8). Available from: https://www.mdpi.com/2072-6694/14/8/1867.
16. Nasimi H, Madsen JS, Zedan AH, Malmendal A, Osther PJS, Alatraktchi FA. Protein biomarker detection in prostate cancer: a comprehensive review of electrochemical biosensors. Sens Actuators Rep [Internet]. 2023;6:100168. Available from: https://www.sciencedirect.com/science/article/pii/S2666053923000310.
17. Numan A, Singh S, Zhan Y, Li L, Khalid M, Rilla K, et al. Advanced nanoengineered—customized point-of-care tools for prostate-specific antigen. Microchim Acta [Internet]. 2021;189(1):27. Available from: https://doi.org/10.1007/s00604-021-05127-y.
18. Bernstein DE, Piedad J, Hemsworth L, West A, Johnston ID, Dimov N, et al. Prostate cancer and microfluids. Urol Oncol Semin Orig Investig [Internet]. 2021;39(8):455–70. Available from: https://www.sciencedirect.com/science/article/pii/S1078143921001204.
19. Khondakar KR, Dey S, Wuethrich A, Sina AAI, Trau M. Toward personalized cancer treatment: from diagnostics to therapy monitoring in miniaturized electrohydrodynamic systems. Acc Chem Res [Internet]. 2019;52(8):2113–23. Available from: https://doi.org/10.1021/acs.accounts.9b00192.
20. Corradini D, Brizi L, Gaudiano C, Bianchi L, Marcelli E, Golfieri R, et al. Challenges in the use of artificial intelligence for prostate cancer diagnosis from multiparametric imaging data. Cancers (Basel). 2021;13(16).
21. Cabello M, Ge H, Aracil C, Moschou D, Estrela P, Manuel Quero J, et al. Extracellular electrophysiology in the prostate cancer cell model PC-3. Sensors. 2019;19(1).
22. Tamada T, Ueda Y, Ueno Y, Kojima Y, Kido A, Yamamoto A. Diffusion-weighted imaging in prostate cancer. Magn Reson Mater Phys Biol Med. 2022;35(4):533–47.
23. Du X, Shen A, Wang X, Feng Z, Deng H. NRD-Net: a noise-resistant distillation network for accurate diagnosis of prostate cancer with bi-parametric MRI images. Multimed Tools Appl. 2024;83(11):33597–614.
24. Maas M, Todenhöfer T, Black PC. Urine biomarkers in bladder cancer — current status and future perspectives. Nat Rev Urol [Internet]. 2023;20(10):597–614. Available from: https://doi.org/10.1038/s41585-023-00773-8.

25. Wang P, Lou J, Yu Y, Sun L, Sun L, Fang G, et al. An ultra-sensitive metasurface biosensor for instant cancer detection based on terahertz spectra. Nano Res [Internet]. 2023;16(5):7304–11. Available from: https://doi.org/10.1007/s12274-023-5386-7.
26. Jarczewska M, Malinowska E. The application of antibody–aptamer hybrid biosensors in clinical diagnostics and environmental analysis. Anal Methods. 2020;12(25):3183–99.
27. Alahdal M, Perera RA, Moschovas MC, Patel V, Perera RJ. Current advances of liquid biopsies in prostate cancer: molecular biomarkers. Mol Ther - Oncolytics [Internet]. 2023;30:27–38. Available from: https://doi.org/10.1016/j.omto.2023.07.004.
28. Qazi S, Raza K. Chapter 4 - Smart biosensors for an efficient point of care (PoC) health management. In: Chaki J, Dey N, De D, editors. Smart biosensors in medical care [Internet], Advances in ubiquitous sensing applications for healthcare. Academic Press; 2020. p. 65–85. Available from: https://www.sciencedirect.com/science/article/pii/B9780128207819000048.
29. Saxena S, Lu Y, Zhang Z, Li Y, Soleymani L, Hoare T. Zwitter-repel: an anti-fouling coating promoting electrochemical biosensing in biological fluids. Chem Eng J [Internet]. 2024;495:153522. Available from: https://www.sciencedirect.com/science/article/pii/S1385894724050113.
30. Jeyaraman M, Jeyaraman N, Ramasubramanian S, Balaji S, Iyengar KP, Jain VK, et al. Nanomaterials in point-of-care diagnostics: bridging the gap between laboratory and clinical practice. Pathol - Res Pract [Internet]. 2024;263:155685. Available from: https://www.sciencedirect.com/science/article/pii/S034403382400596X.
31. Brastianos HC, Murgic J, Salcedo A, Chua MLK, Meng A, Fraser M, et al. Determining the impact of spatial heterogeneity on genomic prognostic biomarkers for localized prostate cancer. Eur Urol Oncol. 2022;5(3):362–5.
32. VanderWeele DJ, Finney R, Katayama K, Gillard M, Paner G, Imoto S, et al. Genomic heterogeneity within individual prostate cancer foci impacts predictive biomarkers of targeted therapy. Eur Urol Focus. 2019;5(3):416–24.
33. Yadav SS, Stockert JA, Hackert V, Yadav KK, Tewari AK. Intratumor heterogeneity in prostate cancer. Urol Oncol Semin Orig Investig. 2018;36(8):349–60.
34. Haffner MC, Zwart W, Roudier MP, True LD, Nelson WG, Epstein JI, et al. Genomic and phenotypic heterogeneity in prostate cancer. Nat Rev Urol [Internet]. 2021;18(2):79–92. Available from: https://doi.org/10.1038/s41585-020-00400-w.
35. Cao K, Arthurs C, Atta-ul A, Millar M, Beltran M, Neuhaus J, et al. Quantitative analysis of seven new prostate cancer biomarkers and the potential future of the 'biomarker laboratory.'. Diagnostics. 2018;8(3).
36. Erickson A, Hayes A, Rajakumar T, Verrill C, Bryant RJ, Hamdy FC, et al. A systematic review of prostate cancer heterogeneity: understanding the clonal ancestry of multifocal disease. Eur Urol Oncol. 2021;4(3):358–69.
37. Cho S, Yang HC, Rhee WJ. Simultaneous multiplexed detection of exosomal microRNAs and surface proteins for prostate cancer diagnosis. Biosens Bioelectron [Internet]. 2019;146:111749. Available from: https://www.sciencedirect.com/science/article/pii/S0956566319308280.
38. Kral M, Kurfurstova D, Zemla P, Elias M, Bouchal J. New biomarkers and multiplex tests for diagnosis of aggressive prostate cancer and therapy management. Front Oncol. 2025;15:1542511.
39. Crocetto F, Russo G, Di Zazzo E, Pisapia P, Mirto BF, Palmieri A, et al. Liquid biopsy in prostate cancer management—current challenges and future perspectives. Cancers (Basel). 2022;14(13):3272.
40. Liu Y, Zhang N, Pan JB, Song J, Zhao W, Chen HY, et al. Bipolar electrode array for multiplexed detection of prostate cancer biomarkers. Anal Chem [Internet]. 2022;94(6):3005–12. Available from: https://doi.org/10.1021/acs.analchem.1c05383.
41. Boehm BE, York ME, Petrovics G, Kohaar I, Chesnut GT. Biomarkers of aggressive prostate cancer at diagnosis. Int J Mol Sci [Internet]. 2023;24(3). Available from: https://www.mdpi.com/1422-0067/24/3/2185.

42. Van Poppel H, Albreht T, Basu P, Hogenhout R, Collen S, Roobol M. Serum PSA-based early detection of prostate cancer in Europe and globally: past, present and future. Nat Rev Urol. 2022;19(9):562–72.
43. Tonry C, Finn S, Armstrong J, Pennington SR. Clinical proteomics for prostate cancer: understanding prostate cancer pathology and protein biomarkers for improved disease management. Clin Proteomics [Internet]. 2020;17(1):41. Available from: https://doi.org/10.1186/s12014-020-09305-7.
44. Lam D, Clark S, Stirzaker C, Pidsley R. Advances in prognostic methylation biomarkers for prostate cancer. Cancers (Basel). 2020;12(10).
45. Couñago F, López-Campos F, Díaz-Gavela AA, Almagro E, Fenández-Pascual E, Henríquez I, et al. Clinical applications of molecular biomarkers in prostate cancer. Cancers (Basel) [Internet]. 2020;12(6). Available from: https://www.mdpi.com/2072-6694/12/6/1550.
46. Paller CJ, Antonarakis ES, Beer TM, Borno HT, Carlo MI, George DJ, et al. Germline genetic testing in advanced prostate cancer; practices and barriers: survey results from the germline genetics working group of the Prostate Cancer Clinical Trials Consortium. Clin Genitourin Cancer. 2019;17(4):275–282.e1.
47. Ashrafizadeh M, Zhang W, Tian Y, Sethi G, Zhang X, Qiu A. Molecular panorama of therapy resistance in prostate cancer: a pre-clinical and bioinformatics analysis for clinical translation. Cancer Metastasis Rev. 2024;43(1):229–60.
48. Ellis SD, Hwang S, Morrow E, Kimminau KS, Goonan K, Petty L, et al. Perceived barriers to the adoption of active surveillance in low-risk prostate cancer: a qualitative analysis of community and academic urologists. BMC Cancer [Internet]. 2021;21(1):649. Available from: https://doi.org/10.1186/s12885-021-08386-3.
49. Suri Y, Yasmeh JP, Basu A. Understanding the uptake and challenges of genetic testing guidelines for prostate cancer patients. Cancer Treat Res Commun [Internet]. 2022;32:100588. Available from: https://www.sciencedirect.com/science/article/pii/S2468294222000788.
50. Bera K, Braman N, Gupta A, Velcheti V, Madabhushi A. Predicting cancer outcomes with radiomics and artificial intelligence in radiology. Nat Rev Clin Oncol. 2022;19(2):132–46.
51. Kwon WA, Joung JY. Precision targeting in metastatic prostate cancer: molecular insights to therapeutic frontiers. Biomolecules. 2025;15(5).
52. Kouspou MM, Fong JE, Brew N, Hsiao STF, Davidson SL, Choyke PL, et al. The Movember prostate cancer landscape analysis: an assessment of unmet research needs. Nat Rev Urol. 2020;17(9):499–512.
53. Wang Y, Tadimalla S, Rai R, Goodwin J, Foster S, Liney G, et al. Quantitative MRI: defining repeatability, reproducibility and accuracy for prostate cancer imaging biomarker development. Magn Reson Imaging. 2021;77:169–79.
54. Schwier M, van Griethuysen J, Vangel MG, Pieper S, Peled S, Tempany C, et al. Repeatability of multiparametric prostate MRI radiomics features. Sci Rep. 2019;9(1):9441.
55. Lee J, Lee YJ, Ahn YJ, Choi S, Lee GJ. A simple and facile paper-based colorimetric assay for detection of free hydrogen sulfide in prostate cancer cells. Sensors Actuators B Chem. 2018;256:828–34.
56. Egevad L, Swanberg D, Delahunt B, Ström P, Kartasalo K, Olsson H, et al. Identification of areas of grading difficulties in prostate cancer and comparison with artificial intelligence assisted grading. Virchows Arch. 2020;477(6):777–86.
57. Bulten W, Kartasalo K, Chen PHC, Ström P, Pinckaers H, Nagpal K, et al. Artificial intelligence for diagnosis and Gleason grading of prostate cancer: the PANDA challenge. Nat Med [Internet]. 2022;28(1):154–63. Available from: https://doi.org/10.1038/s41591-021-01620-2.
58. Fervaha G, Izard JP, Tripp DA, Rajan S, Leong DP, Siemens DR. Depression and prostate cancer: a focused review for the clinician. Urol Oncol Semin Orig Investig. 2019;37(4):282–8.
59. Elmarakeby HA, Hwang J, Arafeh R, Crowdis J, Gang S, Liu D, et al. Biologically informed deep neural network for prostate cancer discovery. Nature. 2021;598(7880):348–52.
60. Lomas DJ, Ahmed HU. All change in the prostate cancer diagnostic pathway. Nat Rev Clin Oncol [Internet]. 2020;17(6):372–81. Available from: https://doi.org/10.1038/s41571-020-0332-z.

61. Merseburger AS, Waldron N, Ribal MJ, Heidenreich A, Perner S, Fizazi K, et al. Genomic testing in patients with metastatic castration-resistant prostate cancer: a pragmatic guide for clinicians. Eur Urol. 2021;79(4):519–29.
62. van der Leest M, Israël B, Cornel EB, Zámecnik P, Schoots IG, van der Lelij H, et al. High diagnostic performance of short magnetic resonance imaging protocols for prostate cancer detection in biopsy-naïve men: the next step in magnetic resonance imaging accessibility. Eur Urol. 2019;76(5):574–81.
63. Smith-Palmer J, Takizawa C, Valentine W. Literature review of the burden of prostate cancer in Germany, France, the United Kingdom and Canada. BMC Urol. 2019;19:1–16.
64. Berenguer CV, Pereira F, Câmara JS, Pereira JAM. Underlying features of prostate cancer—statistics, risk factors, and emerging methods for its diagnosis. Curr Oncol. 2023;30(2):2300–21.
65. Mbugua RG, Oluchina S, Karanja S. Prostate cancer awareness and screening among men in a rural community in Kenya: a cross-sectional study. African J Urol. 2021;27(1):7.
66. Abarghoei S, Fakhri N, Borghei YS, Hosseini M, Ganjali MR. A colorimetric paper sensor for citrate as biomarker for early stage detection of prostate cancer based on peroxidase-like activity of cysteine-capped gold nanoclusters. Spectrochim Acta Part A Mol Biomol Spectrosc. 2019;210:251–9.
67. Sumitha MS, Xavier TS. Recent advances in electrochemical biosensors—a brief review. Hybrid Adv. 2023;2:100023.
68. Bobrowski A, Nayan M, Heimrath O, Goche D, Ludzu E, Singal RK. Supply the demand: assessment of the feasibility of local nonurologists in relieving the burden of chronic indwelling catheters in a low-income country. Can Urol Assoc J = J l'Association des Urol du Canada. 2021;15(5):E261–6.
69. Shete K, Ghoulian J, Hu B, Alsyouf M. Genitourinary cancer care in low- and Middle-Income Countries: disparities in incidence and access to care. Société Int d'Urologie J. 2024;5(5):330–8.
70. Kamaraju S, Drope J, Sankaranarayanan R, Shastri S. Cancer prevention in low-resource countries: an overview of the opportunity. Am Soc Clin Oncol Educ book Am Soc Clin Oncol Annu Meet. 2020;40:1–12.
71. Bosland MC. Prostate cancer in low- and middle-income countries - challenges and opportunities. Prostate Cancer Prostatic Dis. 2024;28:743.
72. Bosland MC, Shittu OB, Ikpi EE, Akinloye O. Potential new approaches for prostate cancer management in Resource-Limited Countries in Africa. Ann Glob Heal. 2023;89(1):14.
73. Mobashir M, Turunen SP, Izhari MA, Ashankyty IM, Helleday T, Lehti K. An approach for systems-level understanding of prostate cancer from high-throughput data integration to pathway modeling and simulation. Cells. 2022;11(24).
74. Zhang H, Guo Y, Li Q, George TJ, Shenkman E, Modave F, et al. An ontology-guided semantic data integration framework to support integrative data analysis of cancer survival. BMC Med Inform Decis Mak. 2018;18(2):41.
75. Young LN, Sherrard A, Zhou H, Shaikh F, Hutchings J, Riggi M, et al. ExoSloNano: multi-modal nanogold tags for identification of macromolecules in live cells & cryo-electron tomograms. bioRxiv Prepr Serv Biol. 2024; https://doi.org/10.1101/2024.10.12.617288.
76. Chowdhury P, Lawrance R, Lu ZY, Lin HC, Chan YH. Recent progress in dual/multi-modal detection modes for improving sensitivity and specificity of lateral flow immunoassays applied for point-of-care diagnostics. TrAC Trends Anal Chem. 2024;177:117798.
77. Yau CN, Hung JTS, Campbell RAA, Wong TCY, Huang B, Wong BTY, et al. INSIHGT: an accessible multi-scale, multi-modal 3D spatial biology platform. Nat Commun. 2024;15(1):10888.
78. Park J, Jeong Y, Kim J, Gu J, Wang J, Park I. Biopsy needle integrated with multi-modal physical/chemical sensor array. Biosens Bioelectron. 2020;148:111822.
79. Perincheri S, Levi AW, Celli R, Gershkovich P, Rimm D, Morrow JS, et al. An independent assessment of an artificial intelligence system for prostate cancer detection shows strong

diagnostic accuracy. Mod Pathol [Internet]. 2021;34(8):1588–95. Available from: https://www.sciencedirect.com/science/article/pii/S0893395222005725.
80. Fransen SJ, Kwee TC, Rouw D, Roest C, van Lohuizen QY, Simonis FFJ, et al. Patient perspectives on the use of artificial intelligence in prostate cancer diagnosis on MRI. Eur Radiol. 2025;35(2):769–75.
81. Baydoun A, Jia AY, Zaorsky NG, Kashani R, Rao S, Shoag JE, et al. Artificial intelligence applications in prostate cancer. Prostate Cancer Prostatic Dis. 2024;27(1):37–45.
82. Harmon SA, Tuncer S, Sanford T, Choyke PL, Türkbey B. Artificial intelligence at the intersection of pathology and radiology in prostate cancer. Diagn Interv Radiol. 2019;25(3):183–8.
83. Alarcón-Zendejas AP, Scavuzzo A, Jiménez-Ríos MA, Álvarez-Gómez RM, Montiel-Manríquez R, Castro-Hernández C, et al. The promising role of new molecular biomarkers in prostate cancer: from coding and non-coding genes to artificial intelligence approaches. Prostate Cancer Prostatic Dis [Internet]s. 2022;25(3):431–43. Available from: https://doi.org/10.1038/s41391-022-00537-2.
84. Tătaru OS, Vartolomei MD, Rassweiler JJ, Virgil O, Lucarelli G, Porpiglia F, et al. Artificial intelligence and machine learning in prostate cancer patient management—current trends and future perspectives. Diagnostics [Internet]. 2021;11(2). Available from: https://www.mdpi.com/2075-4418/11/2/354.
85. Park J, Rho MJ, Moon HW, Park YH, Kim CS, Jeon SS, et al. Prostate cancer trajectory-map: clinical decision support system for prognosis management of radical prostatectomy. Prostate Int. 2021;9(1):25–30.
86. Tan HJ, Spratte BN, Deal AM, Heiling HM, Nazzal EM, Meeks W, et al. Clinical decision support for surgery: a mixed methods study on design and implementation perspectives from urologists. Urology. 2024;190:15–23.
87. Hochstenbach LMJ, Determann D, Fijten RRR, Bloemen-van Gurp EJ, Verwey R. Taking shared decision making for prostate cancer to the next level: requirements for a Dutch treatment decision aid with personalized risks on side effects. Internet Interv. 2023;31:100606.
88. Park J, Rho MJ, Dritschilo A, Choi IY, Mun SK. Prostate clinical outlook visualization system for patients and clinicians considering Cyberknife treatment—a personalized approach. Appl Sci. 2018;8(3).
89. Chen HMHYHHH, Zhang JJJJ, Huang R, Wang DDXDDD, Deng D, Zhang QQQQQQ, et al. Nanomaterial-based electrochemical sensors for the detection of pharmaceutical drugs. Schatten H, editor. Cancers (Basel) [Internet]. 2022;14(1):35. Available from: https://www.sciencedirect.com/science/article/pii/S0039914020305671.
90. Bibault JE, Hancock S, Buyyounouski MK, Bagshaw H, Leppert JT, Liao JC, et al. Development and validation of an interpretable artificial intelligence model to predict 10-year prostate cancer mortality. Cancers (Basel). 2021;13(12).
91. Hueting TA, Cornel EB, Somford DM, Jansen H, van Basten JPA, Pleijhuis RG, et al. External validation of models predicting the probability of lymph node involvement in prostate cancer patients. Eur Urol Oncol. 2018;1(5):411–7.
92. Rasheed S, Kanwal T, Ahmad N, Fatima B, Najam-ul-Haq M, Hussain D. Advances and challenges in portable optical biosensors for onsite detection and point-of-care diagnostics. TrAC Trends Anal Chem [Internet]. 2024;173:117640. Available from: https://www.sciencedirect.com/science/article/pii/S0165993624001225.
93. Sengupta J, Hussain CM. Early detection of cancer utilizing biosensors based on "green graphene": an innovative and sustainable methodology for advancing cancer diagnosis. TrAC Trends Anal Chem [Internet]. 2023;167:117254. Available from: https://www.sciencedirect.com/science/article/pii/S0165993623003412.
94. Pan S, Mao J, Wang L, Dai Y, Wang W. Patient participation in treatment decision-making of prostate cancer: a qualitative study. Support Care Cancer. 2022;30(5):4189–200.
95. Oldenburg J, Aparicio J, Beyer J, Cohn-Cedermark G, Cullen M, Gilligan T, et al. Personalizing, not patronizing: the case for patient autonomy by unbiased presentation of management options in stage I testicular cancer. Ann Oncol. 2015;26(5):833–8.

96. Lomas DJ, Ziegelmann MJ, Elliott DS. How informed is our consent? Patient awareness of radiation and radical prostatectomy complications. Turkish J Urol. 2019;45(3):191–5.
97. Vargas Blasco C, Martin-Fumadó C, Arimany Manso J. Informed consent in urology. Actas Urológicas Españolas (English Ed.). 2024;48(5):340–4.
98. Venderbos LDF. Ethical and legal considerations in active surveillance for prostate cancer. In: Klotz L, editor. Active surveillance for localized prostate cancer: a new paradigm for clinical management. Cham: Springer International Publishing; 2018. p. 31–9.
99. Pereira-Azevedo NM, Venderbos LDF. eHealth and mHealth in prostate cancer detection and active surveillance. Transl Androl Urol. 2018;7(1):170–81.
100. Matos S. Privacy and data protection in the surveillance society: the case of the Prüm system. J Forensic Leg Med. 2019;66:155–61.
101. Paulus JK, Kent DM. Predictably unequal: understanding and addressing concerns that algorithmic clinical prediction may increase health disparities. npj Digit Med. 2020;3(1):99.
102. Haider SA, Borna S, Gomez-Cabello CA, Pressman SM, Haider CR, Forte AJ. The algorithmic divide: a systematic review on AI-driven racial disparities in healthcare. J Racial Ethn Heal Disparities. 2024;13:188.
103. Mahal BA, Gerke T, Awasthi S, Soule HR, Simons JW, Miyahira A, et al. Prostate cancer racial disparities: a systematic review by the prostate cancer foundation panel. Eur Urol Oncol [Internet]. 2022;5(1):18–29. Available from: https://www.sciencedirect.com/science/article/pii/S2588931121001462.
104. Do H, Persily J, Zhong J, Neshatvar Y, Murray K, Nayan M. Mitigating disparities in prostate cancer through fair machine learning models. Urol Oncol Semin Orig Investig. 2025;43(3, Supplement):80.
105. Burnett AL, Nyame YA, Mitchell E. Disparities in prostate cancer. J Natl Med Assoc [Internet]. 2023;115(2, Supplement):S38–45. Available from: https://www.sciencedirect.com/science/article/pii/S0027968423000330.
106. Nyame YA, Cooperberg MR, Cumberbatch MG, Eggener SE, Etzioni R, Gomez SL, et al. Deconstructing, addressing, and eliminating racial and ethnic inequities in prostate cancer care. Eur Urol. 2022;82(4):341–51.
107. Fu J, Fu C, Wang RS, Geynisman DM, Ghatalia P, Lynch SM, et al. Current status and future direction to address disparities in diversity, equity, and inclusion in prostate cancer care. Curr Oncol Rep [Internet]s. 2023;25(7):699–708. Available from: https://doi.org/10.1007/s11912-023-01399-0.
108. Ufuah S, Tallman JE, Moses KA. The pursuit of health equity and equality in urologic oncology: where we have been and where we are going. Eur Urol Focus. 2021;7(5):929–36.
109. Ghose S, Radhakrishnan V, Bhattacharya S. Ethics of cancer care: beyond biology and medicine. Ecancermedicalscience. 2019;13:911.
110. Horgan D, Mia R, Erhabor T, Hamdi Y, Dandara C, Lal JA, et al. Fighting cancer around the world: a framework for action. Healthcare. 2022;10(11).
111. Vakili-Ojarood M, Naseri A, Shirinzadeh-Dastgiri A, Saberi A, HaghighiKian SM, Rahmani A, et al. Ethical considerations and equipoise in cancer surgery. Indian J Surg Oncol. 2024;15(3):363–73.
112. Amorim MLM, Junior OHA, Villarim MR, Gazziro M, Castilho RM, Afonso JA, et al. Early cancer detection biosensors: present situation and future outlooks. IEEE Sensors Rev. 2025;2:209–27.
113. Chowdhury S, Dent T, Pashayan N, Hall A, Lyratzopoulos G, Hallowell N, et al. Incorporating genomics into breast and prostate cancer screening: assessing the implications. Genet Med. 2013;15(6):423–32.
114. Tuffaha H, Edmunds K, Fairbairn D, Roberts MJ, Chambers S, Smith DP, et al. Guidelines for genetic testing in prostate cancer: a scoping review. Prostate Cancer Prostatic Dis. 2024;27(4):594–603.
115. Huang S, Yuan J, Xie Y, Qing K, Shi Z, Chen G, et al. Targeting nano-regulator based on metal–organic frameworks for enhanced immunotherapy of bone metastatic prostate cancer. Cancer Nanotechnol. 2023;14(1):43.

116. Chauhan C. Chapter 12 - Ethical aspects of using artificial intelligence in digital and computational pathology. In: Hameed M, Hanna MG, editors. Digital pathology. Academic Press; 2025. p. 267–75.
117. Mateo J, McKay R, Abida W, Aggarwal R, Alumkal J, Alva A, et al. Accelerating precision medicine in metastatic prostate cancer. Nat Cancer. 2020;1(11):1041–53.
118. Arita Y, Roest C, Kwee TC, Paudyal R, Lema-Dopico A, Fransen S, et al. Advancements in artificial intelligence for prostate cancer: optimizing diagnosis, treatment, and prognostic assessment. Asian J Urol [Internet]. 2025. Available from: https://www.sciencedirect.com/science/article/pii/S2214388225000074.
119. Rabaan AA, Bakhrebah MA, AlSaihati H, Alhumaid S, Alsubki RA, Turkistani SA, et al. Artificial intelligence for clinical diagnosis and treatment of prostate cancer. Cancers (Basel). 2022;14(22).
120. Busby D, Grauer R, Pandav K, Khosla A, Jain P, Menon M, et al. Applications of artificial intelligence in prostate cancer histopathology. Urol Oncol Semin Orig Investig. 2024;42(3):37–47.
121. Baldo TA, de Lima LF, Mendes LF, de Araujo WR, Paixão TRLC, Coltro WKT. Wearable and biodegradable sensors for clinical and environmental applications. ACS Appl Electron Mater. 2021;3(1):68–100.
122. Shajari S, Kuruvinashetti K, Komeili A, Sundararaj U. The emergence of AI-based wearable sensors for digital health technology: a review. Sensors. 2023;23(23).
123. Ho HY, Chung Kasey KS, Kan CM, Wong Cesar SC. Liquid biopsy in the clinical management of cancers. Int J Mol Sci [Internet]. 2024;25(16). Available from: https://www.mdpi.com/1422-0067/25/16/8594.
124. Allen TA. The role of circulating tumor cells as a liquid biopsy for cancer: advances, biology, technical challenges, and clinical relevance. Cancers (Basel) [Internet]. 2024;16(7). Available from: https://www.mdpi.com/2072-6694/16/7/1377.
125. Tayfour Ahmed AE, Dhahi TS, Attia TA, Elhassan Ali FA, Elobaid ME, Adam T, et al. AI optimized electrochemical aptasensors for stable, reproducible detection of neurodegenerative diseases, cancer, and coronavirus. Heliyon [Internet]. 2025;11(1). Available from: https://doi.org/10.1016/j.heliyon.2024.e41338.
126. Papachristou K, Katsakiori PF, Papadimitroulas P, Strigari L, Kagadis GC. Digital twins' advancements and applications in healthcare, towards precision medicine. J Pers Med [Internet]. 2024;14(11). Available from: https://www.mdpi.com/2075-4426/14/11/1101.
127. Chu TN, Wong EY, Ma R, Yang CH, Dalieh IS, Hung AJ. Exploring the use of artificial intelligence in the management of prostate cancer. Curr Urol Rep. 2023;24(5):231–40.
128. Beg S, Handa M, Shukla R, Rahman M, Almalki WH, Afzal O, et al. Wearable smart devices in cancer diagnosis and remote clinical trial monitoring: transforming the healthcare applications. Drug Discov Today. 2022;27(10):103314.
129. Chaabene S, Boudaya A, Bouaziz B, Chaari L. An overview of methods and techniques in multimodal data fusion with application to healthcare. Int J Data Sci Anal. 2025;20:3093.
130. Ma CB, Shang X, Sun M, Bo X, Bai J, Du Y, et al. Emerging multifunctional wearable sensors: integrating multimodal sweat analysis and advanced material technologies for next-generation health monitoring. ACS Sens. 2025;10(4):2388–408.
131. Wang C, He T, Zhou H, Zhang Z, Lee C. Artificial intelligence enhanced sensors - enabling technologies to next-generation healthcare and biomedical platform. Bioelectron Med. 2023;9(1):17.
132. Chu SS, Nguyen HA, Zhang J, Tabassum S, Cao H. Towards multiplexed and multimodal biosensor platforms in real-time monitoring of metabolic disorders. Sensors [Internet]. 2022;22(14). Available from: https://www.mdpi.com/1424-8220/22/14/5200.
133. Arya SS, Dias SB, Jelinek HF, Hadjileontiadis LJ, Pappa AM. The convergence of traditional and digital biomarkers through AI-assisted biosensing: a new era in translational diagnostics? Biosens Bioelectron. 2023;235:115387.

Regulatory Considerations for Biosensor Development for Prostate Cancer

12

Neha Singh Baghel, Veerendra Chaurasia, Shriyansh Srivastava, and Molakpogu Ravindra Babu

Abbreviations

AIM-AHEAD	Artificial Intelligence/Machine Learning Consortium to Advance Health Equity and Researcher Diversity
CADTH	Canadian Agency for Drugs and Technologies in Health
CDER	Center for Drug Evaluation and Research
CDRH	Center for Devices and Radiological Health (FDA)
CDSCO	Central Drugs Standard Control Organization
CMS	Centers for Medicare & Medicaid Services
CPT	Current Procedural Terminology
DHF	design history file
DPC	Diagnosis Procedure Combination
eCTD	Electronic Common Technical Document
EMA	European Medicines Agency
ELISA	Enzyme-Linked Immunosorbent Assay
FDA	Food and Drug Administration
G-BA	Gemeinsamer Bundesausschuss (Federal Joint Committee of Germany)
GDPR	General Data Protection Regulation (EU)
GMLP	Good Machine Learning Practice
HAS	Haute Autorité de Santé (French National Authority for Health)
HIRA	Health Insurance Review and Assessment Service
HTA	health technology assessment

N. S. Baghel · S. Srivastava · M. Ravindra Babu (✉)
Department of Pharmacy, School of Medical and Allied Sciences, Galgotias University, Greater Noida, Uttar Pradesh, India

V. Chaurasia
Babu Mahipat Singh College of Pharmacy, Tiloi, Amethi, Uttar Pradesh, India

S. Srivastava et al. (eds.), *Biosensor Technologies for Prostate Cancer*, https://doi.org/10.1007/978-981-95-8644-8_12

IMDRF	International Medical Device Regulators Forum
IN4ACT	International Network for the Availability of Clinical Trials
IVD	in vitro diagnostic
IVDR	In Vitro Diagnostic Regulation
LOD	limit of detection
LOQ	limit of quantitation
MDR	Medical Device Regulation (EU)
MHLW	Ministry of Health, Labour and Welfare
ML	machine learning
NICE	National Institute for Health and Care Excellence
PATH	Program for Appropriate Technology in Health
PCCP	Predetermined Change Control Plan
PIPEDA	Personal Information Protection and Electronic Documents Act
PMA	premarket approval
PMDA	Pharmaceuticals and Medical Devices Agency
PRIMA	Prostate Cancer Molecular Biomarker Assay
PRO	patient-reported outcome
QALY	quality-adjusted life year
RWE	real-world evidence
SaMD	Software as a Medical Device
SNP	Single Nucleotide Polymorphism
TMPRSS2-ERG	Transmembrane Protease, Serine 2 – ETS-Related Gene
UDI	unique device identification
ZIN	Zorginstituut Nederland (National Health Care Institute of the Netherlands)

12.1 Introduction to Regulatory Frameworks in Biosensor Development

Regulatory guidelines govern the development process of biosensors used for medical diagnostics, including those specific to prostate cancer [1]. Market entry standards establish legal procedures and ensure patient safety by maintaining data reliability and product performance. Biosensors are governed by medical device regulations throughout all global jurisdictions. Under Food and Drug Administration (FDA) regulations in the United States, these devices receive classification as in vitro diagnostic (IVD) devices, and their regulatory oversight depends on risk categories from Class I to Class III (see Fig. 12.1) [2]. These European medical regulations, called Medical Device Regulation (EU 2017/745) and In Vitro Diagnostic Regulation (IVDR) (EU 2017/746), impose stringent requirements on post-market device monitoring through performance assessments, which demand compelling clinical utility and analytical validity data [3]. The submission process for new biosensors becomes more complicated, due to innovative implementations incorporating nanotechnology, artificial intelligence (AI) algorithms, and digital information flows in prostate cancer diagnostic systems [4].

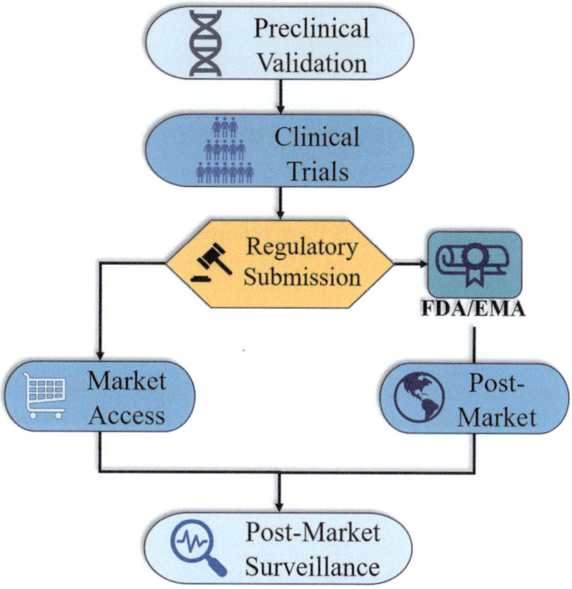

Fig. 12.1 Regulatory pathway for prostate cancer biosensor

12.1.1 Unique Challenges for Prostate Cancer Biosensors

Healthcare professionals employ multiple testing methods, including prostate-specific antigen (PSA) measurement and free/total PSA ratio assessment, with the recent introduction of prostate cancer antigen 3 (PCA3) and TMPRSS2-ERG, as well as exosomal RNAs. Regulatory frameworks now demand [5]: Current measurement thresholds should reach performance levels better than conventional comparators, including ELISA tests and magnetic resonance imaging (MRI)-based biopsies [6]. Performance data should be analyzed by population groups, including age, ethnicity, and genetic profiles, since incorrect positive or negative results can trigger unnecessary treatment or lead to undiagnosed cases [7]. A risk–benefit profiling approach needs to evaluate both the psychological effects of early testing and the effects on subsequent downstream medical procedures. Research has shown that highly sensitive biosensors require thorough real-world testing to assess lot consistency, operator technique, and sample matrix effects between serum and urine [8].

12.1.2 Convergence of Diagnostics and Digital Health

Regulatory authorities transform their regulatory frameworks because digital biosensors, along with wearable diagnostics, enter the market landscape [9]. Traditional medical device assessment protocols are adapting through the programs of the FDA Digital Health Software Precertification and the EU software as a medical device (SaMD) guidance framework [10]. Medical personnel utilizing AI for prostate cancer diagnosis specifically need this approach because AI uses thousands of clinical cases to train machine learning algorithms, which process biosensor results to improve diagnostic accuracy. These combined systems must fulfill two regulatory requirements because they contain hardware together with software elements [11].

12.1.3 Strategic Implications for Developers

The trend indicates that innovators, alongside researchers in prostate cancer biosensor practice, must start their relationship with regulatory bodies right at the beginning of their work [12]. Through programs such as the FDA Q-Submission Program and scientific advice meetings with EU-notified bodies, developers get multiple opportunities for feedback that reduce the chance for non-compliance and minimize necessary product redesigns [13]. Early-stage developers now have faster opportunities to bring innovative prostate cancer diagnostic solutions to market through recent adaptive regulatory frameworks that use real-time review processes combined with conditional approvals and the collaborative pilot programs (such as the UK's NICE MedTech Early Technical Assessment Tool) [14].

12.2 Classification of Biosensors as Medical Devices

The position of a biosensor within regulatory systems determines the needed oversight requirements, along with necessary data specifications and duration of authorization procedures [15]. Diagnostic systems containing microfluidics and nanomaterials, along with integrated AI systems, need accurate regulatory categorization for prostate cancer detection [16].

12.2.1 FDA Classification System: Risk-Based Stratification

Medical devices in the United States receive three classifications (refer to Fig. 12.2) from the FDA, which determine protection measures required for safety and effectiveness [17]: *Class I (Low Risk)*—Medical devices with Low-Risk status (Class I) need general controls and exclude face-to-face testing devices for patients; *Class II (Moderate Risk)*—The majority of prostate cancer diagnostic biosensors belong to Class II (Moderate Risk) category, which necessitates using special controls; and *Class III (High Risk)*—Devices categorized as Class III (High Risk) need premarket approval (PMA) before reaching the market because they include vital devices or inaccurate operations would lead to critical consequences. The regulatory status of most early or differential diagnosis prostate cancer biosensors belongs to Class II [18]. Procedures that contain both new biomarkers and decision-making algorithms and go into Class III classification need to prove their clinical worth, identical to therapeutic products (see Table 12.1 for international classification comparison) [19].

Fig. 12.2 Classification decision tree for biosensors

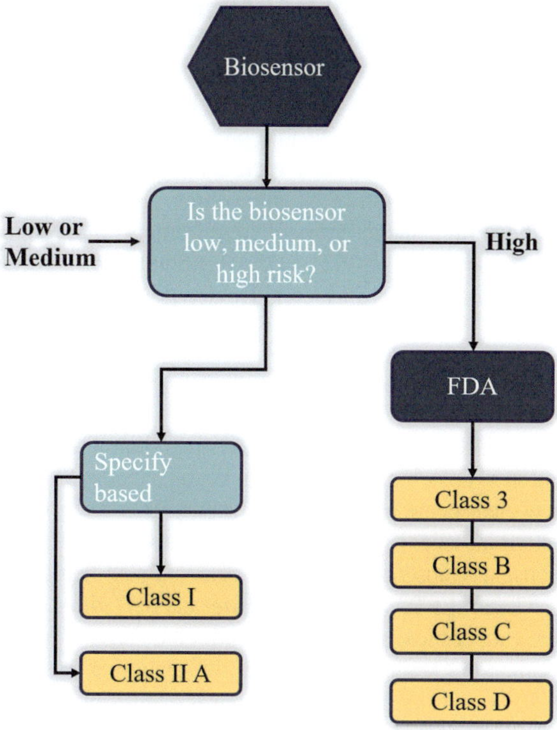

Table 12.1 Comparative regulatory classifications for prostate cancer biosensors

Region/ agency	Classification system	Typical class for PC biosensors	Key submission pathway	Unique notes	References
FDA (United States)	Class I–III (Risk-based)	Class II or III	510(k), De Novo, PMA	AI/ML requires PCCP; SaMD framework	[24]
EMA (EU)	IVDR classes A–D	Class C	Notified body review + performance evaluation report	Stricter clinical performance validation	[22]
Japan (PMDA)	Class I–IV	Class III	STED file or pre-market approval	Requires in-country clinical data	[25]
IMDRF	Harmonized principles	–	–	Provides a global regulatory convergence framework	[26]

12.2.2 Novel Insight: AI-Augmented Devices and Classification Drift

The combination of AI technologies or machine learning systems in biosensor equipment, including AI interpretation of multi-parameter biomarker patterns for risk assessment, can cause regulators to classify devices under stricter control categories [20]. Adaptive AI algorithms generate "Software Pre-Specification" and "Algorithm Change Protocol" requirements that require FDA post-approval regulatory review per the 2021 FDA "Artificial Intelligence/Machine Learning (AI/ML)-Based Software as a Medical Device (SaMD) Action Plan" [21].

12.2.3 EU Regulatory Framework: Transition from IVDD to IVDR

The IVDR 2017/746 regulates the operation of prostate cancer biosensors throughout Europe, replacing the previous In Vitro Diagnostic Directive (IVDD). Under the IVDR, new classification criteria become stricter because they use three core components to determine rules [22]: intended use; impact of diagnostic information on treatment decisions; and biosensors that affect personal well-being and community wellness status.

Under the IVDR's new *four-tier classification system (Classes A–D)*, most prostate cancer biosensors operate under the Class C category because they serve to find biomarkers leading to potential life-changing treatment choices. The revised classification system requires the participation of Notified Bodies to validate performance, together with clinical research, for all medical products, including those which were formerly self-certified [23].

12.2.4 Global Harmonization and the Role of the IMDRF

International Medical Device Regulators Forum (IMDRF) actively engages with the process of creating common medical device classification standards for jurisdictions worldwide [27]. The IMDRF framework establishes a common framework that assists multinational biosensor developers in handling regional regulatory differences across jurisdictions [28]: terminology and classification logic; clinical evaluation standards; and post-market surveillance (PMS) expectations. A white paper from the IMDRF's SaMD Working Group defines how increased regulatory consistency allows disease screening biosensors to be deployed across national and decentralized healthcare settings for prostate cancer testing [29].

12.2.5 Implications for Prostate Cancer Biosensor Innovators

The regulatory classification determines all aspects of biosensor lifecycle development from start to finish [30]: development timelines and budget allocations; clinical trial design and size; labeling, advertising, and claims language; and reimbursement strategies. The safety and effectiveness testing of a Class III (FDA) or Class D (IVDR) biosensor demands thousands of patient involvement in a multi-center prospective clinical trial, which both increases development expenses and extends the commercial release timeline [31].

12.2.6 Emerging Challenge: Hybrid Devices with Diagnostic and Therapeutic Intent

Emerging technological devices represent theranostic biosensors that perform dual detection and therapeutic operations for cancer biomarker recognition and therapeutic drug delivery control, as well as radiation alert generation [32]. Complex regulatory classification, as well as interagency reviews, may occur because theranostic biosensors may require regulatory oversight from both the Center for Devices and Radiological Health-CDER and device and drug/biologic pathways [33].

12.3 Preclinical Requirements and Analytical Validation

A biosensor intended for prostate cancer diagnostics requires thorough preclinical examination, shown in Fig. 12.3, as well as analytical validation before proceeding with clinical evaluation and regulatory submission [34]. During this stage, the fundamental detection technology of the biosensor undergoes evaluations for scientific reliability, repeatability, and solid operation. The preclinical phase holds higher importance for prostate cancer since false diagnostic results may deeply affect patient care practices (see Table 12.2 for validation parameter benchmarks) [35].

12.3.1 The Purpose of Preclinical Testing

Preclinical studies are designed according to the following [36]: The detection mechanism requires confirmation, which exhibits precise identification of PSA or PCA3 or TMPRSS2-ERG fusion genes or exosomal proteins using minimal false reactions; the analytical performance characteristics must be established through the assessment of sensitivity and specificity, as well as the limit of detection (LOD) and dynamic range together with the biomarker concentration linearity; and the biosensor requires validation tests under actual patient sample conditions because lab-only success is not sufficient. Validation protocols should incorporate biological sample characteristics that are present in real-life specimens, including urine, serum, plasma, and semen.

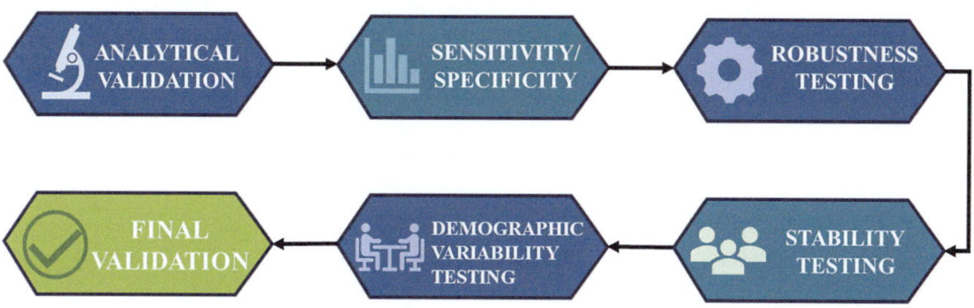

Fig. 12.3 Preclinical validation workflow for prostate cancer biosensors

Table 12.2 Key analytical validation parameters for prostate cancer biosensors

Parameter	Definition	Regulatory thresholds	Notes	References
Sensitivity	Ability to detect true positives	≥85% recommended	Essential for early-stage detection	[36]
Specificity	Ability to avoid false positives	≥90% ideal	Differentiates PC from BPH	[38]
LOD	Minimum detectable concentration	<1 pg/mL with nanotech	Critical for early-stage PC	[39]
LOQ	Lowest quantifiable concentration	Low femtomolar range	Supports quantitative monitoring	[41]
Accuracy	Agreement with the gold standard	Within ±10%	Compare with LC-MS/MS	[40]
Precision	Consistency under the same conditions	CV ≤5%	Reproducibility under the same operator	[40]
Reproducibility	Consistency across sites/labs	CV ≤10%	Inter-laboratory validation	[42]
Interference	Resistance to matrix effects	No false signals in urine/serum	Required per CLSI EP17	[43]
Stability	Sensor durability over time	>6 months storage life	Includes transport simulation	[44]

12.3.2 Key Analytical Performance Metrics

Sensitivity and Specificity: Diagnostic devices rely on two essential metrics, which make up their foundation [37]. The ability of a biosensor to recognize prostate cancer cases as positive represents its sensitivity measurement, but its specificity measurement returns its capacity for excluding benign prostate hyperplasia or prostatitis and alternative medical conditions [38]. The detection system based on PSA measures approximately 80–85% of all present prostate cancer cases, even when it identifies 30–40% of conditions incorrectly as prostate cancer. More diagnostic accuracy is possible when biosensors use multiple biomarkers such as PSA and PCA3. Available multiplex biosensors serve to enhance both biomarker detection parameters through their ability to generate comprehensive diagnostic profiles that use multiple biomarkers.

LOD and Limit of Quantitation (LOQ): The LOD is the smallest amount of biomarker that the biosensor can detect reliably. This is particularly crucial for early-stage prostate cancer, where biomarker concentrations may be extremely low. Nanotechnology-based sensors have demonstrated femtomolar (10^{-15} M) detection limits, a substantial improvement over traditional immunoassays. Gold nanoparticle-enhanced electrochemical biosensors have achieved LODs below 1 pg/mL for PSA, surpassing the performance of standard ELISA [39]. *Accuracy, Precision, and Reproducibility*: A biosensor establishes accuracy levels when test results align with precise biomarker measurements taken through conventional assessment methods, such as LC-MS/MS or standard immunoassay [40]. Research precision indicates how stable test outcomes are during multiple repetitive measurements under uniform procedural conditions. The examination of test performance across various labs, operators, and equipment receivers is known as reproducibility.

Biosensors need to pass clinical use requirements through achieving a coefficient of variation (CV) less than 10% between different test runs and displaying an ideal CV below 5% for high-precision devices [45].

12.3.3 Robustness and Interference Studies

Prostate cancer biosensors must demonstrate stable performance when operating under various physiological conditions. Validation protocols include the following [42]: *Matrix effect studies*: Research on matrix effect aims to test how biosensor operations are affected by different biological fluids that include blood and urine while detecting interference signals during testing. *Cross-reactivity testing*: The testing process should determine if any proteins, enzymes, or antibodies from common samples create incorrect sensor signals. *Stability testing*: Stability testing involves evaluating sensor durability while assessing its behavior during time-based assessments under different storage and transportation situations. The laboratory utilizes detection limits and precision parameters according to Clinical and Laboratory Standards Institute (CLSI) documentation, including EP17, along with EP05 [44].

12.3.4 Biological and Demographic Variability

A highly advanced biosensor needs to incorporate patient-specific variation factors that involve the following [46]: *Genetic polymorphisms*: DNA variations known as SNPs located within the KLK3 gene affect how biomarkers are produced (e.g., SNPs in the KLK3 gene that generate PSA). *Age-related changes*: Hormonal changes related to aging, as well as prostate enlargement, will affect levels of biomarkers in patients. *Ethnic differences*: Ethnic differences in prostate cancer risk and biomarker baseline levels. The PSA levels of African American males might remain high even when prostate pathology reveals no signs of disease. To address these factors, researchers are increasingly creating stratified validation cohorts and utilizing machine learning algorithms to dynamically adjust thresholds and identify confounders during the validation phase [47].

12.3.5 Emerging Trends in Preclinical Validation

Organoid and Microfluidic Models: Prostate organoids and microfluidic "lab-on-a-chip" devices can now be used to replicate actual tumor microenvironments in preclinical testing, thanks to advancements in tissue engineering. This makes it possible for [48]: better approximation of in vivo biomarker secretion profiles;

real-time monitoring of biosensor response in biologically relevant systems; and ethical reduction in animal testing. *Digital Twin Model*: Research teams use in silico models to build digital twins that model how biosensors would manage specific patient data for predicting potential performance outcomes prior to clinical trials [49]. *Multi-Omics Integration*: Current prostate cancer biosensors operate to detect protein biomarkers, circulating miRNAs, DNA methylation patterns, and metabolic signatures [50]. The analysis of multi-omics platforms necessitates new approaches for validating biosensor data, as these platforms handle complex combinations of information while decomposing underlying signals. *Regulatory Expectations and Best Practices*: The FDA, along with European Medicines Agency (EMA), needs preclinical studies to fulfill the following criteria: well-documented and statistically robust, with pre-specified endpoints; the studies took place in enable settings equivalent to Good Laboratory Practice; and the design history file (DHF) maintains its application status as a submitted component that follows the standards of ISO 13485. Developers need to employ standardized reference materials, and they should follow the FDA's Biomarker Qualification Program by contributing to publicly shared data through collaborative consortia to attain biomarker approval [51].

12.4 Clinical Evaluation, Trial Design, and Validation of Biosensors

A biosensor advances toward practical applications during the clinical evaluation stage, enabling it to serve real-world needs. During this phase, testing of prostate cancer diagnostics requires an extremely strict approach because timely, accurate detection leads to better patient results and treatment choices [52]. The FDA, together with the EMA, mandates that developers present evidence about analytical performance alongside clinical validity and clinical utility performance across various population groups. The clinical validation process requires testing biosensors with their innovative designs and unorthodox sampling methods when producing digital clinical outputs in realistic patient scenarios [53]. The first evaluation step involves setting the specific application purpose for the biosensor between screening and diagnosis, staging purposes, or monitoring patients. Design parameters for trials reflect their application, so cohort choice becomes specific to the intended use, and main assessment variables match those endpoints [54]. Applications designed for screening need to enroll large numbers of asymptomatic test subjects, yet staging tools need biopsy-proven groups for evaluation purposes. The requirement for real-world evidence (RWE) causes validation efforts to move from controlled environments into regular clinical spaces to verify device performance when used by general medical staff [55]. The crucial part of demographic representation becomes especially important for prostate cancer due to its divergent occurrences throughout different population groups. The medical needs of African American men require equal recruitment methods because their rates of prostate cancer diagnosis and mortality exceed those of other groups [56]. The performance of biosensor technology for all users requires adequate power along with representative and inclusive trials as per current regulatory demands.

12.4.1 Comparative and Hybrid Validation Models

The current clinical trials devoted to prostate cancer biosensors have progressed past basic biomarker analysis methods. The validation process for prostate cancer biosensors includes new diagnostic criteria that combine the utilization of multiparametric MRI and genomic classifiers on top of PSA and digital rectal exam (DRE) [57]. Yet these complex validation methods present increased requirements to the system but provide superior medical value. The comparison of biosensor outputs to MRI findings and Decipher risk scores generates performance-based evidence that shows the biosensor functions as an add-on or enhances whole testing systems. Testing protocols normally execute separate training and validation stages, especially if AI systems and intricate analytical tools are integrated into biosensors. Performance stability testing needs to finish before validation begins in order to prevent the release of test results to the algorithm [58]. The FDA, together with other regulatory agencies, requires the implementation of a lock phase to ensure that clinical performance accurately represents real-world utilization. Legitimate regulatory submissions that concern adaptive biosensor platforms now need compliance with Good Machine Learning Practice (GMLP) principles [59]. Remote patient recruitment, along with decentralized models, is now more prevalent in the medical field through digital healthcare infrastructure. The methods prove effective for prostate cancer trials because they serve patients across multiple locations and require extended observation periods [60]. The evaluation of usability, together with human factors engineering assessments, has become vital for biosensors meant for use outside health institutions, such as home settings and point-of-care locations [61].

12.4.2 Regulatory Trials and Early Market Access Pathways

Major risk devices require the FDA Investigational New Drug approval to start the regulatory submission process for clinical trials. The medical institutions provide regulatory submissions that combine preclinical evidence with risk assessment reports, procedural documents, and investigator records [62]. Prostate cancer biosensors submitted under EU IVDR requirements require a performance evaluation report (PER) to demonstrate scientific validity and provide test and clinical performance metrics. Regulatory agencies grant expedited approval to biosensors that introduce distinctive functionalities into the market. The FDA's Breakthrough Devices Program facilitates the expeditious regulatory approval of devices that meet critical unmet requirements or offer enhanced diagnostic capabilities [63]. Programs like these have allowed multiple prostate cancer biosensors to reach the market, for which dealers operate with specific requirements related to follow-up research. After a clinical trial concludes, the device labeling statements, along with promotional materials, must match exactly the confirmed research findings. Extending claims past the proven study evidence may lead to regulatory warnings and eventual market withdrawal [64]. Research teams must achieve both scientific accuracy and regulatory future planning at all stages of trial design, from initial planning to final analysis. For biosensors that detect prostate cancer, clinical evaluation serves as the regulatory requirement to achieve translational success while protecting human lives.

12.5 Regulatory Submission, Global Classifications, and Approval Pathways

The diagnostic devices used for prostate cancer fall within the category of IVD medical devices. Their classification and the stringency of the regulatory path depend on their intended use and the potential risk to patients [65]. Prostate cancer biosensors in the United States require 510(k) clearance when they mimic established devices or De Novo review for original moderate-risk equipment or PMA for testing devices that need extensive patient safety scrutiny [66]. Most prostate cancer biosensors within the European Union are classified as Class C by the IVDR, requiring examination by a Notified Body before market approval. The PER considers scientific validity, together with analytical performance and clinical performance in the submission process [67]. The EU AI Act, along with additional safety and transparency requirements, must be adhered to by biosensors that utilize AI.

12.5.1 Harmonized Standards and Technical Documentation

The development of biosensors needs alignment with established international regulatory criteria according to requirements from governing organizations. Medical devices' specific quality management systems follow the guiding standard of ISO 13485:2016 [68]. The standard controls the entire process, encompassing both the selection of acquired materials and the creation of product design, as well as production operations and post-market observation duties. ISO 14971:2019 standards for product risk management enforce detailed methods of hazard analysis alongside failure mode and effects analysis and necessary risk reduction strategies [69]. Biosensors utilizing software components, especially those incorporating AI-driven diagnostics, need to follow IEC 62304 requirements when developing software from planning phases through risk management and validation and maintenance stages [70]. The harmonized standards form an auditable framework for biosensor development, making all design specifications and final products resilient and replicable, along with proof for regulatory assessments. The technical documentation package, known as the Design Dossier, forms the core component of the submission. This comprehensive collection includes the following: device description and specifications; DHF; risk management report; verification and validation data; the device information included documentation for Instructions for Use and labeling material; clinical evidence report; and the submission of AI devices requires documentation about training datasets together with model architecture details and validation evidence of algorithms and evidence that demonstrates generalization ability. The data compilation process of machine learning biosensors must follow both the FDA-created GMLP and the AI/ML SaMD Framework from IMDRF, before receiving approval for clinical use [71].

12.5.2 Regulatory Interaction and Accelerated Approval Pathways

Making contact with regulatory bodies at an early stage ensures developers can prevent submission problems. Argentina presents an alternative method for biosensor developers to seek FDA regulatory feedback on clinical study protocols, analytical methods, and software validation plans through their Q-Submission Program [72]. Through its Scientific Advice procedure, the EMA enables European medical device developers to obtain essential details about IVDR clinical evaluation needs in advance [73]. Novel biosensors reaching the market for prostate cancer diagnosis benefit substantially from accelerated review procedures. Through the FDA's Breakthrough Devices Designation and the EMA's PRIME (Priority Medicines) scheme, developers gain expedited regulatory review benefits, including a combination review process and active governmental authority involvement [74]. The use of these accelerated pathways requires participants to fulfill rising standards of real-world performance assessment, as well as extended safety assessment protocols.

12.5.3 Digital Submissions and PMS

Electronic tools have become the main foundation for contemporary biosensor submissions. Biosensor submissions use the eCTD format as a structured submission system for globally ready documentation supported by cloud-based platforms, enabling efficient team collaboration between regulatory groups, legal departments, and clinical departments [75]. New biosensor developers can track regulatory requirements by using systems that merge regulatory intelligence functions with standards monitoring and regulatory changes tracking. Following market authorization, the biosensor assumes its responsibilities for marketplace operations [76]. PMS plans implemented by developers must contain robust features for adverse event reporting and performance audits, as well as user feedback integration and algorithmic drift monitoring systems when using AI systems [77]. The collection of RWE acquires special importance for validating both new indications and label enhancements.

12.6 Ethical, Legal, and Social Implications of Biosensor Deployment

The existence of biosensors for prostate cancer diagnosis happens independently of broader circumstances [78]. These technologies, when implemented in clinical practice and personal health settings, raise significant questions about ethics, legality, and social implications. Such considerations directly impact regulatory permissions as well as user trust, in addition to determining future integration of these devices into healthcare platforms [79]. Proof-based solutions must be applied to address these issues for responsible innovation to succeed.

12.6.1 Data Privacy, Ownership, and Consent

Personal data obtained through biosensors designed for biomarker-based, physiological, or behavioral pattern assessments frequently includes high-frequency sensitive information. The data wrangled by AI systems serves two simultaneous purposes: enabling quick diagnostics while improving and learning algorithm performance [80]. Research conducted at MIT in 2023 demonstrated that laboratory-made biometric datasets could be identified using open-source genetic information with a 14% success rate, despite being anonymized, which suggests that traditional de-identification methods are ineffective. The practice of obtaining patient consent is facing new challenges due to rapidly evolving data models [81]. Standard consent obtained once is insufficient to protect biosensors that learn and develop their operations from continuous data streams [82]. Approval paradigms known as dynamic consent are currently under development and testing in EU-funded prostate cancer biosensor research programs such as PRIMA and IN4ACT. People continue debating who owns the rights to handle their personal information. The advancement of biosensors that integrate with personal health apps enables patients to manage their health data rights, including access, removal, and payment purposes [83]. New biosensor ecosystems are currently testing the protections provided by the GDPR (EU) and HIPAA (US) through their blurring of the medical research and consumer domains.

12.6.2 Algorithmic Bias and Health Equity

Racial minorities have higher prostate cancer rates than other groups, primarily affecting African American men. The 2022 systematic review of more than 200 AI-based prostate cancer diagnostic models demonstrated that just 15% of them mentioned using race-based performance assessments [84]. The underserved populations face reduced diagnostic accuracy because underreporting becomes a risk factor for algorithmic bias. Through the AIM-AHEAD Program of the NIH, researchers obtain funding together with infrastructure to enhance the diversity of datasets and model transparency with bias auditing capabilities in AI diagnostic systems [85]. The upcoming EU AI Act establishes obligatory documentation requirements for AI system performance statistics within distinct demographic sections, thus affecting biosensor validation procedures. Software developers are implementing bias reduction methods through resampling methods alongside fairness-centric model development algorithms, and after-development performance balancing between socioeconomic and racial demographics [86]. Supporting and reporting these approaches continuously is essential for establishing effective trust in their work.

12.6.3 Legal Liability and Ethical Accountability

Legal responsibilities in diagnostic tasks carried out by automated biosensors remain ill-defined between medical professionals and technology implementers. The delay of proper prostate cancer treatment stemming from unrecognizable early stages by biosensors prompts a legal examination about accountability [87]. Who bears responsibility in this case: the biosensor producer, along with the software engineering team, or the medical practitioners who used the sensor data? Lawmakers currently rely on public liability legislation along with traditional malpractice soot, but these rules seldom protect modern AI-integrated biosensing devices enough [88]. Canada and Germany, along with other jurisdictions, are working on developing joint liability models that combine "explainability clauses," which require AI systems to provide traceable decisions for legal dispute resolution. The ethical principle of accountability by design has begun to gain recognition in various fields [89]. Developers need to incorporate ethical foresight into their design process by predicting potential risks, documenting their assumptions during development, and simulating how their systems will react to misuse or failure [90]. Public health agencies and organizations conducting large biosensor R&D through public–private partnerships now make ethical impact assessments essential components of their programs.

12.7 Market Access, Reimbursement, and Evolving Value Paradigms in Diagnostic Innovation

Current biosensors designed for prostate cancer diagnosis need to prove clinical effectiveness beyond laboratory controls [91]. The payers maintain resistance toward diagnostics until these tools can demonstrate direct effects on treatment selection and patient outcomes duration. The current operating model for health technology assessment (HTA) organizations directs them toward diagnostic solutions that reduce testing times and enhance safety through the avoidance of unnecessary treatments alongside personalized care capabilities [92]. Biosensor developers need to incorporate health economics and outcome research from an early strategic perspective due to present-day market shifts.

12.7.1 Economic Evidence: Beyond Cost Savings

The criterion of cost-effectiveness fails to satisfy present requirements. Modern decision-makers consider biosensor value through three elements, including its contribution to quality-adjusted life years and its influence on clinical decisions and benefits to public populations [93]. The prostate-specific biosensor succeeded in reducing unnecessary biopsies by more than 25%, thus delivering economic advantages up to €4 million for every 10,000 patients screened. Social outcome assessments have gained importance among HTA authorities while directly affecting their reimbursement processes.

12.7.2 HTA Integration and Early Scientific Advice

Public European HTA organizations such as NICE (UK), HAS (France), and ZIN (Netherlands) actively promote biosensor developers to participate in early scientific advice. The collective methodology enables evidence development to match reimbursement requirements from the outset [94]. Multiple clinical trial sites performing successful biosensor evaluations can access expedited healthcare access points or gain restricted reimbursement through evidence advancement cycles.

12.7.3 Country-Specific Reimbursement Pathways

Biosensor reimbursement within the United States requires CPT code structures and Medicare coverage analysis, along with possible qualification under the Advanced Diagnostic Laboratory Tests (ADLTs) framework [95]. Healthcare providers must demonstrate that the implementation of biosensors produces better patient health outcomes through clinical effectiveness assessments. Japan, alongside South Korea and Canada (see Table 12.3 for reimbursement strategies across regions), maintains health technology assessment systems that focus on primary care operations and healthcare technology platforms, thus impacting their approval durations and reimbursement decisions [96].

12.7.4 RWE and Performance-Based Models

Healthcare payers now accept reimbursement based on performance contracts for AI-based and home-usage biosensors, particularly. The reimbursement process under these contracts bases payments on pre-established diagnostic and therapeutic performance targets [101]. The German pilot reimbursement system linked biosensor use to a 15% improvement in prostate cancer detection outcomes in at-risk populations. G-BA evaluates the model for potential implementation at a national level [102].

Table 12.3 Market access and reimbursement pathways by region

Country/ region	Reimbursement model	Key agencies/ tools	Unique biosensor notes	References
United states	CPT codes + ADLT + Medicare	CMS, FDA	Performance-linked reimbursement emerging	[97]
EU	HTA + country-specific assessment	NICE (UK), ZIN (NL), HAS (FR)	PROs increasingly influence decisions	[63]
Japan	DPC system + MHLW approval	PMDA, MHLW	Focus on primary care diagnostics	[98]
South Korea	Value-based assessment	HIRA	Interested in AI-based home tools	[28]
Canada	HTA + provincial coverage	CADTH	Emphasizes rural accessibility	[99]
Germany	Performance-based pilot (15% PC detection boost)	G-BA	Exploring biosensor contracts tied to outcomes	[100]

12.7.5 Patient-Centric Metrics and PRO Integration

Patient-reported outcomes (PROs), along with quality-of-life metrics, now hold significant value for HTA agencies during their evaluation process [103]. Biosensors become more attractive under patient-centered care because they help ease diagnostic anxiety and reduce procedure invasiveness while improving monitoring compliance. Digital patient engagement platforms, which accompany biosensor use, have started to become an essential differentiating factor for access discussions [104].

12.8 Global Market Strategy and the Drive for International Regulatory Harmonization

Developers of biosensors encounter multiple obstacles while attempting to pass through separate regulatory frameworks between different national jurisdictions [105]. Regulatory bodies, such as the U.S. FDA and the EMA, alongside Japan's PMDA and India's CDSCO, maintain different classification parameters, as well as documentation specifications and validation requirements for biosensors. Global deployment slows down due to fragmentation, and development costs rise while duplicate trials are generated [106]. Different global regions have access to medical device and diagnostic regulations because multiple organizations focus on establishing regional compatibility. Standardized regulatory concepts, such as risk-based device categorization, RWE standards, and unique device identification, were created by organizations under the IMDRF [107]. Developers who use harmonization can create a single validation framework for prostate cancer biosensors to operate across various jurisdictions, thus minimizing development timelines and associated costs. EU regulatory authorities elevated requirements for performance documentation and clinical proof when they shifted from IVDD to IVDR. The Medical Device Single Audit Program enables an active EU–FDA partnership, which speeds up international regulatory alignment. Market entry through these harmonization schemes becomes simplified, which provides companies with the opportunity to perform simultaneous launches across multiple countries [108].

12.8.1 Strategic Approaches to Global Market Entry

The successful marketing of biosensors worldwide depends on coordinating regulatory approvals with both local market needs and clinical guidelines in each territory. Software developers choose the "regulatory launch sequencing" strategy by first starting their product launch in countries with clear approval guidelines and high unmet diagnostic requirements before moving to slower approval jurisdictions [109]. The Asia-Pacific market provides entry opportunities through Singapore and Australia because they belong to the Global Harmonization Task Force legacy group and maintain effective approval systems. These geographical areas show an increasing interest from prostate cancer screening services, while reimbursement bodies seek affordable diagnostic solutions at scale [110]. Low- and middle-income countries (LMICs) receive basic biosensor models that require minimal infrastructure, allowing these nations to benefit from the programs. The biosensor manufacturers receive support from PATH and the World Health Organization (WHO) Prequalification Program to develop donor-funded procurement-eligible diagnostic solutions for public health deployment [111]. The harmonization of regulatory standards between nations allows studies to combine their clinical investigations, thus speeding up global data acquisition without repeated evaluations [112]. The EU–Asia consortia conduct simultaneous biosensor testing across different ethnicities and clinical settings through trial evaluations, thereby increasing the external validity of the results and promoting equitable data representation.

12.9 PMS, RWE, and Evolving Regulatory Oversight of Biosensors

The main pillar of regulatory compliance today consists of PMS, which actively tracks newly launched biosensors that surpass their previous reactive status. The regulatory framework now requires prostate cancer diagnostic regulators to monitor sustained safety and ongoing performance, as well as effectiveness maintenance within natural clinical operating environments [113]. The current PMS frameworks focus on continuous monitoring of patient data, including sensors that carry high risk or possess AI capabilities that need updates during their lifecycle across diverse medical scenarios [114]. All Class B and higher diagnostics under the European Union's IVDR must follow strict post-market performance follow-up plans, which require annual reports and the reporting of incidents, while also gathering feedback from users. The U.S. FDA has established post-clearance study requirements, as well as real-world usage evaluation through its 522 postmarket surveillance Program, for specific diagnostic medical devices [115]. Digital biosensors operate within mobile applications and internet-based portals, enabling the remote monitoring of diagnostic devices through automated surveillance methods. Remote tracking capabilities enable these technologies to monitor user patterns while collecting error data and performance benchmarks, thereby establishing an instant information-sharing system for regulators, creators, and end-users [116]. The dynamic oversight capability aligns with the emerging regulatory concept of adaptive regulation, as it enables approval status and clinical guidance to be updated based on new evidence.

12.9.1 RWE as a Regulatory and Clinical Driver

RWE facilitates a shift in the evaluation procedures of prostate cancer biosensors following their regulatory approval. Medical evidence through RWE combines information obtained from clinical registries with electronic health records, as well as claims databases and PROs recorded during normal product usage [117]. The originated evidence shows success in regulatory compliance, as well as sustaining clinical acceptance by payers and guideline incorporation. Multiple biosensor companies have started working with academic medical centers to create real-world performance groups that monitor diagnosis accuracy, together with false results and treatment decision changes through continuous observational studies [118]. A combined U.S.–Canada research project developing urine-based biosensors yielded improved prostate cancer detection results for African American men, which directly promoted regulatory approvals alongside reimbursement parameters [119]. RWE enables scientists to assess biosensor performance by ethnicity, while also considering patient characteristics such as age and comorbidities, as well as healthcare environments, to improve pre-market trial demographics. The recorded data functions as a vital foundation for universal care because it helps screen prostate cancer tools specifically for marginalized populations. The regulatory models employed by Singapore, Australia, and Germany utilize RWE extensively to modify approved indications or add new indications after initial clearance. The regulatory system has launched a new approach for biosensor approvals, which provides provisional acceptance for certain patient clusters to use expanded applications if more RWE information is submitted later. Holding patient access to products can occur rapidly without reducing regulatory control over these systems [120].

12.10 Regulatory Considerations for AI-Driven and Digital Biosensors: Addressing the Challenge of Dynamic Algorithms

The diagnostic biosensors designed by AI operate dynamically for the detection of prostate cancer. Core algorithms undergo development through continual learning arrangements, retraining processes, and the addition of new datasets [121]. The

Table 12.4 Regulatory requirements for AI-enabled biosensors (FDA vs. EMA)

Feature	FDA (USA)	EMA (EU)	References
Approval framework	SaMD Action Plan	IVDR + EU AI Act	[132]
Change control	PCCP	Post-approval AI updates require revalidation	[133]
Training data transparency	Required for submission	Required under the AI Act	[134]
Algorithm bias testing	Encouraged (AIM-AHEAD initiative)	Mandatory across demographics	[135]
Post-market monitoring	Algorithm drift surveillance	Periodic performance update reports	[136]
Explainability tools	SHAP, LIME encouraged	Mandatory for high-risk AI systems (2026 onward)	[137]

established regulatory systems, based on fixed devices and software dependencies, encounter significant difficulties when faced with this situation. The U.S. FDA and other regulatory bodies create a SaMD framework, which identifies two categories of algorithms: locked and adaptive ones. The FDA introduced a Predetermined Change Control Plan (PCCP) in 2023, which serves as a developer tool for specifying system evolution after approval [122]. The conditional clearance mechanisms enable future software upgrade authorization, provided that developers maintain operational boundaries that were initially validated clinically. The introduction of this approach enables biosensors to self-improve their accuracy level throughout their operational period [123]. Researchers test AI-powered urine and blood sensors for their capability to run autonomous threshold adjustments relative to patient demographics, such as age and ethnic origin, or genetic indicators (see Table 12.4 for an AI regulation comparison) [124].

12.10.1 Transparency, Explainability, and Ethical Imperatives

The use of AI-based biosensors becomes challenging because programmers must manage algorithmic biases and data opacity, in addition to feature explanation problems. Prostate cancer AI models that primarily train through European ancestry data show diminished effectiveness within South Asian and African patient populations, thereby creating additional health care inequality [125]. Regulatory bodies require companies to provide explanations about their algorithms as a condition for approving new technology submissions. Commercial AI systems need to provide detailed documentation about the data composition of training datasets, as well as the selection process behind chosen features, in addition to fairness audits [126]. The European Union's AI Act marks 2026 as the full application date for healthcare diagnostics with high-risk categorization that requires bias monitoring alongside human review mechanisms and real-time diagnostics evaluation [127]. The development of biosensors requires firmware features that provide clinical staff, along with patients, the ability to understand their prediction reasoning. SHapley Additive exPlanations (SHAP), along with Local Interpretable Model-Agnostic Explanations (LIME) tools, integrate with biosensor dashboards to generate confidence scores and explain contributing factors and decision processes, which serve vital requirements for medical responsibility assessments as well as regulatory approval standards [128].

12.10.2 Cybersecurity, Data Privacy, and Regulatory Interoperability

Digital biosensors transmit patient data using mobile apps and cloud-based platforms, depending on their network dependency for operation. These devices remain exposed to cyber dangers, for which proper cybersecurity design protections need to be implemented [129]. As of 2024, the U.S. FDA started making Cybersecurity Software Bill of Materials submissions mandatory for companies to report all software components with their security flaws. Several rules, including HIPAA from the United States, GDPR from the EU, and PIPEDA from Canada, demand organizations to maintain strict protection measures for patient data [130]. The developers responsible for biosensors must verify that their products comply with regulatory requirements by adhering to universal standards for privacy protocols, data anonymity procedures, and incident notification systems across all national territories. Globally marketed biosensors require attaining regulatory interoperability to become strategic for their commercial success [131]. The Global Digital Health Partnership, alongside the WHO's Global Digital Health Certification Network, is constructing standards for protection protocols that support data exchange between systems. Biosensor developers who follow these standardized international standards will find faster multi-regional approval processes and gain reliability from worldwide supervisory organizations.

12.11 Case Studies: Regulatory Pathways of Approved Biosensors for Prostate Cancer

12.11.1 Case Study 1: Liquid Biopsy Biosensor for Prostate Cancer Screening

The FDA approved a novel biosensor for detecting prostate cancer biomarkers in blood via the liquid biopsy in 2022 through the De Novo pathway. The biotech company created this device to detect high PCA3 gene levels and TMPRSS2-ERG gene fusion changes, which serve as strong indicators of prostate cancer [138]. The FDA approval of this biosensor represents a significant challenge for non-invasive diagnostic technologies in terms of regulatory issues. The FDA conducted an extensive assessment of clinical trial data, which showed both high accuracy and sensitivity of the prostate cancer detection performance of the liquid biopsy biosensor. A multicenter trial evaluation enabled the determination of Class II device risk classification for the product

[139]. For regulatory approval, the biosensor required extensive testing to prove its uniform operation throughout different sections of the population. The clinical trials received additions of diverse participants because the FDA wanted to eliminate algorithm bias in performance data. The qualification procedure included post-market observation responsibilities from the FDA, requiring organizations to track real-time device operations across larger demographic groups [140]. The biosensor required additional attention to genetic marker variations across multiple demographic populations since this was its core functioning mechanism. The device manufacturer was required to report ongoing statistics about incorrect results to ensure appropriate device usage and prevent unnecessary biopsies [141]. The case illustrates the regulatory shift toward comprehensive assessment, which integrates external evidence and trial participant diversity to achieve safety and broader treatment effectiveness.

12.11.2 Case Study 2: AI-Based Prostate Cancer Detection Biosensor

Medical regulators authorized the implementation of an AI-based prostate cancer biosensor for clinical practice in 2023 throughout the United States and Europe. The biosensor utilizes deep learning algorithms to evaluate DRE imaging in conjunction with multiparametric MRI for identifying abnormalities and determining cancer risk levels [142]. The AI tool performs automated examinations and measurements of prostate abnormalities, providing results that offer objective and standardized assessments that surpass traditional methods. The development of this AI biosensor followed the SaMD framework established by the FDA, as both aim to support innovative AI technologies [143]. The algorithm needed to demonstrate its ability to correctly detect prostate cancer throughout diverse clinical situations during the approval process through extensive performance testing. The 510(k) pathway allowed U.S. FDA approval because the device proved equivalent to previously cleared products. The testing of the AI biosensor included standard biopsy examination and evaluation of existing multiparametric MRI methods [144]. The device went through complete testing at different stages during the regulatory approval process, showing its precision alongside reliability features and its accomplishment in decreasing unneeded biopsies. Throughout the approval procedure, multiple obstacles that particularly affect AI technologies gained recognition. The regulatory authority required the company to continuously monitor algorithm performance after obtaining device clearance [145]. The manufacturer needed to report regular updates to show that the AI system maintained its accuracy while preventing bias development during its lifespan as an essential demonstration of adaptive AI device regulation.

12.11.3 Case Study 3: Urine-Based Biomarker Detection Biosensor

The EMA gave its approval to a prostate cancer diagnosis biosensor based on biomarkers in urine during 2021, thus advancing non-invasive diagnostic tools [146]. The biosensor detects elevated PCA3 and TMPRSS2-ERG gene fusion biomarkers in urine samples, providing an alternative to invasive biopsy procedures. EU medical device regulations distinguished the regulatory process for this biosensor since it fell within the Class III medical device category [147]. The medical device classification provides an extensive evaluation mechanism. Multiple tests on the device revealed its performance capacity to identify various stages of prostate cancer from early through advanced clearances. The EMA used a new adaptive method for approving this device. The medical device needed to complete post-market clinical follow-up studies following initial clearance to receive final approval for monitoring its performance within real-world clinical practices [148]. The EMA demonstrates a new regulatory practice that reflects expanded programs for real-time biosensor collection of evidence and performance tracking. Patient education materials needed to meet requirements as part of the approval process to explain that this non-invasive test provides patients with different options instead of biopsy procedures [149]. The presented case illustrates how regulatory changes aim to integrate patient-welcoming product development with genuine field data throughout biosensor product life cycles.

12.12 Future Outlook: Evolving Regulatory Science and the Emergence of Dynamic Frameworks for Next-Gen Biosensors

A urine-based biomarker detection biosensor for prostate cancer diagnosis received approval from the EMA in 2021, making it a new non-invasive diagnostic tool [150]. The biosensor detects elevated PCA3 and TMPRSS2-ERG gene fusion biomarkers in urine samples, providing an alternative to invasive biopsy procedures. EU medical device regulations distinguished the regulatory process for this biosensor since it fell within the Class III medical device category [151]. The medical device classification provides an extensive evaluation mechanism. Multiple tests on the device revealed its performance capacity to identify various stages of prostate cancer from early through advanced clearances [152]. The EMA used a new adaptive method for approving this device. The medical device required completion of post-market clinical follow-up studies following initial clearance to receive final approval for monitoring its performance within real-world clinical practices [153]. The EMA demonstrates a new regulatory practice that reflects expanded programs for real-time biosensor collection of evidence and performance tracking. Patient education materials are needed to meet the requirements as part of the approval process, explaining that this non-invasive test provides patients with different options instead of biopsy procedures [154]. Patient-centered design integration and real-world data collection now play an important role in regulatory screening processes that develop biosensors.

12.12.1 Integration of AI and Machine Learning in Regulation

In 2021, the EMA approved a biosensor based on urine biomarker detection, demonstrating enhanced capabilities for prostate cancer diagnosis. The biosensor identifies elevated PCA3 and TMPRSS2-ERG gene fusion biomarkers present in urine samples, thus offering an alternative solution to invasive biopsy procedures [155]. EU medical device regulations distinguished the regulatory process for this biosensor since it fell within the Class III medical device category. The medical device classification provided it with an extensive evaluation mechanism [156]. Multiple tests on the device revealed its performance capacity to identify various stages of prostate cancer from early through advanced clearances. The EMA used a new adaptive method for approving this device. The medical device needed to complete post-market clinical follow-up studies following initial clearance to receive final approval for monitoring its performance within real-world clinical practices [157]. The EMA demonstrates a new regulatory practice that reflects expanded programs for real-time biosensor collection of evidence and performance tracking. Patient education materials needed to meet requirements as part of the approval process to explain that this non-invasive test provides patients with different options instead of biopsy procedures [158]. The regulatory situation highlights an ongoing trend to integrate patient-led design and authentic data collection into the biosensor creation process.

12.12.2 Global Harmonization of Regulatory Standards

The growth of international prostate cancer detection biosensors requires active global standardization efforts for regulatory purposes [159]. The implementation of AI and machine learning diagnostic technologies extends beyond European and American territories because countries like India, along with China and Latin America, are establishing new innovative biosensors and AI applications for early cancer detection. The absence of standardization across different areas results in trade obstacles and makes it harder to integrate clinical activities [160]. The IMDRF continues to establish global medical device regulations, which will include recommendations for AI-based device development throughout member countries. Through this common pathway program, manufacturers gain quicker access to markets, and better borderless partnerships become possible [161]. The combination of standardized practices will grant prostate cancer biosensors international acceptance without compromising security measures for patients. The WHO focuses on implementing biosensors as part of its worldwide health programs to benefit specifically those areas classified as LMICs [162]. The WHO works to create uniform regulatory standards that will increase worldwide accessibility of early cancer diagnostics to achieve better health results for disadvantaged patient populations.

12.13 Conclusion

The chapter analyzed essential rules that guide the development and use of biosensors for diagnosing prostate cancer. Current biosensor technology innovations compel regulatory institutions to develop new procedures that protect safety while also facilitating advances in this field using nanomaterials, AI, and machine learning, as well as real-time tracking capabilities. Regulatory approvals for biosensors depend on proactive authority relations, demanding clinical assessments, and expanding evidence needs from real-world settings for initial authorizations and market surveillance. This research demonstrates that regulatory agencies, including the FDA and EMA, along with their global equivalents, are moving toward adaptable risk-based approaches for next-generation diagnostic assessment. The discussion focused on evaluating both ethical aspects and AI-based biosensor particular challenges while highlighting the need to standardize regional standards for worldwide diagnostic access control. The chapter explored real-life case examples that demonstrated how regulatory navigation impacts the modern medical landscape, while also highlighting potential pitfalls and available benefits for practitioners. The successful advancement of prostate cancer biosensors requires both technological progress and skilled regulatory compliance, while maintaining patient welfare. The development of life-saving tools will continue to depend on regulatory science because its advancing role remains indispensable for clinical delivery through laboratory research.

12.14 Summary

This chapter examines the changing regulatory environment for biosensors designed for the detection of prostate cancer. It highlights the need for new regulatory frameworks resulting from the transformation of diagnostic tools brought about by technological advancements, including AI integration, digital health applications, and nanomaterials. The chapter examines the classification schemes, validation procedures, and approval routes of significant organizations such as the FDA, EMA, and IMDRF. Case studies illustrate the successful regulatory journeys of real-world biosensors, demonstrating how innovation and compliance can coexist. A forward-looking viewpoint on dynamic regulatory frameworks and global harmonization initiatives concludes the discussion, which covers ethical, legal, and PMS aspects.

Glossary

Biosensor A device that uses biological molecules to detect chemical or biological markers and convert them into measurable signals.

IVD Tests performed outside the body to detect diseases or conditions, often using samples like blood or urine.

SaMD Software as a Medical Device software intended for medical use without being part of a physical medical device.

Nanotechnology Technology that operates at the nanoscale (1–100 nm), often used in sensors for increased sensitivity.

Clinical Validation The process of confirming that a device accurately detects or predicts a clinical condition.

PMS Ongoing monitoring of a device's performance after it has been approved and released into the market.

Algorithmic Drift Degradation or unintended behavior in AI model performance over time due to changes in data patterns.

Risk Classification Regulatory categorization based on the level of risk a medical device poses to patients.

RWE Data collected from real-world settings (outside of clinical trials) to assess safety and effectiveness.

Regulatory Harmonization The process of aligning regulatory requirements across jurisdictions to streamline global approval.

References

1. Damborský P, Damborská D, Belický Š, Tkáč J, Katrlík J. Sweet strategies in prostate cancer biomarker research: focus on a prostate specific antigen. BioNanoScience. 2018;8(2):690–700. https://doi.org/10.1007/s12668-017-0397-z.
2. Garg S, Sachdeva A, Peeters M, McClements J. Point-of-care prostate specific antigen testing: examining translational progress toward clinical implementation. ACS Sens. 2023;8(10):3643–58. https://doi.org/10.1021/acssensors.3c01402.
3. Mummareddy S, Pradhan S, Narasimhan AK, Natarajan A. On demand biosensors for early diagnosis of cancer and immune checkpoints blockade therapy monitoring from liquid biopsy. Biosensors. 2021;11(12):500.
4. Falkowski P, Lukaszewski Z, Gorodkiewicz E. Potential of surface plasmon resonance biosensors in cancer detection. J Pharm Biomed Anal. 2021;194:113802. Available from: https://www.sciencedirect.com/science/article/pii/S0731708520316885.
5. Sánchez-Salcedo R, Gómez-Meijide P, Miranda-Castro R, de-los-Santos-Álvarez N, Lobo-Castañón MJ. Electrochemical sensors using oligonucleotides as recognition ligands for liquid biopsy in prostate cancer. Biosens Bioelectron X. 2022;12:100227.
6. Sanko V, Kuralay F. Label-free electrochemical biosensor platforms for cancer diagnosis: recent achievements and challenges. Biosensors. 2023;13(3). Available from: https://www.mdpi.com/2079-6374/13/3/333.
7. Mishra S, Kim ES, Sharma PK, Wang ZJ, Yang SH, Kaushik AK, et al. Tailored biofunctionalized biosensor for the label-free sensing of prostate-specific antigen. ACS Appl Bio Mater. 2020;3(11):7821–30. https://doi.org/10.1021/acsabm.0c01002.
8. Lin J, Chen Y, Liu X, Jiang H, Wang X. Engineered intelligent electrochemical biosensors for portable point-of-care diagnostics. Chem. 2025;13(4):146.
9. Fountzilas E, Pearce T, Baysal MA, Chakraborty A, Tsimberidou AM. Convergence of evolving artificial intelligence and machine learning techniques in precision oncology. npj Digit Med. 2025;8(1):75.
10. Vasudevan S, Saha A, Tarver ME, Patel B. Digital biomarkers: convergence of digital health technologies and biomarkers. npj Digit Med. 2022;5(1):36.
11. Xu R, Hu J. The role of JNK in prostate cancer progression and therapeutic strategies. Biomed Pharmacother. 2020;121:109679.
12. Testa U, Castelli G, Pelosi E. Cellular and molecular mechanisms underlying prostate cancer development: therapeutic implications. Medicine. 2019;6(3). Available from: https://www.mdpi.com/2305-6320/6/3/82.
13. Cunningham JJ, Brown JS, Gatenby RA, Staňková K. Optimal control to develop therapeutic strategies for metastatic castrate resistant prostate cancer. J Theor Biol. 2018;459:67–78.

14. Oczkowski M, Dziendzikowska K, Pasternak-Winiarska A, Włodarek D, Gromadzka-Ostrowska J. Dietary factors and prostate cancer development, progression, and reduction. Nutrients. 2021;13(2). Available from: https://www.mdpi.com/2072-6643/13/2/496.
15. Alharthi SD, Bijukumar D, Prasad S, Khan AM, Mathew MT. Evolution in biosensors for cancers biomarkers detection: a review. J Bio-and Tribo-Corrosion. 2021;7:1–17.
16. Lino C, Barrias S, Chaves R, Adega F, Martins-Lopes P, Fernandes JR. Biosensors as diagnostic tools in clinical applications. Biochim Biophys Acta Rev Cancer. 2022;1877(3):188726. Available from: https://www.sciencedirect.com/science/article/pii/S0304419X22000518.
17. Hoyle AP, Ali A, James ND, Cook A, Parker CC, de Bono JS, et al. Abiraterone in "High-" and "Low-risk" metastatic hormone-sensitive prostate cancer. Eur Urol. 2019;76(6):719–28.
18. Sharma PK, Kamini, Jain A, Shukla VK. Innovative biomedical equipment for diagnosis of cancer. In: Malviya R, Sundram S, editors. Targeted cancer therapy in biomedical engineering. Singapore: Springer Nature Singapore; 2023. p. 405–36.
19. Baumgartner C, Schröttner J, Müllner PS. Regulatory framework for medical devices and IVDs in Europe. In: Baumgartner C, Johann H, Schröttner J, editors. Medical devices and in vitro diagnostics: requirements in Europe. Cham: Springer International Publishing; 2022. p. 1–37.
20. Rusanov B, Ebert MA, Sabet M, Rowshanfarzad P, Barry N, Kendrick J, et al. Guidance on selecting and evaluating AI auto-segmentation systems in clinical radiotherapy: insights from a six-vendor analysis. Phys Eng Sci Med. 2025;48(1):301–16.
21. Bahadir CD, Omar M, Rosenthal J, Marchionni L, Liechty B, Pisapia DJ, et al. Artificial intelligence applications in histopathology. Nat Rev Electr Eng. 2024;1(2):93–108.
22. Kahles A, Goldschmid H, Volckmar AL, Ploeger C, Kazdal D, Penzel R, et al. Structure and content of the EU-IVDR. Die Pathol. 2023;44(2):73–85.
23. Taryma-Leśniak O, Sokolowska KE, Wojdacz TK. Current status of development of methylation biomarkers for in vitro diagnostic IVD applications. Clin Epigenetics. 2020;12(1):100.
24. Mooghali M, Rathi VK, Kadakia KT, Ross JS, Dhruva SS. Medical device risk (re)classification: lessons from the FDA'S 515 program initiative. BMJ Surg Interv Heal Technol. 2023;5(1):e000186.
25. Tazawa Y. Perspective for the development of companion diagnostics and regulatory landscape to encourage personalized medicine in Japan. Breast Cancer. 2016;23(1):19–23. https://doi.org/10.1007/s12282-015-0586-y.
26. Sah H, Ramesh M, Amrutha C. Regulating Software as Medical Device (SaMD): a Comprehensive Overview of The International Medical Device Regulators Forum (IMDRF) Framework and Gap Analysis of Indian Medical Devices Rules, 2017. In: 2025 Emerging Technologies for Intelligent Systems (ETIS); 2025. p. 1–6.
27. Rimpi, Verma SJ, Pinky, Baldi A. Evidence-based recommendations for comprehensive regulatory guidelines in medical devices: the imperative for global harmonization. Naunyn Schmiedeberg's Arch Pharmacol. 2025; https://doi.org/10.1007/s00210-025-03843-3.
28. Lim K, Heo TY, Yun J. Trends in the approval and quality management of artificial intelligence medical devices in the Republic of Korea. Diagnostics. 2022;12(2):355.
29. Minghetti P, Musazzi UM, Manellari S, Pagella V, Rocco P. Patient-managed digital medical devices: do we need further regulation? Informatics Med Unlocked. 2024;47:101506.
30. Chai K, Xu C, Man J, Deng Y, Yang L. Evolving paradigms in prostate cancer screening: a decade of bibliometric insights and technological advancements. Front Oncol. 2025;15:1511880.
31. Alshehri S, Imam SS, Rizwanullah M, Akhter S, Mahdi W, Kazi M, et al. Progress of cancer nanotechnology as diagnostics, therapeutics, and theranostics nanomedicine: preclinical promise and translational challenges. Pharmaceutics. 2021;13(1):24.
32. Jain S, Naicker D, Raj R, Patel V, Hu YC, Srinivasan K, et al. Computational intelligence in cancer diagnostics: a contemporary review of smart phone apps, current problems, and future research potentials. Diagnostics. 2023;13(9):1563.

33. Correia ET d O, Baydoun A, Li Q, Costa DN, Bittencourt LK. Emerging and anticipated innovations in prostate cancer MRI and their impact on patient care. Abdom Radiol. 2024;49(10):3696–710.
34. Sailer V, von Amsberg G, Duensing S, Kirfel J, Lieb V, Metzger E, et al. Experimental in vitro, ex vivo and in vivo models in prostate cancer research. Nat Rev Urol. 2023;20(3):158–78.
35. Li J, Yin L, Li Y, Xue Y, Wang X, Xu W, et al. Development and validation of an LC–MS/MS method for quantitative determination of LXT-101 sustained-release suspension, a novel drug in treating prostate cancer, in beagle plasma. Sci Rep. 2025;15(1):11868.
36. Okpua NC, Okekpa SI, Njaka S, Emeh AN. Clinical diagnosis of prostate cancer using digital rectal examination and prostate-specific antigen tests: a systematic review and meta-analysis of sensitivity and specificity. Afr J Urol. 2021;27(1):32. https://doi.org/10.1186/s12301-021-00129-x.
37. Jones D, Friend C, Dreher A, Allgar V, Macleod U. The diagnostic test accuracy of rectal examination for prostate cancer diagnosis in symptomatic patients: a systematic review. BMC Fam Pract. 2018;19(1):79. https://doi.org/10.1186/s12875-018-0765-y.
38. Merriel SWD, Pocock L, Gilbert E, Creavin S, Walter FM, Spencer A, et al. Systematic review and meta-analysis of the diagnostic accuracy of prostate-specific antigen (PSA) for the detection of prostate cancer in symptomatic patients. BMC Med. 2022;20(1):54. https://doi.org/10.1186/s12916-021-02230-y.
39. Liang H, Wang X, Li F, Xie Y, Shen J, Wang X, et al. Label-free plasmonic metasensing of PSA and exosomes in serum for rapid high-sensitivity diagnosis of early prostate cancer. Biosens Bioelectron. 2023;235:115380.
40. Wasserman NF, Niendorf E, Spilseth B. Measurement of prostate volume with MRI (A guide for the perplexed): Biproximate method with analysis of precision and accuracy. Sci Rep. 2020;10(1):575.
41. Loguercio LF, Griep J, Demingos PG, Morawski R, Brolo AG, Andrade GFS, et al. Enhanced enzymatic electrochemical detection of an organophosphate pesticide: achieving wide linearity and femtomolar detection via gold nanoparticles growth within polypyrrole films. Talanta. 2025;281:126714. Available from: https://www.sciencedirect.com/science/article/pii/S0039914024010932.
42. Song S, Li N, Bai L, Gai P, Li F. Photo-assisted robust anti-interference self-powered biosensing of MicroRNA based on Pt–S bonds and the inorganic–organic hybridization strategy. Anal Chem. 2022;94(3):1654–60.
43. Dolnicar S, Chapple A. Scholar (6). Annals of Tourism Research. 2015. Available from: http://www.sciencedirect.com/science/article/pii/S0160738315000444.
44. Malla B, Aebersold DM, Dal Pra A. Protocol for serum exosomal miRNAs analysis in prostate cancer patients treated with radiotherapy. J Transl Med. 2018;16(1):223.
45. Zhuo Y, Wang Y, Gao R, Zhan C, Liu H, Liu Y, et al. Novel simultaneous separation and detection of CTCs and PSA on an integrated multistage microfluidic chip for early diagnosis of prostate cancer. Microchem J. 2025;212:113330. Available from: https://www.sciencedirect.com/science/article/pii/S0026265X2500685X.
46. Cooperberg MR, Erho N, Chan JM, Feng FY, Fishbane N, Zhao SG, et al. The diverse genomic landscape of clinically low-risk prostate cancer. Eur Urol. 2018;74(4):444–52.
47. Farashi S, Kryza T, Clements J, Batra J. Post-GWAS in prostate cancer: from genetic association to biological contribution. Nat Rev Cancer. 2019;19(1):46–59.
48. Saranyutanon S, Deshmukh SK, Dasgupta S, Pai S, Singh S, Singh AP. Cellular and molecular progression of prostate cancer: models for basic and preclinical research. Cancers (Basel). 2020;12(9). Available from: https://www.mdpi.com/2072-6694/12/9/2651.
49. Basak D, Gregori L, Johora F, Deb S. Preclinical and clinical research models of prostate cancer: a brief overview. Life. 2022;12(10):1607.
50. Mohler ML, Sikdar A, Ponnusamy S, Hwang DJ, He Y, Miller DD, et al. An overview of next-generation androgen receptor-targeted therapeutics in development for the treatment of prostate cancer. Int J Mol Sci. 2021;22(4). Available from: https://www.mdpi.com/1422-0067/22/4/2124.

51. Virgolini I, Decristoforo C, Haug A, Fanti S, Uprimny C. Current status of theranostics in prostate cancer. Eur J Nucl Med Mol Imaging. 2018;45(3):471–95.
52. Soares JC, Soares AC, Rodrigues VC, Melendez ME, Santos AC, Faria EF, et al. Detection of the prostate cancer biomarker PCA3 with electrochemical and impedance-based biosensors. ACS Appl Mater Interfaces. 2019;11(50):46645–50. https://doi.org/10.1021/acsami.9b19180.
53. Chiou YE, Yu KJ, Pang SN, Yang YL, Pang ST, Weng WH. A highly sensitive urinary Exosomal miRNAs biosensor applied to evaluation of prostate cancer progression. Bioengineering. 2022;9(12). Available from: https://www.mdpi.com/2306-5354/9/12/803.
54. Rusling JF, Forster RJ. Biosensors designed for clinical applications. Biomedicine. 2021;9(7). Available from: https://www.mdpi.com/2227-9059/9/7/702.
55. Takita S, Nabok A, Lishchuk A, Mussa MH, Smith D. Enhanced performance electrochemical biosensor for detection of prostate cancer biomarker PCA3 using specific Aptamer. Eng. 2023;4(1):367–79.
56. Mavrikou S, Moschopoulou G, Zafeirakis A, Kalogeropoulou K, Giannakos G, Skevis A, et al. An ultra-rapid biosensory Point-of-Care (POC) assay for Prostate-Specific Antigen (PSA) detection in human serum. Sensors. 2018;18(11):3834.
57. Morakis D, Adamopoulos A. Hybrid machine learning algorithms to evaluate prostate cancer. Algorithms. 2024;17(6):236.
58. Lapa P, Castelli M, Gonçalves I, Sala E, Rundo L. A hybrid end-to-end approach integrating conditional random fields into CNNs for prostate cancer detection on MRI. Appl Sci. 2020;10(1):338.
59. Chen T, Hu W, Zhang Y, Wei C, Zhao W, Shen X, et al. A multimodal deep learning nomogram for the identification of clinically significant prostate cancer in patients with gray-zone PSA levels: comparison with clinical and radiomics models. Acad Radiol. 2025;32(2):864–76.
60. Zamboglou C, Carles M, Fechter T, Kiefer S, Reichel K, Fassbender TF, et al. Radiomic features from PSMA PET for non-invasive intraprostatic tumor discrimination and characterization in patients with intermediate- and high-risk prostate cancer a comparison study with histology reference. Theranostics. 2019;9(9):2595–605.
61. Sushentsev N, Rundo L, Blyuss O, Nazarenko T, Suvorov A, Gnanapragasam VJ, et al. Comparative performance of MRI-derived PRECISE scores and delta-radiomics models for the prediction of prostate cancer progression in patients on active surveillance. Eur Radiol. 2022;32(1):680–9.
62. Uyl-de Groot CA, Heine R, Krol M, Verweij J. Unequal access to newly registered cancer drugs leads to potential loss of life-years in Europe. Cancers (Basel). 2020;12(8):2313.
63. Martin T, Hervias A, Armoiry X, Martelli N. Early access programs for medical devices in France: overview of recent reforms and outcomes (2015–2022). Health Policy (New York). 2024;148:105146.
64. Raith F, O'Donovan DH, Lemos C, Politz O, Haendler B. Addressing the reciprocal crosstalk between the AR and the PI3K/AKT/mTOR signaling pathways for prostate cancer treatment. Int J Mol Sci. 2023;24(3):2289.
65. Jaratlerdsiri W, Jiang J, Gong T, Patrick SM, Willet C, Chew T, et al. African-specific molecular taxonomy of prostate cancer. Nature. 2022;609(7927):552–9.
66. Parolia A, Cieslik M, Chu SC, Xiao L, Ouchi T, Zhang Y, et al. Distinct structural classes of activating FOXA1 alterations in advanced prostate cancer. Nature. 2019;571(7765):413–8.
67. Simão DC, Zarrabi KK, Mendes JL, Luz R, Garcia JA, Kelly WK, et al. Bispecific T-cell engagers therapies in solid tumors: focusing on prostate cancer. Cancers (Basel). 2023;15(5):1412.
68. Noris Chiorda B, Zollo F, Magnani T, Badenchini F, Gatto L, Claps M, et al. How to implement the requirements of a quality assurance system for prostate cancer. World J Urol. 2021;39(1):41–7.
69. Wirth M, Fossati N, Albers P, Bangma C, Brausi M, Comperat E, et al. The European prostate cancer centres of excellence: a novel proposal from the European Association of Urology Prostate Cancer Centre Consensus Meeting. Eur Urol. 2019;76(2):179–86.

70. Mayo CS, Feng MU, Brock KK, Kudner R, Balter P, Buchsbaum JC, et al. Operational ontology for oncology (O3): a professional society-based, multistakeholder, consensus-driven informatics standard supporting clinical and research use of real-world data from patients treated for cancer. Int J Radiat Oncol. 2023;117(3):533–50.
71. Russo A, Incorvaia L, Capoluongo E, Tagliaferri P, Gori S, Cortesi L, et al. Implementation of preventive and predictive BRCA testing in patients with breast, ovarian, pancreatic, and prostate cancer: a position paper of Italian Scientific societies☆. ESMO Open. 2022;7(3):100459.
72. Tortorella E, Giantulli S, Sciarra A, Silvestri I. AR and PI3K/AKT in prostate cancer: a tale of two interconnected pathways. Int J Mol Sci. 2023;24(3):2046.
73. Salem O, Hansen CG. The hippo pathway in prostate cancer. Cells. 2019;8(4):370.
74. He Y, Xu W, Xiao YT, Huang H, Gu D, Ren S. Targeting signaling pathways in prostate cancer: mechanisms and clinical trials. Signal Transduct Target Ther. 2022;7(1):198.
75. Beckers R, Kwade Z, Zanca F. The EU medical device regulation: implications for artificial intelligence-based medical device software in medical physics. Phys Med. 2021;83:1–8.
76. Geaney A, O'Reilly P, Maxwell P, James JA, McArt D, Salto-Tellez M. Translation of tissue-based artificial intelligence into clinical practice: from discovery to adoption. Oncogene. 2023;42(48):3545–55.
77. Mulla SJ, Patel M. Global regulatory perspectives on sensor-enabled and biomaterial-integrated medical devices: a focus on India, Canada, and Australia. Biomed Mater Devices. 2025;4:1303.
78. Qazi S, Raza K. Chapter 1: Translational bioinformatics in healthcare: past, present, and future. In: Raza K, Dey N, editors. Translational bioinformatics in healthcare and medicine, Advances in ubiquitous sensing applications for healthcare, vol. 13. Academic; 2021. p. 1–12.
79. Qazi W, Sharma A, Qazi S. Computational intelligent systems in oncology: a way toward translational healthcare. In: Raza K, editor. Computational intelligence in oncology: applications in diagnosis, prognosis and therapeutics of cancers. Singapore: Springer Singapore; 2022. p. 55–64.
80. Adams LC, Makowski MR, Engel G, Rattunde M, Busch F, Asbach P, et al. Prostate158 – an expert-annotated 3T MRI dataset and algorithm for prostate cancer detection. Comput Biol Med. 2022;148:105817.
81. Golubnitschaja O, Topolcan O, Kucera R, Costigliola V, Akopyan M, Akulov SN, et al. 10th anniversary of the European Association for Predictive, Preventive and Personalised (3P) medicine – EPMA World Congress Supplement 2020. EPMA J. 2020;11(1):1–133.
82. Calais J, Czernin J, Fendler WP, Elashoff D, Nickols NG. Randomized prospective phase III trial of 68Ga-PSMA-11 PET/CT molecular imaging for prostate cancer salvage radiotherapy planning [PSMA-SRT]. BMC Cancer. 2019;19(1):18.
83. Auffenberg GB, Ghani KR, Ramani S, Usoro E, Denton B, Rogers C, et al. askMUSIC: leveraging a clinical registry to develop a new machine learning model to inform patients of prostate cancer treatments chosen by similar men. Eur Urol. 2019;75(6):901–7.
84. Puri D, Pandit K, Choi N, Rose BS, McKay RR, Bagrodia A. Striving for equity: examining health disparities in urologic oncology. Cancers (Basel). 2024;16(21):3559.
85. Taber P, Armin JS, Orozco G, Del Fiol G, Erdrich J, Kawamoto K, et al. Artificial intelligence and cancer control: toward prioritizing justice, equity, diversity, and inclusion (JEDI) in emerging decision support technologies. Curr Oncol Rep. 2023;25(5):387–424.
86. Dankwa-Mullan I, Ndoh K, Akogo D, Rocha HAL, Juaçaba SF. Artificial intelligence and cancer health equity: bridging the divide or widening the gap. Curr Oncol Rep. 2025;27(2):95–111.
87. Adhikari K, Naik N, Hameed BMZ, Raghunath SK, Somani BK. Exploring the ethical, legal, and social implications of ChatGPT in urology. Curr Urol Rep. 2024;25(1):1–8.
88. Taylor S, Johnson H, Peat S, Booker J, Yorke J. Exploring the experiences of patients, general practitioners and oncologists of prostate cancer follow-up: A qualitative interview study. Eur J Oncol Nurs. 2020;48:101820.

89. Imber BS, Varghese M, Ehdaie B, Gorovets D. Financial toxicity associated with treatment of localized prostate cancer. Nat Rev Urol. 2020;17(1):28–40. https://doi.org/10.1038/s41585-019-0258-3.
90. Kim H, Goodall S, Liew D. Health technology assessment challenges in oncology: 20 years of value in health. Value Health. 2019;22(5):593–600.
91. De Abreu Lourenco R, Williams S. Health technology assessment and health care utilisation in the management of early prostate cancer. Eur Urol Focus. 2019;5(2):134–6.
92. Hospodková P, Husár T, Klíčová B, Severová L, Šrédl K, Svoboda R. Cost analysis of selected Radiotherapeutic modalities for prostate cancer treatment—Czech Republic case study for the purposes of hospital based HTA. Healthcare. 2021;9(1):98.
93. Lawlor A, Beyer K, Russell B, Steinbeisser C, Bjartell A, De Meulder B, et al. PIONEER big data platform for prostate cancer: lessons for advancing future real-world evidence research. Nat Rev Urol. 2025;22(2):116–24.
94. Kiselova Bilekova B, Gavurova B, Rogalewicz V. Application of the HTA Core Model for complex evaluation of the effectiveness and quality of Radium-223 treatment in patients with metastatic castration resistant prostate cancer. Health Econ Rev. 2018;8(1):27.
95. Ngcamphalala C, Östensson E, Ginindza TG. The economic burden of prostate cancer in Eswatini. BMC Health Serv Res. 2022;22(1):483.
96. Gratzke C, Aggarwal H, Kim J, Chaignaud H, Oskar S. A cross-sectional survey of physicians to understand biomarker testing and treatment patterns in patients with prostate cancer in the USA, EU5, Japan, and China. Eur Urol Open Sci. 2025;71:148–55.
97. Smart D, Schreier J, Singh IR. Inappropriate laboratory testing: significant waste quantified by a large-scale year-long study of Medicare and commercial payer reimbursement. Arch Pathol Lab Med. 2024;149(3):253–61. https://doi.org/10.5858/arpa.2023-0486-OA.
98. Matsumoto T, Strachan L, Oyama S, Ishiguro Y, Lee SS. Current medical technology reimbursement system in Japan. Value Heal Reg Issues. 2023;34:118–24. Available from: https://www.sciencedirect.com/science/article/pii/S2212109922002060.
99. Lexchin J. Reimbursement recommendations before and after adoption of application fees by the Canadian Agency for Drugs and Technologies in Health: a cross-sectional study. J Pharm Heal Serv Res. 2025;16(1):rmaf004. https://doi.org/10.1093/jphsr/rmaf004.
100. Conrad DA, Grembowski D, Hernandez SE, Lau B, Marcus-Smith M. Emerging lessons from regional and state innovation in value-based payment reform: balancing collaboration and disruptive innovation. Milbank Q. 2014;92(3):568–623. Available from: https://onlinelibrary.wiley.com/doi/abs/10.1111/1468-0009.12078.
101. de Pouvourville G, Cunningham D, Fricke FU, Lindgren P, Mantovani L, Murphy LA, et al. Across-country variations of real-world data and evidence for drugs: a 5-European-country study. Value Health. 2023;26(4, Supplement):3–10.
102. Low CA, Bartel C, Fedor J, Durica KC, Marchetti G, Rosso AL, et al. Associations between performance-based and patient-reported physical functioning and real-world mobile sensor metrics in older cancer survivors: a pilot study. J Geriatr Oncol. 2024;15(2):101708.
103. Patalano F, Gutzwiller FS, Shah B, Kumari C, Cook NS. Gathering structured patient insight to drive the PRO strategy in COPD: patient-centric drug development from theory to practice. Adv Ther. 2020;37(1):17–26.
104. Aloia TA. Chapter 53: Value proposition in cancer care: quantifying patient-centered value in a comprehensive cancer care center. In: Hagberg C, Gottumukkala V, Riedel B, Nates J, Buggy D, editors. Perioperative care of the cancer patient. New Delhi: Elsevier; 2023. p. 549–56.
105. Tran HH, Yamaguchi A, Manning HC. Radiotheranostic landscape: A review of clinical and preclinical development. Eur J Nucl Med Mol Imaging. 2025;52:2685.
106. da Silva J, Chaker J, Martail A, Costa Moreira J, David A, Le Bot B. Improving exposure assessment using non-targeted and suspect screening: the ISO/IEC 17025: 2017 quality standard as a guideline. J Xenobiotics. 2021;11(1):1–15.
107. Corti C, Cobanaj M, Dee EC, Criscitiello C, Tolaney SM, Celi LA, et al. Artificial intelligence in cancer research and precision medicine: applications, limitations and priorities

to drive transformation in the delivery of equitable and unbiased care. Cancer Treat Rev. 2023;112:102498.
108. Zeković M. Metabolic reprogramming as a prostate cancer hallmark. In: Kocic G, Hadzi-Djokic J, Simic T, editors. Prostate cancer: advancements in the pathogenesis, diagnosis and personalized therapy. Cham: Springer Nature Switzerland; 2024. p. 123–43.
109. Al-Worafi YM. Prostate cancer management in developing countries. In: Al-Worafi YM, editor. Handbook of medical and health sciences in developing countries: education, practice, and research. Cham: Springer International Publishing; 2023. p. 1–19.
110. Hao R, Namdar K, Liu L, Haider MA, Khalvati F. A comprehensive study of data augmentation strategies for prostate cancer detection in diffusion-weighted MRI using convolutional neural networks. J Digit Imaging. 2021;34(4):862–76.
111. Mahal BA, Gerke T, Awasthi S, Soule HR, Simons JW, Miyahira A, et al. Prostate cancer racial disparities: a systematic review by the prostate cancer foundation panel. Eur Urol Oncol. 2022;5(1):18–29. Available from: https://www.sciencedirect.com/science/article/pii/S2588931121001462.
112. Sumanasuriya S, Omlin A, Armstrong A, Attard G, Chi KN, Bevan CL, et al. Consensus statement on circulating biomarkers for advanced prostate cancer. Eur Urol Oncol. 2018;1(2):151–9.
113. Liu S, Xu Y, Jiang X, Tan H, Ying B. Translation of aptamers toward clinical diagnosis and commercialization. Biosens Bioelectron. 2022;208:114168.
114. Kasoju N, Remya NS, Sasi R, Sujesh S, Soman B, Kesavadas C, et al. Digital health: trends, opportunities and challenges in medical devices, pharma and bio-technology. CSI Trans ICT. 2023;11(1):11–30.
115. Amen MT, Pham TTT, Cheah E, Tran DP, Thierry B. Metal-oxide FET biosensor for point-of-care testing: overview and perspective. Molecules. 2022;27(22):7952.
116. Kumar PS, Ramasamy M, Varadan VK. Transforming healthcare technologies with wearable, implantable, and ingestible biosensors and digital health. In: Chandra P, Mahato K, editors. Miniaturized biosensing devices: fabrication and applications. Singapore: Springer Nature Singapore; 2022. p. 177–204.
117. Leith A, Ribbands A, Kim J, Clayton E, Gillespie-Akar L, Yang L, et al. Impact of next-generation hormonal agents on treatment patterns among patients with metastatic hormone-sensitive prostate cancer: a real-world study from the United States, five European countries and Japan. BMC Urol. 2022;22(1):33.
118. Booth CM, Karim S, Mackillop WJ. Real-world data: towards achieving the achievable in cancer care. Nat Rev Clin Oncol. 2019;16(5):312–25.
119. Lin Y, Zhao X, Miao Z, Ling Z, Wei X, Pu J, et al. Data-driven translational prostate cancer research: from biomarker discovery to clinical decision. J Transl Med. 2020;18(1):119.
120. Hommerding M, Hommerding O, Bernhardt M, Kreft T, Sanders C, Tischler V, et al. Real-world data on the prevalence of BRCA1/2 and HRR gene mutations in patients with primary and metastatic castration resistant prostate cancer. World J Urol. 2024;42(1):491.
121. Pathmanathan AU, van As NJ, Kerkmeijer LGW, Christodouleas J, Lawton CAF, Vesprini D, et al. Magnetic resonance imaging-guided adaptive radiation therapy: a "game changer" for prostate treatment? Int J Radiat Oncol. 2018;100(2):361–73.
122. Cetnar A, Ayan AS, Graeper G, Weldon M, Woods K, Klamer B, et al. Prospective dual-surrogate validation study of periodic imaging during treatment for accurately monitoring intrafraction motion of prostate cancer patients. Radiother Oncol. 2021;157:40–6.
123. Nturubika BD, Guardia CM, Gershlick DC, Logan JM, Martini C, Heatlie JK, et al. Altered expression of vesicular trafficking machinery in prostate cancer affects lysosomal dynamics and provides insight into the underlying biology and disease progression. Br J Cancer. 2024;131(8):1263–78.
124. Johnson LA, Harmon SA, Yilmaz EC, Lin Y, Belue MJ, Merriman KM, et al. Automated prostate gland segmentation in challenging clinical cases: comparison of three artificial intelligence methods. Abdom Radiol. 2024;49(5):1545–56.

125. Metta C, Beretta A, Pellungrini R, Rinzivillo S, Giannotti F. Towards transparent healthcare: advancing local explanation methods in explainable artificial intelligence. Bioengineering. 2024;11(4):369.
126. Aktar SF, Andrei S. Bias, ethical concerns, and explainable decision-making in medical imaging research. In: Zheng B, Andrei S, Sarker MK, Gupta KD, editors. Data driven approaches on medical imaging. Cham: Springer Nature Switzerland; 2023. p. 179–205.
127. Subasi ID, Özçelik ŞB. Artificial intelligence in breast imaging: opportunities, challenges, and legal-ethical considerations. Eurasian J Med. 2023;55(1):114–9.
128. Jha D, Durak G, Sharma V, Keles E, Cicek V, Zhang Z, et al. A conceptual framework for applying ethical principles of AI to medical practice. Bioengineering. 2025;12(2):180.
129. Kondylakis H, Kalokyri V, Sfakianakis S, Marias K, Tsiknakis M, Jimenez-Pastor A, et al. Data infrastructures for AI in medical imaging: a report on the experiences of five EU projects. Eur Radiol Exp. 2023;7(1):20.
130. Abernethy A, Adams L, Barrett M, Bechtel C, Brennan P, Butte A, et al. The promise of digital health: then, now, and the future. NAM Perspect. 2022;2022. https://doi.org/10.31478/202206e.
131. Pugliese R, Regondi S, Marini R. Machine learning-based approach: global trends, research directions, and regulatory standpoints. Data Sci Manag. 2021;4:19–29.
132. Mahler M, Auza C, Albesa R, Melus C, Wu JA. Chapter 11: Regulatory aspects of artificial intelligence and machine learning-enabled software as medical devices (SaMD). In: Mahler M, editor. Precision medicine and artificial intelligence. Academic; 2021. p. 237–65. Available from: https://www.sciencedirect.com/science/article/pii/B9780128202395000103.
133. Scholar (7).
134. Flannery BP., Teukolsky SA., Vetterling WT., Leckenby J, Li H, Bruns A, et al. Scholar (8). Vol. 26, Convergence in the information industries. Telecommunications, broadcasting and data processing 1981–1996. 2004. pp. 125–50. Available from: http://www.sciencedirect.com/science/article/pii/S0160738315000444%0A, http://eprints.lancs.ac.uk/48376/%5Cn, https://doi.org/10.1002/zamm.19630430112.
135. Yus, Bruns a, Turnbull CHS and D, Dolnicar S, Chapple A, et al. Scholar 下午9. Vol. 10, Mass Communication and Society. 1974. pp. 349–83. Available from: http://www.sciencedirect.com/science/article/pii/S0160738315000444.
136. Bruns a, Turnbull CHS and D, Dolnicar S, Chapple A, Adorno T, Horkheimer M, et al. Scholar (10). Vol. 3, Mass Communication and Society. 1974. p. 349–83. Available from: http://www.sciencedirect.com/science/article/pii/S0160738315000444.
137. Turnbull CHS, D., Dolnicar S, Chapple A, Adorno T, Horkheimer M, et al. Scholar (11). Vol. 10, Why We Need the Journal of Interactive Advertising. 2004. p. 349–83. Available from: http://www.sciencedirect.com/science/article/pii/S0160738315000444
138. Welch EC, Yu H, Barabino G, Tapinos N, Tripathi A. Electric field facilitated rapid and efficient dissociation of tissues into viable single cells. Sci Rep. 2022;12(1):10728.
139. Wright S, Burkholz SR, Zelinsky C, Wittman C, Carback RT, Harris PE, et al. Survivin expression in luminal breast cancer and adjacent Normal tissue for Immuno-oncology applications. Int J Mol Sci. 2023;24(14):11827.
140. Shi J, Zhang H, Cui Y, Xing J, Wang W, Chen J, et al. Extracellular vesicles for breast cancer diagnosis and therapy. Extracell Vesicle. 2024;3:100039.
141. Glud EN, Rasmussen M, Zhang Y, Mandrup OA, Salachan PV, Borre M, et al. Identification of a high-risk immunogenic prostate cancer patient subset as candidates for T-cell engager immunotherapy and the introduction of a novel albumin-fused anti-CD3 × anti-PSMA bispecific design. Br J Cancer. 2022;127(12):2186–97.
142. Mishra KN, Mishra A, Ray S, Kumari A, Waris SM. Enhancing cancer detection and prevention mechanisms using advanced machine learning approaches. Inform Med Unlocked. 2024;50:101579.
143. Tang S, Cheng H, Zang X, Tian J, Ling Z, Wang L, et al. Small extracellular vesicles: crucial mediators for prostate cancer. J Nanobiotechnol. 2025;23(1):230. https://doi.org/10.1186/s12951-025-03326-w.

144. Tortora F, Guastaferro A, Barbato S, Febbraio F, Cimmino A. New challenges in bladder cancer diagnosis: how biosensing tools can Lead to population screening opportunities. Sensors. 2024;24(24):7873.
145. Zhou Z, Xu T, Zhang X. Empowerment of AI algorithms in biochemical sensors. TrAC Trends Anal Chem. 2024;173:117613.
146. Chen CK, Liao J, Li MS, Khoo BL. Urine biopsy technologies: cancer and beyond. Theranostics. 2020;10(17):7872–88.
147. Bax C, Lotesoriere BJ, Sironi S, Capelli L. Review and comparison of cancer biomarker trends in urine as a basis for new diagnostic pathways. Cancers (Basel). 2019;11(9):1244.
148. Sequeira-Antunes B, Ferreira HA. Urinary biomarkers and point-of-care urinalysis devices for early diagnosis and management of disease: a review. Biomedicine. 2023;11(4):1051.
149. Wiesel O, Sung SW, Katz A, Leibowitz R, Bar J, Kamer I, et al. A novel urine test biosensor platform for early lung cancer detection. Biosensors. 2023;13(6):627.
150. Bolis M, Bossi D, Vallerga A, Ceserani V, Cavalli M, Impellizzieri D, et al. Dynamic prostate cancer transcriptome analysis delineates the trajectory to disease progression. Nat Commun. 2021;12(1):7033.
151. Doultsinos D, Mills IG. Derivation and application of molecular signatures to prostate cancer: opportunities and challenges. Cancers (Basel). 2021;13(3). Available from: https://www.mdpi.com/2072-6694/13/3/495.
152. Pomerantz MM, Qiu X, Zhu Y, Takeda DY, Pan W, Baca SC, et al. Prostate cancer reactivates developmental epigenomic programs during metastatic progression. Nat Genet. 2020;52(8):790–9.
153. Zhou M, Ko M, Hoge AC, Luu K, Liu Y, Russell ML, et al. Patterns of structural variation define prostate cancer across disease states. JCI Insight. 2022;7(17):e161370.
154. Zahir N, Sun R, Gallahan D, Gatenby RA, Curtis C. Characterizing the ecological and evolutionary dynamics of cancer. Nat Genet. 2020;52(8):759–67.
155. McIntosh C, Conroy L, Tjong MC, Craig T, Bayley A, Catton C, et al. Clinical integration of machine learning for curative-intent radiation treatment of patients with prostate cancer. Nat Med. 2021;27(6):999–1005.
156. Suarez-Ibarrola R, Hein S, Reis G, Gratzke C, Miernik A. Current and future applications of machine and deep learning in urology: a review of the literature on urolithiasis, renal cell carcinoma, and bladder and prostate cancer. World J Urol. 2020;38(10):2329–47.
157. Chaddad A, Tan G, Liang X, Hassan L, Rathore S, Desrosiers C, et al. Advancements in MRI-based Radiomics and artificial intelligence for prostate cancer: a comprehensive review and future prospects. Cancers (Basel). 2023;15(15):3839.
158. Liberini V, Laudicella R, Balma M, Nicolotti DG, Buschiazzo A, Grimaldi S, et al. Radiomics and artificial intelligence in prostate cancer: new tools for molecular hybrid imaging and theragnostics. Eur Radiol Exp. 2022;6(1):27.
159. Zippel C, Ronski SC, Bohnet-Joschko S, Giesel FL, Kopka K. Current status of PSMA-radiotracers for prostate cancer: data analysis of prospective trials listed on ClinicalTrials.gov. Pharmaceuticals. 2020;13(1):12.
160. Kanesvaran R, Castro E, Wong A, Fizazi K, Chua MLK, Zhu Y, et al. Pan-Asian adapted ESMO Clinical Practice Guidelines for the diagnosis, treatment and follow-up of patients with prostate cancer. ESMO Open. 2022;7(4):100518.
161. Oudard S, Courbon F. Controversies and consensus in the innovation access for cancer therapy in the European countries: on the subject of metastatic prostate cancer. Ann Oncol. 2017;28(2):421–6.
162. Pallari E, Lewison G. The evidence base of international clinical practice guidelines on prostate cancer: a global framework for clinical research evaluation. In: Daraio C, Glänzel W, editors. Evaluative Informetrics: the art of metrics-based research assessment: festschrift in honour of Henk F Moed. Cham: Springer International Publishing; 2020. p. 193–212.

MIX
Papier aus verantwortungsvollen Quellen
Paper from responsible sources
FSC® C105338

FSC
www.fsc.org

If you have any concerns about our products,
you can contact us on
ProductSafety@springernature.com

In case Publisher is established outside the EU,
the EU authorized representative is:
Springer Nature Customer Service Center GmbH
Europaplatz 3, 69115 Heidelberg, Germany

Printed by Libri Plureos GmbH
in Hamburg, Germany